Making Sense of Interventions for Children with Developmental Disorders

© 2017 J&R Press Ltd

All rights reserved. No part of this publication may be reproduced, stored in a retrieval system or transmitted in any form or by any means, electronic, mechanical, photocopying, recording, scanning or otherwise, except under the terms of the Copyright Designs and Patents Act 1988 or under the terms of a licence issued by the Copyright Licensing Agency Ltd, without the permission in writing of the Publisher. Requests to the Publisher should be addressed to J&R Press Ltd, Farley Heath Cottage, Albury, Guildford GU5 9EW, or emailed to rachael_jrpress@btinternet.com

The use of general descriptive names, registered names, trademarks, etc. in this publication does not imply, even in the absence of a specific statement, that such names are exempt from the relevant protective laws and regulations and therefore free for general use.

British Library Cataloguing in Publication Data
A catalogue record for this book is available from the British Library

Cover design: Jim Wilkie
Cover image: by 'Tanor' used under license from Shutterstock.com
The artwork by Emina McLean, Eloise Retallick, and Helen Rippon was originally created for this work.

Project management, typesetting and design: J&R Publishing Services Ltd, Guildford, Surrey, UK; www.jr-publishingservices.co.uk

The Publisher and the Authors present the information in this book in good faith, but ultimately decisions regarding intervention rest with the reader.

Printed and bound by CPI Group (UK) Ltd, Croydon, CR0 4YY

Making Sense of Interventions for Children with Developmental Disorders
A Guide for Parents and Professionals

Caroline Bowen and Pamela Snow

J&R Press Ltd

Dedication

This little book is dedicated to the children we have assessed, thought about, planned treatment for, worked with, researched, agonized over, enjoyed, and bid farewell. Without Abbie, Jack, Kim, Pattie, Robert-Louis, Tomás and the others, we would not have had the privilege of knowing their amazing families for a while. In working with them through thick and thin, their skills, insights and problem-solving ingenuity deepened our understanding of children with developmental disorders, reinforcing our respect for anyone doing the most complicated job in the world: parenting.

Caroline Bowen and Pamela Snow

Contents

Foreword vii

Acknowledgements xi

Acronyms and abbreviations xiii

1 Goldfields and minefields 1

2 The baby business: Accelerating typical development ... 19

3 Executive control, attention, and working memory 31

4 Children with autism spectrum disorders 59

5 Behaving, feeling, and getting along with others 105

6 AAC: Controversies, contradictions, and change 149

7 Voice, language, speech, and fluency 171

8 Auditory processing and learning 199

9 Reading 219

10 Diets, supplements, and nutrition: What's on the menu? ... 255

11 Parents navigating the marketplace 291

12 Treatment choices in everyday practice 303

   Epilogue 335

   References 343

   Index 379

Foreword

If your child is diagnosed with a developmental disorder, your first question is likely to be, "What treatments are available?" The professional who made the diagnosis will probably have suggested some source of help: perhaps from a paediatrician, speech-language therapist/pathologist or psychologist. But what if the interventions on offer seem unsatisfactory? The temptation these days is to go on the web to look for other, better options. But the catch is that there are so many options out there, and many of them are worse rather than better. Caroline Bowen and Pamela Snow are professionals with extensive experience of this dilemma, and in this book they distil their wisdom from years of talking to parents and practitioners to help both groups navigate the maze of possibilities.

The stance of this book is scientific and evidence-based. Thus, the primary approach to evaluating an intervention is to ask, "What is the evidence?" The answer is not always straightforward. Some interventions are easy to dismiss: any educated person is likely to have doubts about "psychological astrology" or "spiritual nutrition" just because of the name. But many interventions sound plausible and may be promoted by apparently reputable people in the media or elsewhere. Furthermore, there are examples of interventions that appear to have a plausible basis and have been widely taken up by mainstream practitioners, but are then subsequently found to be based on inadequate evidence. And, sadly, it is clear that conflicts of interest play a major role in promotion of interventions for children with developmental disorders. Sometimes this is blatantly financial but, as the authors note, the conflict often involves belief systems and reputation: many practitioners of dubious interventions are sincere people who genuinely believe in what they are promoting. And we cannot regard scientists as free from such influences; anyone who has invested a large amount of time in developing and testing an intervention will find it painful to relinquish it when clinical trials prove disappointing.

As this book makes clear, there is no clear dividing line between pseudoscientific rubbish and scientifically respectable interventions. There is a continuum, ranging from the frankly whacky ideas that no scientist would endorse, through to plausible but unproven approaches, right up to interventions with a clear scientific rationale that have been shown to be effective in well-designed trials. Part of the problem, though, is that, for many developmental disorders, there are relatively few interventions in that latter category, and fewer still that can lead to a marked improvement. The same, of course, is true for much of mainstream medicine; some conditions can be totally cured by dramatic treatments such as surgery or antibiotics, but in many cases, medicine helps us treat a condition to make its symptoms more manageable and less severe. If we accept that, in our current state of knowledge, this is a realistic goal for most interventions for developmental disorders, this helps avoid falling prey to those who offer "miracle cures".

Bowen and Snow note some other general pointers that can help us decide whether a treatment is worth considering. A warning sign is the absence of any scientific research to back up the claims. Stories of satisfied parents saying how their child was transformed are the mainstay of advertising claims by those who want to promote a non-evidence-based treatment. It is human nature to take interest in such stories, especially if they provide hope. But without proper clinical trials, such accounts are worthless because we are never told about the children who did not succeed – and there may be 999 of those to every one who reports success. And indeed, we cannot always rule out the possibility that the glowing endorsement is a fake. Another warning sign is the treatment that is proposed for a very wide range of conditions. If someone is proposing a radical new method that will cure autism, ADHD, language disorders, dyslexia, migraine and schizophrenia, the odds are it is an over-hyped placebo.

An important point made by Bowen and Snow is that one needs to look at potential harms as well as benefits of interventions. In some cases, children are put at considerable risk. There have been rare reports of infants dying after craniosacral manipulations by chiropractors whose methods have their origins in pseudoscientific ideas formulated by a grocer, Daniel David Palmer (Todd et al., 2015). Other methods may involve restricting children's diets or keeping them unvaccinated and at risk of serious illnesses. Facilitated communication, which is covered in detail in this book, is ethically unacceptable because it involves putting words into the mouths of individuals who cannot speak for themselves, and who may be seriously damaged as a consequence. Many methods seem relatively harmless; for instance, wearing coloured lenses cannot treat "Irlen syndrome", as this is a fictitious construct, but it is unlikely to damage the child – the main harm it will do will be to the parents' bank balance. But, as the authors note, other, supposedly innocuous, interventions do carry considerable opportunity costs. I remember being astonished at reading a thesis by a proponent of the Arrowsmith Program, who noted that she failed to find the expected improvements in academic attainments, but justified this by saying: "*The Arrowsmith program itself does not focus on academic instruction, although some of these students did receive some academic instruction apart from their Arrowsmith programming. The length of time away from academic instruction could increase the amount of time needed to catch up with the academic instruction these students have missed.*" (Kemp-Koo, 2013, p. 35). The fact that many schools in Australia are buying into this programme illustrates the importance of Bowen and Snow's message!

This brings me to a final refreshing feature of this book: it offers advice not just for parents but also for professionals, noting the ethical issues that can arise when an evidence-based practitioner is confronted with colleagues in their own or an allied discipline who are using discredited or unevidenced methods. Does one keep one's head down to avoid damaging relationships, or speak out and run the risk of appearing arrogant and controlling? And what should one do when working with a child whose parent insists on supplementing conventional treatment with complementary methods of dubious validity? These are thorny issues that are often encountered in clinical practice, yet I have never before seen them discussed. The final chapter, outlining some common dilemmas and suggesting ways of resolving them, will give confidence to those who have come across these issues but felt uncertain how to respond.

References

Kemp-Koo, D. (2013). A case study of the Learning Disabilities Association of Saskatchewan (LDAS) Arrowsmith Program. Doctor of Philosophy thesis, University of Saskatchewan, Saskatoon.

Todd, A.J., Carroll, M.T., Robinson, A. & Mitchell, E.K.L. (2015). Adverse events due to chiropractic and other manual therapies for infants and children: A review of the literature. *Journal of Manipulative and Physiological Therapeutics*, 38(9), 699–712. http://dx.doi.org/10.1016/j.jmpt.2014.09.008

Professor Dorothy V.M. Bishop
Department of Experimental Psychology
University of Oxford
OX1 3UD, UK
29 December 2016

Acknowledgements

> "If we teach only the findings and products of science—no matter how useful and even inspiring they may be—without communicating its critical method, how can the average person possibly distinguish science from pseudoscience? Both then are presented as unsupported assertion."
>
> Carl Sagan, 1996

The collegial experience of taking *Making Sense of Interventions for Children's Developmental Disorders* from concept, to collaborative co-authorship, to completion represents a "first" for us, as newcomers to writing a book with just one other person. We divided the workload evenly, explored our topics eagerly, resolved intellectual differences easily, fussed over edits endlessly, celebrated breakthroughs enthusiastically, and stuck to our timeline exactly. It was hard work, but uncomplicated – made enjoyable by our effortless meshing as writers, and the loving support and soundingboard skills of our husbands, Don Bowen and Stuart Snow. We are truly appreciative of each other, and of them. We will probably miss the midnight messages author-to-author, and they probably will not.

Thanks, too, to: our wonderful publishers, the skilled and unflappable Rachael Wilkie and cover design specialist extraordinaire Jim Wilkie of J&R Press; Dorothy Bishop, Bronwyn Hemsley, and contributors to the Developmental Disorders of Language and Literacy (DDOLL) network including James Chapman, Max Coltheart, Molly de Lemos, Kerry Hempenstall, Yvonne Meyer, Roslyn Neilson, Linda Siegel, and Kevin Wheldall, for inspiring us; Suze Leitão and other fabulous Speech Pathology Australia friends for spurring us on; our multitalented illustrators Emina McLean , one of whose many talents turned out to be indexing, and Eloise Retallick; and our eternally willing and creative cartoonist Helen Rippon.

Family, friends, colleagues, and @TxChoices followers around the world contributed incalculably to our goal of revealing the theories, methods and findings of the science behind interventions that work or show promise, while elucidating the notions, schemes and claims of pseudoscience and why the products it spawns do not or cannot work (Sagan, 1996). For this, we must thank Pauline Ackermann, Kristin Anthian, Greg Ashman, Richard Armstrong, Jennifer Bekins, Heidi Bibby, Philippa Brandon, Jennifer Buckingham, Luke Buesnel, Alli Campbell, Anne Castles, Simon Chapman, Julie Cichero, Louise Coigley, Kate Crosher, Eileen Devaney, Nikia Dower, Susan Ebbels, Tatyana

Elleseff, Edzard Ernst, Miriam Fein, Kamini Gadhok, Susan Gosland, Linda Graham, Shafaq Hassan, Alan Henson, Debbie Heppelwhite, Belinda Hill, Kerry Holland, Mary Huston, Victoria Joffe, David Kinnane, Katie Kirby, Megan Leece, Tracie Lindblad, Maria Luscombe, Rosalind Merrick, Patricia McCabe, Gabrielle Miller, Louisa Moats, Zoe Morris, Avril Nicoll, Fiona O'Neill, Claire Oldham, Stephen Parsons, Frederick Patchell, Nina Pedersen, Joy Pénard, John Pierce, Suzanne Purdy, St. Amant Research, Jacqueline Roberts, Rochdale ICAN, Susan Rvachew, Katherine Sanchez, Janette Sedgebeer, Holly Shapiro, Judy Singer, Katie Snow, Darren Stops, Nathaniel Swain, Haley Tancredi, Kathryn Thorburn, Peter Tierney, James Todd, Robyn Wheldall, Grant Williams, and Shaun Ziegenfusz, for sending (or writing) articles, feedback, opinions, positive Tweets, and good cheer.

Acronyms and abbreviations

AAC	Augmentative and Alternative Communication
AAI	Animal-assisted intervention
AAT	Animal-assisted therapy
ABA	Applied Behaviour Analysis
ABI	Acquired Brain Injury
ADD	Attention Deficit Disorder
ADHD	Attention Deficit Hyperactivity Disorder
ADL	Activities of Daily Living
AHP	Allied Health Professional
AHPRA	Australian Health Practitioner Regulation Agency
AIT	Auditory Integration Treatments (or Training)
ALS	Amyotrophic Lateral Sclerosis (Lou Gehrig's Disease)
APD/CAPD	Auditory Processing Disorder/Central Auditory Processing Disorder
App	Application (mobile application)
ASD	Autism Spectrum Disorder(s)
ASHA	American Speech-Language-Hearing Association
ASL	American Sign Language
BED	Body Ecology Diet
BCBA	Board Certified Behaviour Analyst
BG	Brain Gym® (Educational Kinesiology)
C-BOS	Competency-Based Occupational Standards
CAM	Complementary and Alternative Medicine
CAS	Childhood Apraxia of Speech
CASANA	Childhood Apraxia of Speech Association of North America
CBT	Cognitive Behaviour Therapy
CCC	Certificate of Clinical Competence
CD	Coeliac Disease
CD	Compact Disc
CD	Conduct Disorder
CD-ROM	Compact Disc Read-Only Memory
CDC	Centers for Disease Control and Prevention
CE	Continuing Education
CEU	Continuing Education Unit
CF	Casein Free

CNS	Central Nervous System
CPD	Continuing Professional Development
CPSP	Certified Practising Speech Pathologist
DLD	Developmental Language Disorder (aka LLI; SLI)
Ds	Down syndrome
DSM-IV	Diagnostic and Statistical Manual of Mental Disorders, Fourth Edition
DSM-5	Diagnostic and Statistical Manual of Mental Disorders, Fifth Edition
DTT	Discrete Trial Training
DVD	Digital Video Disc
DVD	Developmental Verbal Dyspraxia
EBE	Evidence-Based Education
EBP/E3BP	Evidence-Based Practice
ECT	Electro-Convulsive Therapy
ED	Emergency Department
EEG	Electroencephalogram
EDTA	Ethylenediaminetetraacetic acid
EFA	Essential fatty acids (Omega-3 fatty acids)
EFT	Electronic Funds Transfer
EI	Early Intervention
EIBI	Early Intensive Behavioural Intervention
ENT	Ear Nose and Throat (specialist)
ERIC	Education Resource Information Center
ESSA	Every Student Succeeds Act
FAQ	Frequently Asked Questions
FASD	Foetal Alcohol Spectrum Disorder
FC	Facilitated Communication
FFW	Fast ForWord®
fMRI	Functional Magnetic Resonance Imaging (Functional MRI)
FODMAPs	Fermentable, oligo-, di-, monosaccharides, and polyols
FPIES	Food Protein-Induced Enterocolitis syndrome
G-tube	Gastric Tube
GAPS	Gut and Psychology Syndrome; Gut and Physiology Syndrome
GcMAF	Globulin component Macrophage Activating Factor
GF	Gluten Free
GFCF	Gluten Free Casein Free
GP	General Practitioner (medical doctor)

Acronyms and abbreviations

HCP	Health Care Professional
HCPC	Health and Care Professions Council
IAHAIO	International Association of Animal-Human Interactions Organizations
IASLT	Irish Association of Speech and Language Therapists
ICD	International Classification of Diseases
ICF	International Classification of Functioning, Disability and Health
ICP	International Communication Project
ICT	Information and Communication Technology
ID	Intellectual Disability
IE	Feuerstein Instrumental Enrichment
IEP	Individual Education Plan/Individualized Education Program
IM	Interactive Metronome
IQ	Intelligence Quotient
ISAAC	International Society for Augmentative and Alternative Communication
K-BIT	Kaufman Brief Intelligence Test
IT	Information Technology
LiPS	Lindamood Phoneme Sequencing
LLI	Language Learning Impairment (aka DLD; SLI)
LS	Learning Styles
MBA	Master of Business Administration (degree)
MI	Multiple Intelligences
MH	Mental Health
MMR	Measles, Mumps and Rubella (vaccine)
MND	Motor Neurone Disease (includes Lou Gehrig's Disease)
MRA	Mutual Recognition (of Professional Association Credentials) Agreement
MSD-NOS	Motor Speech Disorder Not Otherwise Specified
MT	Music Therapy
MUSEC	Macquarie University Special Education Centre
NCLB	No Child Left Behind Act (USA)
NGO	Non-government Organization
NHS	National Health Service (UK)
NIH	National Institutes of Health (USA)
NIH	Not Invented Here (IKEA effect)
NORD	National Organization for Rare Disorders
NOS	Not Otherwise Specified

NQR	Not Quite Right
NS-OME	Non-speech Oral Motor Exercises
NS-OMT	Non-Speech Oral Motor Therapy
NS-OMT	Non-Speech Oral Motor Treatment
NSOM	Non-speech Oral Motor Movement
NZSTA	New Zealand Speech-language Therapists' Association
ODD	Oppositional Defiant Disorder
OG	Orton-Gillingham
OMT	Oral Motor Therapy
OPT	Oral Placement Therapy
OT	Occupational Therapist; Occupational Therapy
PA	Phonological Awareness
PBR	Practice-Based Research
PBE	Practice-Based Evidence
PC	Personal Computer
PD	Professional Development
PDD-NOS	Pervasive Developmental Disorder Not Otherwise Specified
PEG	Percutaneous Endoscopic Gastrostomy (tube)
PhD	Doctor of Philosophy
Pro-D	Professional Development
PSR	Professional Self-Regulation
RCSLT	Royal College of Speech & Language Therapists
RCT	Randomized Controlled Trial
RPM	Rapid Prompting Method
RR	Reading Recovery
RTI	Response to Intervention
SAC-OAC	Speech-Language & Audiology Canada— Orthophonie et Audiologie Canada
SASLHA	South African Speech-Language-Hearing Association
SCT	Sluggish Cognitive Tempo
SFBT	Solution-Focussed Brief Therapy
SGD	Speech Generating Device
SIT	Sensory Integration Therapy
SLD	Specific Learning Disability
SLI	Specific Language Impairment (aka DLD; LLI)
SLP	Speech-Language Pathologist; Speech-Language Pathology
S-LP	Speech-Language Pathologist; Speech-Language Pathology (Canada)

SLT	Speech and Language Therapist; Speech and Language Therapy
SP	Speech Pathologist
SPA	Speech Pathology Australia
SSD	Speech Sound Disorder(s)
STM	Short Term Memory
TBI	Traumatic Brain Injury
TD	Typical Development; Typically Developing
Tx; T_x	Treatment
UNDRDP	United Nations Declaration of the Rights of Disabled Persons
VAK	Visual, Auditory, or Kinaesthetic/tactile
VML	Verbal Motor Learning
VPM	Voice-Place-Manner
W3C®	Web Content Accessibility Guidelines
WHO	World Health Organization
WISC	Wechsler Intelligence Scale for Children®
WL	Whole Language
WM	Working Memory
WWC	What Works Clearinghouse

1 Goldfields and minefields

> "I regard (parenting) as the hardest, most complicated, anxiety-ridden, sweat-and-blood producing job in the world. Succeeding requires the ultimate in patience, common sense, commitment, humor, tact, love, wisdom, awareness, and knowledge. At the same time, it holds the possibility for the most rewarding, joyous experience of a lifetime, namely, that of being successful guides to a new and unique human being."
> Virginia Satir, 1972, p. 197

All parents guide their children, want the best for them, and work hard to satisfy their needs. When outside help for a child's developmental difficulty is needed, they seek intervention gold in the form of practices that are widely recognized as the best available. "Recognized" and "best" mean different things to different parents. Some rely on mainstream professionals whose interventions are generally based in science; some prefer other practitioners whose methods are described as "complementary and alternative" (CAM); and some hedge their bets, combining the two (Cirik & Efe, 2015) in regimens that they see as "integrative" and holistic.

Metaphorically, goldfields are a source of wealth, valuable information, or resources, while minefields hold hidden hazards. Exploring options, parents swiftly discover that in the landscape of treatment and tuition, goldfields and minefields coexist in confusing and troubling ways. Pseudoscience masquerades as science; fact competes with fad; gold standards, if they exist, are hard to identify; crank interventions persist and proliferate.

The motley mix can confound parents, families, and professionals. Recognizing this, our aim in *Making Sense of Interventions for Children with Developmental Disorders* is to help all readers distinguish the worthwhile from the whacky, and to help practitioners to formulate constructive responses to ethical dilemmas (Chabon, Morris, & Lemoncello, 2011) around assessment and intervention practices.

The content spans issues in typical development and hothousing (Chapter 2); difficulties with executive control, attention, and working memory (Chapter 3); autism spectrum disorders (Chapter 4); trouble with behaviour, feelings, and getting along with other people (Chapter 5); nonverbal or minimally verbal children and the complex issues that exist around alternative and augmentative communication systems (Chapter 6); voice, language, speech and fluency disorders (Chapter 7); auditory processing and learning problems (Chapter 8); reading and spelling difficulties (Chapter 9); and controversies around eating and drinking and diet (Chapter 10). We address Chapter 11 to parents, and Chapter 12 to mainstream professionals, with a summation of the issues raised, the consequences of ignoring them, and suggestions for addressing ethical dilemmas and distress. Finally, there is a brief section called Epilogue, rather than Conclusion, because fad interventions come, go, and rebadge, but never quite go away, and we know that it is impossible to cover everything in one little book.

Parents, practitioners, publishers, presenters and writers

This chapter begins with a quotation from Satir (1972) about the most important "guides" in a child's world: parents. The primary motivation for *Making Sense of Interventions for Children with Developmental Disorders* is to provide a guide for the guides. True to its subtitle, *A Guide for Parents and Professionals*, it also speaks to professionals in allied health, education, medicine and psychology; CAM practitioners; and education, health, wellness and CAM authors, commentators, editors, journalists, producers, publishers, and TV and radio presenters. We describe interventions supported only by anecdotal evidence, contrasting them with those that are backed by scientific evidence, albeit of varying quality, believing that no-one can make reasoned treatment choices without access to reliable, clearly stated information.

Anecdotal evidence or "anecdata" is unscientific "proof" drawn from interpretations of unique events, the significance of which has often been distorted, inflated, simplified, or over-interpreted. Anecdata may be based around some combination of myth (e.g., eating bird-pecked fruit cures stuttering), false "medical" findings (e.g., sun-gazing improves eyesight), a home-remedy (e.g., Arnica reduces bruising), coincidence (e.g., wearing a copper bracelet or a magnetic wrist strap eases arthritis symptoms), or pseudoscience (e.g., mouth exercises improve speech clarity). Joan's story is a case in point. Joan confided to her good friends Mal and Erica that she was worried about her 4-year-old grandson, Guy, who was speaking only in 3-word grabs and whose behaviour was difficult. Mal and Erica said that Guy sounded alarmingly like their niece who was diagnosed with autism. Her development "went backwards" after receiving the MMR vaccination at 15 months. Increasingly anxious and upset, Joan conflated this information, recalling that Guy also had his first MMR shot at 15 months, and was due for the next in a few weeks. What if he went backwards too? Her dread intensified when she joined an "anti-vaxxer" Facebook group where friends shared devastating vaccination stories. When Joan alerted Guy's parents, they quickly pointed out that Joan's real-life and social media friends trusted anecdote, correlation fallacies and coincidence, shored up by confirmation bias. On the other hand, they as parents were more influenced by scientific research evidence in deciding how best to help Guy, *and* they had irrefutable evidence (Taylor, Swerdfeger, & Eslick, 2014) that the MMR does not cause autism.

Parents and family

By *parents* we mean a child's family: mother, father or primary caregiver, who may or may not be supported by grandparents and a wider circle of family and friends: the *significant others* in the child's community. Children, families and communities are interconnected, each influencing the other. Child development cannot unfold without *family*, irrespective of what that word implies for a particular child in our world of diverse family hierarchies and forms. Family types include adoptive, blended, dislocated, extended, foster, nuclear, reconstituted, same-sex, and sole parent forms. Across cultures, elders, ancestors and recently-deceased family members influence family functioning, and expectations of child-rearing, even after they are dead, with the family regrouping around the missing one, as in cases of sudden infant death, or a parent's or grandparent's passing.

Mainstream professionals

"Mainstream professionals" or "professionals" denote properly credentialed academics, audiologists, behaviour analysts, clinical psychologists and neuropsychologists, dentists, dieticians, educational and developmental psychologists, medical practitioners, nurses, occupational therapists, oral health practitioners, orthoptists, pharmacists, physiotherapists, researchers, social workers, speech-language pathologists/speech and language therapists (SLPs/SLTs), teachers and other education and allied health personnel. Usually, professionals graduate university after years of study. They are eligible (if not mandated) to join a *bona fide* professional association, or to register with a regulatory body such as the Health and Care Professions Council (HCPC) in the UK, and the Australian Health Practitioner Regulation Agency (AHPRA) in Australia. They are bound by a Code of Ethics, strict standards of practice, and rigorous expectations of ongoing professional development (or continuing education). Many achieve advanced credentials, in their speciality or in a related field. Non-medical professionals who can call themselves "doctor" have a doctorate, such as an AuD, DPhil, EdD, or PhD, from a recognized university. This requires a minimum of three (but typically more) years of postgraduate study.

Professionals mostly administer conventional assessments and interventions, with some incorporating CAM methods. Certain complementary assessment protocols and treatments become so widely used by clinicians and teachers that they move from trial status ("is this is a promising direction to take?"), to becoming fads ("everybody's doing it") and on to being considered "mainstream", without adequate evaluation. Similarly, it is common for professionals to receive training in a new therapeutic intervention or teaching methodology, well ahead of a scientific basis being established. This creates long-term difficulties, as ideas and doctrine are often presented by engaging trainers as "facts", and enter the practice realm aided and abetted by the bandwagon effect, with no, or skimpy piloting and refinement. Some that do not belong in the practice repertoire are "there" because of negligible surveillance.

Professionals may produce, and usually value, up-to-date literature, particularly in the form of peer-reviewed research articles in scholarly journals. When professionals refer to "the literature", "refereed literature" or "juried literature", they mean a mix of articles in scientific journals and chapters in authoritative textbooks. Peer review is designed to exercise quality-control assurance over what is published in journals and texts, and overall the process serves the research community, and its consumers, well. It can fall down in two ways, however. First, peers who carry out such reviews (usually anonymously) do so voluntarily in their own time. They do their best, but sometimes they, and editors, miss important gaps or flaws in a study and it is published, warts and all. Increasingly, such shortcomings are identified and discussed by science bloggers in an activity known as "post-publication peer review", but this is not ideal. Once an article is peer reviewed and published, it gains an almost hallowed status. Journals seldom publish retractions, except in instances of identified fraud or significant errors. Second, scientific journals do not share equal status in academe. *Nature*, for example, receives over 10,000 manuscripts annually, accepting around 800. A lesser-known journal in a field like education or a clinical science might struggle to attract submissions so, to ensure survival, lowers the bar, publishing a higher percentage of the papers it receives than *Nature*'s 8 percent and, inevitably, the laws of supply and demand dictate what seeps through to the consumer. So, peer review is necessary, but not enough in itself to assure readers of the quality of a treatment.

Professionals may also write *about* research-and-practice in popular print and electronic media, in plain language for a mixed readership. In addition to what these authors garner from the literature, their knowledge comes from textbooks, conferences, meetings and professional development courses where the content is focused on an understanding of accepted scientific principles and evidence-based practice. They question eminence-based practice – mediated by the perceived high profile of those who produce it – and disdain celebrity-based practice fuelled by stars of stage, screen, sport, cooktop and catwalk, and the odd royal. Professionals' reputations grow via word-of-mouth rather than self-promotion, and although flowery endorsements can be found on practice websites, professional associations tend to counsel against such tactics, or explicitly instruct their members not to publish testimonials (e.g., Speech Pathology Australia, 2015) or ban their use altogether. The dim view of testimonials is borne out by the requirement by the Australian Health Practitioner Regulation Agency (2014, p. 10) that:

> *"A practitioner must take reasonable steps to have any testimonials associated with their health service or business removed when they become aware of them, even if they appear on a website that is not directly associated and/or under the direct control or administration of that health practitioner and/or their business or service. This includes unsolicited testimonials."*

Scientific research

By "scientific research" we mean inquiry that (a) is based on a theoretical model and (b) has followed a rigorous and replicable line of inquiry. Broadly, there are two main approaches to conducting social sciences research – qualitative and quantitative – and with the application of appropriate quality checks and balances, both have a place in informing the body of knowledge and professional practice.

Quantitative methodologies: These are derived from the physical sciences, and employ data collection approaches such as direct measurement (e.g., of skills or attitudes, or of bodily attributes such as height or blood pressure) using carefully fashioned tools that derive numerical values which are then subjected to statistical summary and analysis. Quantitative approaches have traditionally been favoured in medicine and psychology. Researchers seek to be as objective as possible, though the extent to which this is achieved can be open to challenge.

Qualitative methodologies: These come from sociology and anthropology, and employ data collection approaches such as in-depth interviews, focus groups, Delphi-techniques, and document analysis, using protocols that are developed from published research. Fundamentally, such approaches aspire to gain an in-depth understanding of an issue from a stakeholder perspective, rather than trying to measure it. In qualitative inquiry, the researchers are explicit about their stance and acknowledge the influence of it on their data interpretation.

Many research questions are best addressed using both approaches in a meticulous and reasoned balance, and this is referred to as *Mixed Methods research*. What matters is the quality of the rigour, auditability and replicability in the write-up, so that consumers of the research can assess its merit, and fellow researchers can attempt to reproduce the findings in similar studies. All scholarly research, regardless of paradigm, therefore needs to pass through a verifiability filter in order to be considered evidence-based.

CAM practitioners

For want of better terms, the "other practitioners", or "CAM practitioners", provide *alternative* services, using non-mainstream approaches *in place of* the conventional approaches favoured by mainstream professionals. Among them are astrologers, behavioural optometrists, chiropractors, herbalists, homeopaths, lifestyle coaches, naturopaths, osteopaths, spiritual healers[1], and wellness experts; also *self-styled* authorities, consultants, educators, nutritionists, parenting gurus and tutors; and CAM and education entrepreneurs. They may have pursued studies of unknown duration and quality in unaccredited institutes or training centres in order to call themselves "practitioners", and they

---

1 Ernst (2015) reports that in the early 1990s there were about 14,000 registered spiritual healers in the UK, outnumbering all the acupuncturists, chiropractors, herbalists, homeopaths and osteopaths put together, noting that by 2015 the number exceeded 15,000, even though spiritual healing fares no better than placebos in well-controlled studies.

may belong to associations, some bearing impressive- or plausible-sounding names, that are not recognized alongside mainstream national peak bodies.

Some other practitioners publish, or are published in, books promoting their approaches. They also write advice for parents and the general public in newspapers, magazines, newsletters and pamphlets, social media, and elsewhere online. Some are people with personal experience of developmental disorders, who have "found" or contrived remedies. Take, for instance, Barbara Arrowsmith-Young: *The Woman Who Changed Her Brain*, whose "multiple learning disabilities" dogged her through school, and who espouses her own instructional method (Arrowsmith-Young, 2013) based on the philosophy that it is possible to treat specific learning disabilities by identifying and strengthening cognitive capacities; and Dave McGuire who asserts that he cured his own stutter with what eventually became The McGuire Programme (McGuire, 2003; revised, updated and reissued under the same title in 2015).

Rather than delivering interventions based on published and peer-reviewed scientific studies, and building their reputations conservatively via word-of-mouth, the other practitioners, and their promotors, employ hard-hitting marketing techniques, including endorsement by mainstream professionals, celebrity endorsement, and endorsement by implication.

Physics Nobel laureate Arthur Schawlow (b. 1921 d. 1999) was won over by Facilitated Communication for his son with autism, and actively promoted its use. Children's authors, Mem Fox, a retired university lecturer in an Education faculty, and Paul Jennings, a one-time school teacher and SLP, campaign for *Whole Language* literacy instruction (Fox, n.d.; Jennings, 2004). British SLT Janet O'Keefe (www.janetokeefe.co.uk) lends credibility to, promotes and sells Juice Plus+® "whole food based nutrition" (www.janetokeefe.juiceplusvirtualfranchise.com/contact-us) which is relentlessly promoted by some franchisees, with outrageously improbable claims, to parents of children with ADHD, ASD, eczema, psoriasis and the sniffles. Singer-songwriter Gareth Gates advocates and trains for The McGuire Programme. Prominent among the new-age-faithful, HRH Prince Charles pleads insistently for CAM (Gorski, 2015), notably Rudolf Steiner Biodynamic Agriculture (Paull, 2011), "natural" medicine and homeopathy (Ernst, 2015). British sisters, lifestyle bloggers and "nutridense" superfood believers, Jasmine and Melissa Hemsley (www.hemsleyandhemsley.com) put Dr Natasha Campbell-McBride's GAPS first on a list of the five books that shaped their philosophy. The GAPS diets are magic bullet regimens claimed to help with everything from ADHD to autism to schizophrenia to blotchy skin. Third on the list is the *Body Ecology Diet* by Donna Gates (www.bodyecology.com) of "Autism Recovery" note.

CAM therapies fall under five headings: (1) biologically-based practices involving herbal and other nutrient and non-nutrient substances such as aromatic essences, fish oils, and vitamin and mineral supplements; (2) mind-body therapies that include support groups and counselling; (3) manipulative and body-based practices such as acupuncture, "body work", chiropractic, craniosacral therapy, kinesiology, and osteopathy; (4) energy therapies like Pulsed Magnetic Field therapy, Qigong, and Reiki; and (5) traditional and holistic medical systems like Acupuncture, Anthroposophy, Ayurveda, homeopathy, Kanpō, naturopathy, and Traditional Chinese Medicine.

Publishers and producers, authors, editors, journalists and presenters

Among readers of *Making Sense of Interventions for Children with Developmental Disorders* will be: publishers and authors of wellness and self-help books; the skilled journalists and editors whose job is to translate technical health and medical information from quality journals for a lay readership; and producers, reporters and presenters on radio and TV health channels and science programmes. Some journalists courageously challenge pseudoscience, like Simon Singh who says that his greatest inspiration is "James 'The Amazing' Randi, a magician who became a father of the modern sceptic/rationalist movement. My writing career started by championing great science, but Randi made me realise that it's equally important, perhaps even more so, to challenge pseudoscience" (BMJ, 2016). Dr Singh is an author, journalist, and TV producer who was famously sued for libel in 2008 by the British Chiropractic Association – a case he ultimately won. His books include *Trick or Treatment*, a critical analysis of CAM co-authored with Dr Edzard Ernst (Singh & Ernst, 2008).

When a child's developmental disorder is suspected, the first person that many parents turn to is their GP or family doctor. Others seek a mainstream professional attached to a Community NHS Trust (UK), a Community Health Centre (Australia), an independent professional practice, an Early Intervention Program (USA) and the like. Some start with the self-help shelves of a bookshop or its online counterpart, where books may or may not be written by authorities with relevant qualifications. Others head to the Internet, tapping into health, education and news sites: e.g., *Croaky Blog*: http://blogs.crikey.com.au/croakey/tag/health-journalism; *Huffington Post*:

www.huffingtonpost.com/healthy-living; *Science Daily*: www.sciencedaily.com; *NHS*: www.nhs.uk/News/Pages/NewsArticles.aspx; *The Conversation*: www.theconversation.com; and the work of members of the Association of Health Care Journalists: www.healthjournalism.org in the US, and the Guild of Health Writers: www.healthwriters.com in the UK. Yet others rely on TV health, science, education and lifestyle programmes and child health and development video channels such as Healthy Child on YouTube™: www.youtube.com/user/HealthyChild. Wherever they turn, newcomers to these realms may be swamped by contradictory information and advice.

Mainstream and other professionals and alternative practices

Children – some sporting tinted specs to keep them focused, or weighted vests to keep them squeezed – in schools around the world limber up with Brain Gym®, on days that start with "great tasting, chewable fish oil capsules for kids" (Google™ that with quotes, when you've googled weighted+vests+squeeze, without) and a glassy-eyed stint on a whole-brain training App with a yellow overlay, all in the name of optimizing their capacity to learn.

Some mainstream professionals adopt suspect interventions, honestly believing they are legitimate ingredients for children to progress (Travers, Ayres, Simpson, & Crutchfield, 2016). For example, in parts of North America up to 85% of speech-language pathologists purchase "oral motor tools and toys" and administer Non-Speech Oral Motor Treatments (NS-OMT), in their practice with children with speech sound disorders. These techniques have good *face validity*: looking like something that *could* work, but there is no evidence to support their use. Probably most of the 85% see these activities not as an alternative, but rather as a complement, to mainstream techniques, but because they absorb valuable "therapy time" that could be better spent, they come with an opportunity cost. Many education authorities, school districts and teachers adopt literacy instruction methods devoid of scientific credentials, such as the Arrowsmith Program™, Cellfield™, Reading Recovery™, Switch-On Reading, and Whole Language-based programs. The long-since debunked Learning Styles concept (which is as silly and as widespread as left-brain-right-brain dominance theory) pervades Education, and to a lesser extent, OT, Psychology and SLP/SLT.

Evidence-based practice: EBP/E³BP

Evidence-based practice is abbreviated EBP, or E³BP with the superscript 3 denoting that it is an arrangement involving (1) the client and family, (2) the clinician, and (3) the evidence. E³BP has its roots in clinical medicine, but has extended its reach to become a conventional aspect of allied health, psychology, and public health practice. Dollaghan (2007, p. 2) defines E³BP as "the conscientious, explicit, and judicious integration of best available external evidence from systematic research, best available evidence internal to clinical practice, and best available evidence concerning the preferences of a fully informed patient". Where children are concerned, and depending on the child's capabilities and age, we can modify her definition, so that it ends with, "…and best available evidence concerning the preferences of a fully informed patient[2] and/or the patient's family". Dollaghan continues, "E³BP requires honest doubt about a clinical issue, awareness of one's own biases, a respect for other positions, a willingness to let strong evidence alter what is already known, and constant mindfulness of ethical responsibilities to patients" (p. 3). Developing this point, and encouraging practitioners to aim for balance between absolute acceptance of their customary practice and a willingness to survey and accept new ideas, Kamhi (2011a, p. 59) argues that, "…the scientific method and evidence-based approaches can provide guidance to practitioners but will not lead to a consensus about best clinical practices".

There is no binary distinction between "evidence-based" and "non-evidence-based" practice, and no EBP has an "effectiveness and effects" guarantee that it *will* work. A client's response to treatment that is genuinely evidence-based, for a research sample, will vary in terms of factors such as their age, the severity of their disorder, their motivation and capacity to cooperate, cultural factors, and the degree of family support, so that Client-A may respond more positively to a particular EBP than Client-B. However, using an EBP maximizes the probability that it will be more effective, confer more benefits, and minimize potential harms[3], than would an unverified intervention, because it has undergone some degree of stringent scientific assessment.

EBP is a process and a responsibility. It is located at the intersection between the clinician's expertise, experience and educated engagement with scientific theory and research on one hand, and their appreciation of the client's

---

2 Within SLP/SLT, and across other professional groups, "patients" are referred to as clients, consumers of clinical services, patients, and students.

3 Gambrill (2012, pp. 123–158) discusses "a rogue's gallery of harms" in the helping professions.

world, including their beliefs, values and wishes, on the other. The obligation for *adopting* EBP rests with individual clinicians, and in the occasionally shambolic clinical reality, it is a responsibility that can be difficult to sustain.

EBP has a less prominent parallel in Education. Evidence-based education (EBE) is an approach to all aspects of education – from policy-making to classroom practice – where the methods used are based on significant and reliable evidence. EBE is a late entrant and still has an emergent profile in education (see Travers, 2016, for discussion of EBE in special education). There is considerable unevenness in how EBE is defined, and the extent to which education undergraduates are schooled in its principles as a basis for their later classroom practice and lifelong professional learning.

Education, as a paradigm, has historically not placed the premium on scientifically-derived evidence that is so strong in clinical and public health, with educators continually debating "what counts as evidence". This has led to premature practice changes, while others are delayed or prevented, and it remains a significant tension.

> *"A tradition is a ritual, belief or object passed down within a society, maintained in the present, with origins in the past. A scientist embarking on a research trend inherits the tradition of preceding scientists, along with their conclusions and critical discussion. A sense of such a crucial inheritance of tradition is what sets apart the best scientists; those who change their fields through their embrasure ("widening") of tradition."*
> Kuhn, 1977

Academic researchers construct the evidence aspect of EBP or EBE. They develop, evaluate, systematically modify, synthesize, report, and teach new research, theory, therapy or teaching, and best practice, and integrate it into the existing body of knowledge, explaining where it fits. Whether it physically takes place in a lab, clinic or classroom, research is usually done under somewhat *controlled* "laboratory conditions".

Clinicians or teachers translate, sometimes modify, and then apply the outcomes of research, not under tight, researcher-controlled conditions, but in the messy, *uncontrolled* and unpredictable real world. Intervention sessions may proceed swimmingly, but clinics or "speech rooms" are places where children, usually treated individually or in small groups, can miss or arrive late for appointments, exhibit varying motivation and cooperation, encounter good days and bad days, and have distracting "things" happen that interrupt the flow, or simply not like what they are being asked to do, and respond accordingly. Comparable factors influence EBE where children are usually taught in large or small groups, and rarely individually, and then only for short periods. They can also miss or be late for school, have changeable motivation and cooperation, have good days and bad days, and have distracting "things" happen that interrupt the flow, and respond accordingly.

A perverse aspect of E^3BP is that the burden of converting a mainstream profession into an evidence-based discipline is frequently allocated to practitioners, without factoring-in to their workloads the necessary *skills*, *time*, and *resources* to keep up with the available evidence and integrate it into practice. This can lead to a mindset among clinicians, and possibly teachers too, that equates "research findings" with "impossible to operationalize" or "impracticable".

Parents, E^3BP, and being "fully informed"

Thinking about E^3BP specifically, we wonder what proportion of parents "involved in it" (from the professional's perspective) already have, or quickly gain through explanation and discussion, a clear understanding of what it means for them, and for their child's management. It is fair to assume that many parents looking for a provider do not think about E^3BP in the first instance.

Their priorities may well be to find a professional in a convenient location, with space in their schedule, who can accommodate them at a mutually convenient time for affordable fees (if fees are involved), and whose services – where relevant – are covered by the right insurance plan, and in culturally and linguistically diverse settings: one who speaks the same language.

They may not ask what *kind* of intervention is offered, let alone what its evidence base is. It may be important to them to feel at ease with the provider without querying credentials, and to be confident in an intervention that "seems right" without checking its validity. Similarly, the top criteria parents use to select a school – if they are in a position to select – may not see EBE high on the list, if it is there at all.

Respect

> *So, did you hear the one about the chiropractor?*
> *It will crack you up.*

It is easy for mainstream professionals, steeped in E^3BP or EBE, to joke about

CAM, ridicule it, and to be dismissive at their mere mention by a client, parent, student or colleague. It is easy, too, to develop a judgmental good-vs-evil (EBP-vs-CAM) and an arrogant rational-vs-gullible (those who follow EBP versus those who do not) outlook. But the effect of jokey remarks, negativity and scorn may be to alienate, humiliate or insult the person asking, and that is counterproductive and unkind. As well, it is a missed opportunity to ease into a grown-up conversation that might alert them to aspects of EBP or EBE they have not considered (or understood).

In *Making Sense of Interventions for Children with Developmental Disorders* our aim is not to shoot contentious interventions down in flames unthinkingly, without consideration for the parents who access them – or indeed for the professionals and other (CAM) practitioners who embrace them. Rather, the topic is approached with respect, and a mature understanding of, and empathy for those who are: doubtful about conventional treatments; disappointed with the mainstream professionals associated with them; and attracted to controversial interventions because of the hope they offer to their child. Moreover, we agree that most "other practitioners" are likely to be sincere, honourable and fervent believers that their interventions are genuinely helpful.

Speaking personally: The book's raison d'être

Professional and personal factors drove the decision to write this book. Dr Bowen is an SLP, family therapist, parent and grandparent. Having worked professionally with over 3000 children and their families she is well acquainted with the issues that arise – for everyone concerned – around unscientific, scientific-sounding approaches to children's difficulties. She is a veteran of hundreds of "expert opinions" where many of the parents who brought their children for reassessment were caught up in unhelpful, detrimental, and even dangerous CAM practices. Professor Snow is an SLP, psychologist, academic, parent, and grandparent. She also has a sister with a severe congenital disability, so has some personal understanding of the vulnerabilities of families, and their aspirations for their offspring. As an academic, she has taught prospective practitioners in the fields of medicine, teaching, psychology, nursing, midwifery, speech-language pathology, physiotherapy, occupational therapy, pharmacy, and social work. She encourages all future clinicians to adopt a position of humility and respectful curiosity when dealing with parents' anxieties and hopes for their children, and warns that the therapeutic alliance is ever vulnerable to internal and external threats.

About a month before we signed an agreement with Jim and Rachael Wilkie, the J&R of J&R Press, Rachael asked us to "outline your reasons for proposing a new book in this area". We answered individually, Caroline from a clinician's perspective and Pamela from an academic's.

CAROLINE
Candidly, it arises from years of steering clients, students and colleagues, in conversation or in written Assessment Reports, towards more mainstream, evidence-based approaches, without the benefit of a "sensible" book or other source that was not hysterical, dogmatic, patronizing or self-serving. I foresee clinicians across disciplines, teachers and academics recommending Making Sense of Interventions for Children with Developmental Disorders *to clients, students and colleagues in pursuit of accurate information and down-to-earth advice.*

PAMELA
I am conscious of the fact that talk of "a lack of research evidence" can be dry and almost irrelevant to family members who just want to invest in some kind of optimistic belief system. If we take away this optimism by debunking myths and exposing unrealistic promises, then we have a responsibility to provide something that does still meet parents' needs – for accurate information about their child's disorder (or at least where to go for this) and for emotional and practical support about how to effectively parent in a family unit where there is a child with special-needs.

We both had concerns about the marketing strategies associated with questionable interventions, noting that sometimes teachers and allied health professionals themselves are so caught up in the hype that they fail to adequately question the evidence (or lack of) behind them. We were also eager to acknowledge, in this book, the undeniable challenges of parenting a child with special needs, noting that mainstream health-providers and the systems in which they work often fall short, or fail, with respect to meeting the informational, practical, and emotional needs of parents. Appreciating this is important, because if the mainstream did a better job, the conditions under which crank interventions flourish would be stifled.

We hope our backgrounds as practised clinician-researchers enable us to speak directly to parents and professionals, with noticeable warmth, respect and empathy. We think that if readers have key questions to ask practitioners when they are concerned about aspects of an intervention, they will be better equipped to make their own decisions – at all points of the process:

initial inquiry, signing up, and seeking to end a contract. We also encourage practitioners to maintain a questioning stance on their practice and to feel empowered to act when concerns arise.

Twitter

Readers can follow Caroline @Speech_Woman, Pamela @PamelaSnow2 and *Making Sense of Interventions for Children with Developmental Disorders* in Twitter @TxChoices.

Children

Some children receive treatment, tuition or coaching, but are developing typically. The interventions their parents choose are designed to "accelerate" the normal maturation process, to make the children smarter than their peers, or more advanced in the academic sense. This is sometimes called "hothousing", and it may occur ambitiously, with the aim of nurturing talents, gifts, and IQ or other test-performance so as to gain entry to a certain school, a gifted and talented academic extension programme, or to win a scholarship. It may also be done to assuage parents' feelings of guilt or inadequacy, and a desire to give their children opportunities they themselves missed out on.

Children who *are* experiencing difficulties may have conditions including: autism spectrum disorders (ASD), behavioural or conduct issues, communication disorders, global developmental delay, intellectual disability (the term generally used in Australia, New Zealand, the Republic of Ireland and North America) or learning disability (the preferred term in the UK), language disorder, Developmental Language Disorder (DLD), or reading difficulties. Some of them will be "syndromal", with physical and cognitive characteristics that are known to occur with particular chromosomal variations, e.g., Down, Fragile-X, Klinefelter, Prader-Willi, Rett, and Williams syndromes.

Many children who are the focus of this book do not have medically diagnosable syndromes. Instead, they have a constellation of difficulties and strengths, or a "symptom cluster" that fits the profile of a widely understood disorder such as ADHD and Childhood Apraxia of Speech (CAS). There are usually no laboratory tests or medical imaging tools that diagnose, classify or "label" them. Diagnosis rests instead on expert opinion and the application of detailed interviews, observation protocols, and standardized measurement tools, in a process that sees parents as key participants.

Then, there will be a minority of children with rare or "low prevalence" (less than 5 per 10,000 of population in the community) diseases, disorders and syndromes such as those listed in the National Organization for Rare Disorders (NORD) database (www.rarediseases.org). These children have one-off profiles of skills and needs, presenting particular challenges to the implementation of E^{3}BP principles, and often their parents are better-informed than the health and education professionals involved with the child.

Diagnostic labels

Diagnostic labels can be a mixed blessing for children, their families, and for clinicians. They are helpful when they are right, but that is not always the case. They are more likely to be accurate in situations where an objective process exists for their application, as in the case of genetically-based disorders where a blood-test can confirm or exclude the presence of a particular disorder. On the plus side, it can be reassuring to be given a (correct) label that comes with explanations for an otherwise confusing collection of difficulties, often after drawn-out searching for information and answers. A label can provide entrée to much-needed support groups, whether face-to-face or online, and access to help with advocacy for better services. Sometimes, a diagnostic label assigned by a credentialed professional is the "anointment" needed in order to access publicly-funded services. On the other hand, diagnostic labels make good servants and poor masters. In the case of most developmental disorders, diagnostic labels involve clinical judgement and are hence open to challenge by *other* clinicians. This can be bewildering and exasperating for families. We caution that diagnostic labels can impose preconceived ideas about a child's potential, and that such ideas may be inaccurate.

Crank interventions

Crank interventions for children's developmental disorders range from diets and dietary supplements to alleviate speech problems; to spectacles with coloured lenses, coloured overlays, and special fonts to combat the effects of dyslexia; to music CDs and super foods to boost literacy skills, academic performance and social relationships; to weighted clothing to ameliorate the behavioural manifestations of autism and hyperactivity; to curricula that remediate specific learning difficulties; and so on. These thrive alongside a motherlode of other pseudoscientific treatments and even "cures" and "scientific breakthroughs" for

ADHD, ASD, ankyloglossia, apraxia, and the rest of the dictionary of *known* conditions, as well as remedies for a number of *made-up* conditions: Amalgam Illness, Cerebellar Developmental Delay (CDD), Functional Disconnection syndrome, Gameboy Disease, Gut and Physiology syndrome (GAPS), Gut and Psychology syndrome (GAPS again), Irritable Baby syndrome, Irlen® Syndrome, Magnetic Field Deficiency syndrome, Multiple Chemical Sensitivity, Nonverbal Learning Disability, Retained Neonatal Reflexes™, Retained Reflex syndrome, Sensory Integration Disorder, Wilson's Temperature syndrome, etcetera, etcetera.

Classically, crank interventions are marketed, spruiked and talked-up to parents and professionals without a whisker of scientific evidence. Proponents often come with elaborate, authoritative-looking websites, questionnaires and online DIY assessments that hoodwink potential clients into "diagnosing" their own or their children's "problems", clever social media, celebrity seals of approval, highly publicized philanthropic donations, testimonials or sciency-sounding endorsements (e.g., vague claims that "research shows" and "experts agree") often spoken by a beautiful person in a white coat holding an important-looking clipboard.

The interventions can come at considerable and sometimes escalating cost to users who may become ensnared in "a plan". For example, professionals may commit to accreditation courses with taster, introductory, practitioner, advanced and trainer levels, with each tranche greater than the last. Some products are marketed directly to advocacy organizations (e.g., parent-led Down syndrome, Prader-Willi syndrome, or Cleft Lip and Palate associations), concerned and well-motivated to give children with a specified diagnosis the best chances in life.

Predictably, initial assessments employ a range of manipulative, pseudoscientific ploys that can appear valid and proper to the non-expert – but are actually designed to "confirm" a parent's possibly unfounded home-diagnosis, and/or their belief that a specific intervention will be beneficial. Once their child has "failed", parents may hear more medical or quasi-medical terms, and with high anxiety levels about hitherto unsuspected *additional* conditions, are prone to agree with the indisputable proposition that their child merits every possible chance to achieve his or her potential (and they wouldn't want to *fail* darling little Alex, *would* they?).

To a degree, parents' susceptibilities may have been fostered by mainstream practitioners' dismissive, jargon-loaded, or otherwise unhelpful responses to their anxieties about their child. By being attentive and responsive (and sometimes charismatic), crank practitioners cleverly meet needs that qualified professionals often overlook. Feeling relieved at finally being *heard*, parents are now vulnerable to signing on the dotted line.

While the crank interventions are not supported by solid theory or empirical evidence, they have the capacity to compete strongly with interventions that are. This is because they can appear to the parents and professionals who are attracted to them to be more scientific, more efficient, more exciting, more "natural", and trendier than mainstream approaches. They often have explanations that appeal to "magical thinking" and do not require any scientific knowledge for buy-in. Magical thinking is an understandable human tendency to dismiss well-grounded doubts in favour of unrealistic and unquestioning optimism that an approach has merit. Its flip-side, scientific knowledge, is a distinct, though not fail-safe, protective factor that some fortunate parents can swing into action.

The hype is persuasive, the advertising seductive, the lure of the quick fix often irresistible, and the endorsements emotive and plausible – often playing to a parent's insecurities, anxiety and guilt over their child's predicament. Among those who are not quite convinced about the benefits, there are those who purchase them on an it-might-work-and-it-can't hurt basis. After all, what parent would not want to give their child every possible chance of success?

2 The baby business: Accelerating typical development

The air steams with eager anticipation as the *Child Prodigy School of Hothousing* auditorium fills for the annual *Society for Children as Money-spinners* awards. Competition has been intense with strong contenders in the edu*SCaM*, neuro*SCaM* and thera*SCaM* categories from countries as diverse as Egypt, Japan, Russia, Scotland and the US. Onstage are three frontrunners in each category, their hearts pounding as *SCaM's* Founder strides to the spotlit podium. "*Good* evening, friends, contestants, sponsors, and happy *SCaM*sters. Before revealing our *amazing* winners – and *really,*" Dr Credible radiates a sunny combination of compliments and italics, "everyone who competed is a winner. Our judges' task in picking tonight's *very wonderful* finalists was *so especially* difficult." He smiles incandescently at the nervous nine.

"I won't keep you in suspenders…" Appreciative chuckles from the darkness "…very much longer, but want to remind you of the *stringent* judging criteria: our threefold formula for a lucrative *SCaM*: a carefully constructed blend of *pseudoscience, marketing* and *novelty*. Eligible entries must *appear* to be…" "SCIENTIFIC", they bellow. "They must come with *lavish* testimonials and evoke…" "CONFIDENCE" shrills half the gathering; "guilt" croons the other. "And in order to *triumph*, every new intervention must have…" They are on their feet now, "A different name, logo, website and corporate colours from any similar one that's gone before! In a word, any new edu*SCAM*, neuro*SCAM* or thera*SCAM* must be…" "NOVEL". His expressive hands will them to descend, so they sink, tense and sweaty, merging with the velvety plush.

Applause thunders as Dr Credible calls the winners. First up, edu*SCAM* – Bronze: superlative vis-à-vis guilt, but slightly unpersuasive in the other two areas; Silver: lost precious points by having someone else write her testimonials; and Gold: successful on all counts! Then, neuro*SCAM* – Bronze: meticulous use of neuroscientific-sounding jargon and poignant case vignettes in an entry marred only by a substandard info-graphic that did not *quite* capture the concentric swirls of the *Geniusificating Your Kid's Cortex Vortex*; Silver: trailing the winner by a point; and Gold: top marks for epic pseudoscience, guilt and novelty; and finally, the thera*SCAM* winners in a dazzling tie for Gold, Gold, Gold. The winners wallow rapturously in the crowd's adulation; bronze, silver and gold Toddlers-In-Mortarboards Oscars held aloft.

Better and brighter

There are multitudes of baby media, enrichment programmes, interventions, tutoring methods and supercharged education systems on offer. Their common claim is that they fast-track the motor skills, cognitive development and language acquisition of typical babies and children beyond the progress expected with age, thereby giving them an emotional, physical, intellectual and academic edge. There are intriguing book titles: *Teach Your Baby to Read*, and *How to Raise a Brighter Child* from the 1960s, alongside present-day websites: *Brainy-Child: How to Improve Your Child's IQ*, and *Can your Child's Diet Boost her Intelligence?* Web headers scream, *Your Child Can Learn Faster, Easier and Earlier*, and *Sign up for Great Information, Offers and Discounts*, drawing consumers to Baby Einstein™, The Brainy Baby Company, Jones Geniuses, Mercury, The Infant Learning Company and more. And it all seems terribly scientific (to some).

Baby Einstein™

In 1997, an entrepreneurial former high-school English teacher and self-described "stay at home mom", Julie Aigner-Clark, and her husband and business partner Bill Clark invested $US18,000 to start the first baby media company in their Alpharetta, Georgia home. Unique in the early childhood marketplace, their initial product was a VHS (videotape cassette) called Baby Einstein™, and the company soon bore the same name. It would be another eleven years before the Apple App Store launched with just 500 apps in July 2008, a year after the release of the first iPhone, heralding the current dominance of the native mobile application. The original Baby Einstein™ video, and subsequent media (VHS, DVDs, Music CDs and Apps), featured toys with well-known brands (e.g., Ambi® Toys, Brio®, Chimes, Dakin, TOMY). These were intermixed with "visuals" of old masters (Monet, Da Vinci, Van Gogh), music (Bach, Beethoven, Mozart, Vivaldi), maths and science (Da Vinci, Einstein, Galileo, Newton), words from many languages (English, French, German, Hebrew, Italian, Japanese, Russian, Spanish), stories and poetry (Shakespeare and Wordsworth), and "nature" (Dr Dolittle, Neptune, Noah, Old Macdonald).

Baby Einstein™ became a multimillion-dollar franchise, and was sold to the Walt Disney Company in 2001, inspiring a 2005 *Playhouse Disney* TV series called *Little Einsteins*. By 2009, the brand's revenues were worth $US400 million. Because "Einstein" and "Albert Einstein" are licensed trademarks of the Hebrew University of Jerusalem, the company paid royalties so huge that

Einstein holds the posthumous distinction of being on Forbes's dead rich list, along with Theodor Geisel (Dr Seuss), Michael Jackson, John Lennon, Marilyn Monroe, Elvis Presley, Yves Saint Laurent, Charles Schultz, and Elizabeth Taylor, earning millions beyond the grave.

Owned by Kids II Inc. since 2013, Baby Einstein™ is franchised globally as "interactive" multimedia products for babies, toddlers and threes. Probably mindful of litigation around false advertising and misleading testimonials, bad press (Lewin, 2009; Paul, 2006), and widely-publicized articles in scholarly journals between 2006 and 2013 (e.g., DeLoache, Chiong, Sherman, Islam, Vanderborght, Troseth, & O'Doherty, 2010; Zimmerman, Christakis, & Meltzoff, 2007; and see Ferguson & Donnellan, 2014), carefully worded product-aims-and-benefits appear on the Kids II Inc. site (www.kidsii.com/brands/baby-einstein). Carefully worded they may be, but they are also absurd, or impossible to substantiate, or both.

For their Art range, the improbable come-on is that, "real images [of classical artworks] and beloved baby Einstein characters" will "help build baby's visual pathways". The Language products promise to entertain (they may well do) and "inspire baby's language development" (unlikely) through object identification in multiple languages. The Music series will "enrich playtime" (maybe) and, inarguably, "expose baby to rhythm, pitch, and harmony". For Nature, baby is taught about the world and its habitants through exposure to images of animals in various settings. The site tells, "How to raise a cultured baby" through free "expert approved activities". The expertise of the experts is unclear and the definition of a "cultured baby" remains a mystery.

Baby media and music

Baby Einstein™ imitators proliferated, amid extravagant assurances of faster progress, high IQs ("IQ"is explained on pages 268–269,) and bright futures, advising that an early start is best. A parallel music industry grew up, typified by Music for Babies™, in The Listening Program® range from Advanced Brain Technologies (see Chapter 8): CDs with "special" arrangements of classical, folk and nursery tunes "to enhance a baby's brain development while providing a nurturing environment".

Jones Geniuses Accelerated Education

The Early Learning READING Accelerated Homeschool Curriculum Kit, the Early Learning MATH Accelerated Homeschool Curriculum Kit and Digital Early Learning READ, among other products from Dr Chris Jones of Jones Geniuses Accelerated Education (www.jonesgeniuses.com), are aimed at typically developing children aged 2 to 6, with an Internet marketing focus on families who home school. Dr Jones's Early Learning non-evidence-based online course, delivered via www.blackboardcollaborate.com, is for parents of 2–6-year olds who want to "learn how to teach phonics, letter and number formation, counting, naming of numbers and letters, quantity, addition and subtraction, and reading", assuring customers that, "in a series of easy steps your child will soon be adding, subtracting and reading" exclamation mark.

The Infant Learning Company (Your Baby Can Learn)

Dr Robert Titzer of *The Infant Learning Company* (www.yourbabycanlearn.com) writes that he is "trying to change the way societies view early literacy and early learning despite legal and political resistance in the United States". A search of the site for "products by age" reveals 16 DVD boxed sets for infants aged 3–12 months through which your baby can *learn* (it does not say *speak*) Dutch, French, Japanese, Spanish and Vietnamese, five lift-the-flap books, the redubbed *Your Baby Can Learn* (formerly *Your Baby Can Read*) DVD boxed set, and one set of vocabulary "teaching cards" (words in English printed on flash cards to use with the DVDs). Dr Titzer says, "I recommend playing with the words for a few seconds hundreds of times a day rather than having one longer session". The other age categories are 1–4 years (here baby still can *learn* Dutch, French, Japanese, Spanish and Vietnamese, and *speak* German), and plus where baby *learns* the same five languages, *speaks* German, and *speaks* Spanish.

The Brainy Baby® Company

The Kiddly Company (www.thekiddlycompany.com) owns The Brainy Baby® Company (www.thebrainystore.com). This is the hype, with their caps, not ours: "Brainy Baby® is UNIVERSITY STUDIED AND PEER REVIEWED with positive results that says (sic) children can learn 22x more with Brainy Baby® DVDs." Note the use of the plural, in DVDs. Hidden in a downloadable pdf brochure for parents (www.thebrainystore.com/parents/resources.html) it says of the study, "The results showed that toddlers between 18 and 33 months, in the experimental group, were 22 times more successful identifying the crescent shape in a book, after being exposed to the crescent in the DVD, than those in the control group." To be fair, this now refers to just the DVD that Vandewater, Barr, Park, and Lee (2010) devised specifically for the study, rather than the entire *Brainy Baby®* DVD range, but it does not represent the modest nature of their actual findings. The toddlers in the experiment viewed a 10-minute video, using the same techniques as, and excerpts from *Brainy Baby®* videos, about different shapes, at least once daily for 15 days, with no parent participation. The experimental-group video included the novel word and shape "crescent", while the control-group video did not. The experimental group was significantly more likely to correctly point to the crescent shape at test than children in the control group. The children in the experimental group were also more likely to *say* "crescent" than the control group children. The research team concluded that, "Though this study suggests that some learning from video is possible among children under age 2, additional empirical research on the effect of different types of learning strategies and specific content on learning from video is necessary". So, the study did *not* show that "children can learn 22x more with *Brainy Baby®* DVDs" but rather that children could learn a new, unusual word after repeated exposure over many days. This finding is remarkable, but only in the sense that children are remarkable at 18 to 33 months, when they soak up new vocabulary *anyway* – from people and media in their environments, including radio and TV – like thirsty little sponges.

Hemispheres apart

Among the neuromyths cleverly and attractively packaged for schoolteachers, is the mistaken belief that "traditional education" feeds the left "academic" hemisphere while neglecting the right "creative" or "artistic" hemisphere, supposedly leaving one half of a student's brain undereducated. It is further suggested that students will become better learners if educators employ tasks and exercises that engage either the entire brain (in "whole-brain" techniques), or the purportedly overlooked "right brain" (in "right-brain" techniques), which is popularly said to deal with colour, creativity, expressing emotions, face recognition, images, intuition, music, and reading emotions.

Champions – including university-educated professionals whose crammed undergraduate curricula left little space for training as critical consumers of new knowledge and paradigms – of whole-brain and right-brain philosophies have participated in the development of a range of untested educational theories, tools, and systems. These approaches are covered in depth in Chapter 3, but Brainy Child, Mercury Learning Systems, Shichida™ and HEGL (pronounced "heguru" in Japanese, and always followed by the Heguru trade mark) belong here because they are intended for typically developing children from birth in the case of the first two, and in utero through to adulthood for Shichida™ and HEGL/Heguru™.

Brainy Child

The marketing approaches of Brainy Child and Mercury Learning Systems, probably make many parents say "whoa", and "caveat emptor" in the same breath – at least, we hope so. The Brainy Child (www.brainy-child.com) store is packed with appealing, competitively priced, colourful toys that claim to "make your child smarter". Its website houses a "library" (online bookstore) and scores of articles so breathtakingly neuromythological that they defy serious analysis: so we will not try. They include: *How to give your child encyclopaedic knowledge*, *Boost your child's intelligent with baby sign* (that *is* what it says), *Enhancing right brain learning*, and *What is brain balancing?*

Mercury Learning Systems

The Mercury Learning Systems site (www.acceleratedlearningmethods.com) is similarly implausible, to anyone who studied basic scientific method at school, in its quest for "higher learning for young children". A product that may get right up your nose is Mercury's Olfactory Stimulation Kit of 25 essential oil essences for upwards of age *3 months*. "Some experts tell us inhalation is the most direct route between the outside world and our brains. Our right brains have the ability to trigger extremely fast memory recall and other accelerated brain functions. In many children, this potential goes untapped or underdeveloped because the pathways between their right- and left-brains haven't been properly stimulated to form strong connections. This kit helps build and strengthen these connections and is an excellent way to teach your child to recognize objects and their associated scents." Then, for one year and up: Right Brain/Left Brain Memory Writing: "This lesson can be done for as little as a few seconds a day up to several minutes depending on your child's attention span and interest. It's the same type of lesson given at the Shichida™ Child Academies throughout Asia. It's an excellent way to train your child to quickly take in information (a right brain function) and practice writing from memory (a left brain function)." One-year-olds *writing*? We don't think so.

Shichida™: Success beyond imagination

> *"They were able to read 'Edison', a biography for elementary school children which is close to two hundred pages long, in five minutes and later in two minutes. There is a noticeable difference in the results when we do meditation, deep breathing, suggestion and image training first and when we don't."*
> Shichida parent, writing about children aged 6 and 8
> www.shichidamethod.com

Almost all-available information on Shichida™ is on its remarkably similar company websites. Turning to blogs, social media and Wikipedia® as a last resort, we found Shichida™ has a low profile in Facebook, Instagram, Pinterest and Twitter, and no Wikipedia® entry suggesting that franchisees might have been told not to go there. Information from other sources – predominantly Shichida™ imitators, and an outraged blogger who says he wasted his money – is contradictory and lacking in detail.

Like the Institutes for the Achievement of Human Potential methods initiated by Glenn Doman™ and Carl Delacato in 1955, and Dr Paul Dennison's Brain Gym® International and Educational Kinesiology Foundation dating from the 1960s, the Shichida™ Child Academy's Shichida™ Method founded in 1978 is a "whole brain" instructional approach that emphasizes the importance of right-brain learning. It rests on one principle, expounded by its Japanese founder, Dr Makoto Shichida (b. 1929 d. 2009), that every child is born a genius. He said, "The genius is in the right brain, not in the left brain. Every child between zero and six has innate abilities in their right hemispheres of the brain. However, if ignored, these abilities will diminish and vanish by the age of six." Dr Shichida's half-baked but gentle, plausible education and "brain development" philosophy is widely admired and embraced by parents, particularly in Indonesia, Japan, Korea, Malaysia, and Singapore; and increasingly in Australia, the UK and US.

> *"The purpose of education in the future will not be to create people with heads crammed full of knowledge, but to rear children who know how to efficiently use the whole brain. Rearing children with enormous ability, rich creativity, and*

> *the capability to make use of high proportion of their brain should be the goal of child rearing."*
>
> Makoto Shichida
> www.shichidamethod.com

A child attends Shichida™ once weekly, with one parent, for a fast-paced 50-minute session, with no more than five other children in a class, and does 30 minutes' daily practice with the parent at home. In Phase 1 (Age 0 to 3) "The basic functions of the two brain hemispheres are enriched for the maturity of 6 innate abilities". The innate abilities include: "photographic memory, creativity, perfect pitch in music, multi-languages mastery and lightning rapid calculation abilities". Working at this level from birth is explained thus: "An infant has incredible learning abilities. Even though an infant may not be able to display his/her learning abilities or potential, the cells in the brain are connecting fast for future brain usage".

In Phase 2 (Ages 4 and 5) "The parent has developed a higher awareness of the child's abilities and character" and in Phase 3 (Age 6 and above) "Elite Brain Foundation 1 to 3: The children progress on to strengthen higher abilities for both academic and non-academic areas of learning".

Answers to parents' questions are on Shichida's site (www.shichidamethod.com/faq.html) along with an alarming warning about its right-brain imitators: "You need to be careful and check the source of other programs as the brain of a young child is very delicate and once wired wrongly, is difficult to undo any damage".

HEGL/Heguru™ from the Henmi Educational General Laboratory

The HEGL method, developed in Japan over a 30-year period by Mr Hirotada and Ms Ruiko Henmi, focuses on training adults how to "grow the abilities" of foetuses, babies and children to "acquire education", with promises that they will learn to "draw out the genius in your child", "awaken their sleeping talents" and unleash "their right brain creativity". The first step in HEGL is Hado Reading, contrived by Ms Henmi in 1997, the year that Baby Einstein™ was born. Hado Reading lets those who achieve it read, memorize and comprehend a whole book in one second, by simply riffling through the pages, making it possible to read 10,000 books in a month. Candidly, seeing that far-fetched claim marked the point at which we lost all interest. Three hundred and twenty-two books a day over 31 days? Pull the other one. On the www.heguru.com home page, Ms Henmi writes: "Anyone can achieve this ability if they commence their training with the Heguru™ program at an early age". Those proficient in Hado Reading can become members of Ichimankai (literally "the 10,000 group"): "the starting line for the serious development of your right brain", triggering the gradual surfacing of "excellent abilities in both sports and arts" and the ability to control the right and left brains simultaneously.

Called Heguru™ beyond Japan, because foreigners mispronounce HEGL, it is promoted as *the* way to make the most of right-brain learning, with two teachers conducting each fast-paced weekly lesson: 42×50 minutes per year from age 6 months to the 4th birthday; 42×90 minutes for 4–6-year-olds; and a more advanced programme of 42×90 minutes for 7–11-year-olds. It is said to assist children to "attain greater brain power and learning capabilities, increase sensitivity and empathy towards others", "gain age appropriate physical competence", and "lead a happy life". The activities include: Right Brain Training, Left Brain Training, Heart Education "for higher emotional intelligence", Physical Activities, and Music and Rhythm "to stimulate imaging abilities".

HEGL/Heguru™ is available in multiple locations in Australia, China, Indonesia, Kuwait, Malaysia, Singapore, and Thailand. Our advice: keep well clear.

Baby Sign

There is a distinct contrast between promotional messages delivered by Canada-based WeeHands™, and Baby Sign Language "based out of Southlake, Texas" (email correspondence, December 17, 2015). In 2001 Sara Bingham, a former Applied Behaviour Analysis practitioner and Communicative Disorders Assistant, founded WeeHands™ (www.weehands.com), teaching families, child care staff, teachers and others how to use American Sign Language (ASL) with infants, toddlers and children, 0–5 years, who have normal hearing. WeeHands™ became a division of Morneau Shepell (www.morneaushepell.com) in early 2014, and Ms Bingham is now its Product Manager. Her LinkedIn™ (www.linkedin.com) profile says her responsibilities in that role include marketing, content development, and "product development of curriculum for Morneau Shepell's baby, toddler and preschool students; supervision of students; development and implementation of online course both for WeeHands™ instructors and for early childhood educators, teachers and caregivers". As well, she "plans, creates and publishes relevant, engaging content for WeeHands™ social media platforms".

While the FAQ section of the website affirms that "no studies have shown that sign actually enhances a baby's language development", elsewhere on the site there are powerful little anecdotes, relating to Ms. Bingham's own "wee ones", Sabrina and Joshua, which insinuate that early signing will enhance early language and literacy. For example, "At 16 months, Sabrina had a vocabulary of more than 80 words, a combination of her signs and verbal words. Babies who are not signed to at this age typically have 10–15 verbal words. Signing allows babies to develop larger vocabularies!" and, "my almost 6-year-old son, Joshua, is starting to learn to read and his ability to sign is really helping him develop literacy skills. Signing the alphabet has really helped him learn his letters".

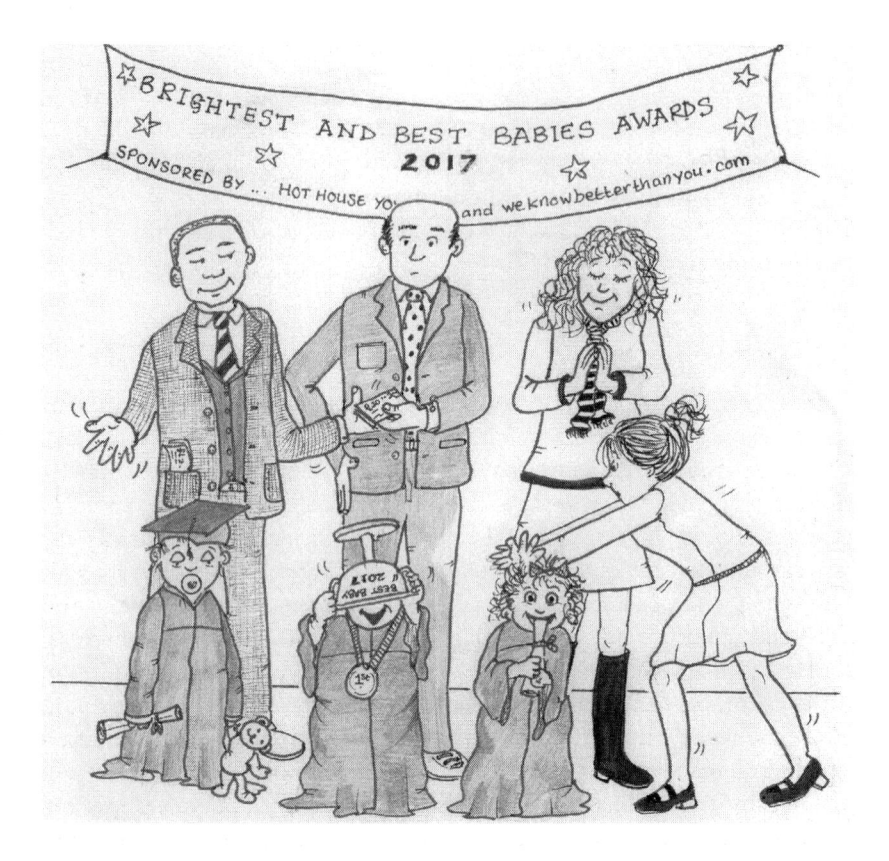

Helen Rippon

WeeHands™ style is persuasive, but the message is soft compared with the inflated claims of Baby Sign Language (www.babysignlanguage.com). In a nutshell: "Baby Sign Language has three types of benefits (sic): 1. Practical: less fussing and more fun 2. Emotional: creates a closer parental bond 3. Cognitive: boosts brain development." They declare that "studies show" Baby Sign Language will lead to fewer tantrums, closer parent-child relationships, higher parental self-esteem, a "+12 IQ point advantage, larger speaking vocabulary and ability to form longer sentences, earlier reading and larger reading vocabulary, and better grades in school".

Is hothousing beneficial?

The focus of *Making Sense of Interventions for Children with Developmental Disorders* is children who actually *have* developmental difficulties, and approaches – mainstream and otherwise – that purport to address those difficulties. So we will not waste the reader's time with a lengthy critique of hothousing approaches. Remember Dr Credible, and his formula of pseudoscience, marketing and novelty? The interventions described in this chapter meet all those criteria, and they have the potential to tap into any (likely irrational) anxious or guilty thoughts parents might have of not doing enough for their children.

Hothousing is unnecessary and does not produce accelerated development. Play and playthings are essential to normal progress, but parents don't need to spend their resources on special "acceleration" toys, programmes and materials in order for their typically developing children to thrive and achieve their potential. If parents and their children enjoy educational toys, then by all means go for them, remembering that identical benefits are inherent in some combination of being talked to, listened to, and read to interactively, and played with; and, the babyproof contents of a pots-and-pans cupboard, a dressing-up basket, a large sheet of butchers' paper, a garden hose on a hot day, a nature ramble or walk in a park, and getting to know other animals: two- and four-legged!

Right-brain-left-brain-whole-brain approaches are nonsensical and redundant. There is no evidence to support the ideas that: traditional education systems and the teachers therein neglect the right hemisphere; it is possible for a healthy individual, including babies, to lopsidedly favour one side of the brain; or, that an educational approach can activate or enhance the performance of one hemisphere. The cerebral hemispheres have some specialized roles, but this is no simple demarcation and they are richly connected with each other so that we humans can go about our business with ready access to a full deck of mental functions. Baby Sign is not all it is cracked up to be. Signing with a baby and sign classes may be good fun, but will not lead to speedier speech and language development, earlier or stronger literacy skills, fewer tantrums and tussles, increased IQ, amplified self-esteem or enhanced parent-child bonding.

Way to go!

> *"Parenthood remains the greatest single preserve of the amateur."*
>
> Alvin Toffler

Save your money and enjoy interacting with your child in a variety of ways through everyday experiences, outings, objects, activities and developmentally appropriate toys. Put down your own screen, if you are a little hooked on it away from work, and be led by your child's bids for engagement, their questions, and their natural ingenuity and curiosity about the world around them. Give your child space enough to enjoy solitary, imaginative play and to learn the art of being content in his or her own company, without continual "special" stimulation. Take a break yourself from time to time, modelling enjoyment of family relationships, friends, conversation, humour, silliness, forthright debate and discussion, reading, writing, creativity (e.g., arts and crafts, cooking, building, gardening, "making", and sewing), and quiet reflection. If your culture is one where "instructing children" comes more naturally than imaginative play, do what is comfortable, without feeling pressured into signing up for classes, programmes or baby media.

Although it is difficult to remember in some situations, you are not in competition with other parents to raise the brightest, most popular and cup-and-medal-winning child in your circle. Forget the Toddlers-In-Mortarboards people, avoid the *Society for Children as Money-spinners* types, and value the ups-and-downs, and the extraordinary, and ordinary, rewards of parenthood.

3 Executive control, attention, and working memory

If you know infants, you know that gaining their attention is generally a breeze, and that keeping it focused is a whole different thing. The distractibility of infants, toddlers and young children is a characteristic that crafty parents can sometimes (not always) use to advantage, e.g., by pointing out a dog, or some other exciting thing nearby, to divert the attention of a toddler in full tantrum, thereby instating calm (more on this in Chapter 5) until the next outburst. The skills of focusing and sustaining attention over time develop over a long period, from infancy through to early adulthood. Vital to the process of acquiring, consolidating, and using new information, they also rely on interest and motivation, and are fragile in the context of most developmental disorders.

Executive control and attention

"Attention" denotes a complex set of skills that are present at birth in only the most rudimentary ways but which develop apace in the first few years of life, continuing to undergo refinement well into late adolescence and early adulthood. There are several ways to conceptualize attention and to categorize its component parts, along with its close relative, *executive function*, which we also consider in this chapter.

According to Rueda, Posner and Rothbart (2005), there are three key attentional systems: alerting, orienting, and executive control. Present at birth, the *alerting* system underwrites our states of wakefulness and arousal. The *orienting* system matures rapidly in the first six months of life, supporting our ability to select information from an array of multisensory inputs. *Executive control of attention* develops last, emerging just before the third birthday, to support our capacity to take voluntary control over focusing and sustaining attention. Executive control is more effortful, and hence more tenuous in the face of challenges such as competing demands, stress, and/or fatigue; and executive control difficulties are commonly observed in children with developmental disorders.

Focusing, sustaining, and strategically shifting attention play central roles in cognitive, language, emotional, social, and behavioural development, providing critical support to academic success. Consequently, they are skills that teachers constantly strive to cultivate in the 25–30 children of varying developmental levels and aptitudes in their classes. The development of attentional skills reflects maturation in underlying brain systems (particularly in the late-to-mature prefrontal regions), and the nature, frequency, and quality of interactions and experiences that children have. According to Loher and Roebers (2013), the executive functions needed to support attention include *switching* (the ability to flexibly respond and adapt to change in the environment), *inhibition* (the ability to suppress an urge to focus on and process irrelevant information), and *working memory* (the ability to temporarily hold information in mind and use it to perform a mental operation). In short, we are dealing here with high-level, complex, late-to-develop, and often brittle skills.

The "anterior" prefrontal areas of the brain, at the forefront of the cerebral cortex, support attentional and executive function skills, and are among its later maturing regions, typically remaining under-construction until early adulthood (Blakemore & Choudhury, 2006). Parents may use different terms to describe it, but they know from experience that the functions supported by the prefrontal regions (planning, organization, self-regulation, curbing impulses, complex problem-solving, thinking in the abstract, and focusing and sustaining attention) are clearly the latest to mature, requiring scaffolding and support from adults well into adolescence and early adulthood. Unsurprisingly, attention, and its conscious control, is related to the child's ability to *self-regulate* behaviourally, emotionally, and socially. Self-regulation supports the ability to comply with adult requests, to wait, take turns, delay gratification, and to empathize with others (Graziano, Calkins, & Keane, 2011; Rueda et al., 2005). These skills are all critical to psychosocial, academic, and vocational success, and interact closely with a related cognitive process: working memory.

Working memory

Working memory (WM) – sometimes described as mental "notepads" – is the brain's short-term storage system that lets us retain information long enough to work with, or mentally *manipulate,* it. For example, when logging into a secure website on your computer, you might be sent a 4–6-digit password by phone. You look at the numbers on your phone screen, and might mutter them aloud or "say" them in your head, to retain them – in sequence – long enough to type them. Unless you consciously decide, and work, to remember them, they will be gone without trace moments later, because they have served their purpose, thanks to your WM.

WM grew out of the concept of short-term memory (STM), but differs from STM in the sense that it is used when more than simple temporary storage (as in a classic digit-span task) is required, and some kind of concurrent mental operation must be performed, without succumbing to distraction or interference. At the heart of this system sits the "central executive", a limited attentional control mechanism supported by two "slave" systems: the phonological loop and the visuospatial sketchpad (Baddeley & Hitch, 1974). The phonological loop supports temporary storage of verbal (heard) information and, as the name suggests, the visuospatial sketchpad supports temporary storage of visual (seen) and spatial (where objects are relative to each other) information. Together, the central executive and slave systems support considerable everyday cognitive activity, especially the kinds of mental operations children are regularly asked to perform at school, e.g., when completing mathematical operations such as adding, subtracting, dividing, and multiplying, or when reading or listening to a story. In recent times, the idea of poor WM in instructional settings has been considered from the viewpoint of *cognitive load* — a theory that "...is concerned with the learning of complex cognitive tasks, in which learners are often overwhelmed by the number of interactive information elements that need to be processed simultaneously before meaningful learning can commence" (Paas, Van Gog, & Sweller, 2010, p. 116).

It stands to reason that children with poor WM capacity often underachieve in reading and/or maths (Gathercole & Alloway, 2008), but this does not mean that all reading or maths difficulties reflect poor underlying WM. Similarly, WM deficits are commonly (though not invariably) seen in children diagnosed with Attention Deficit Hyperactivity Disorder (ADHD), and hence they are a particular focus of some interventions aimed at reducing ADHD symptoms.

ADHD

Attentional problems of various forms are commonly identified in children with developmental disorders, but not all of them will have a formal diagnosis of Attention Deficit/Hyperactivity Disorder (ADHD). According to the current version of Diagnostic and Statistical Manual of the American Psychiatric Association (DSM-5, 2013), ADHD is "...a neurodevelopmental disorder defined by impairing levels of inattention, disorganisation, and/or hyperactivity-impulsivity" (p. 32). Accordingly, for a diagnosis of ADHD to be made, six of the features listed in Table 3.1 must be present before age 12

Table 3.1 DSM-5 ADHD Diagnostic criteria.

Inattention	Hyperactivity/impulsivity
Lack of attention to detail; careless mistakes	Often fidgets, taps, squirms
Difficulty sustaining attention	Frequently leaves seat
Does not seem to listen	Often runs about or climbs in situations where it is not appropriate
Does not follow through on instructions (easily sidetracked)	Often unable to play or engage in other leisure activities quietly
Difficulty organizing tasks and activities	Seemingly always "on the go" and perceived by others as restless
Avoids sustained mental effort	Often talks excessively
Loses and misplaces objects	Often blurts out answers
Easily distracted	Often has difficulty waiting in turn
Forgetful in daily activities	Often interrupts or intrudes on others

(in DSM-IV, it was age 7), have persisted over a period of six months, and be directly negatively impacting on social and academic/occupational activities (for adolescents and adults to be diagnosed according to DSM-5's criteria, only five features need to be present).

It is usual for clinicians to consider three subtypes of ADHD: *inattentive*, *hyperactive*, and *combined*. The DSM-5 also stipulates that these features must not be better accounted for by a diagnosis of oppositional defiant disorder, but a diagnosis of autism spectrum disorder (ASD) no longer excludes a diagnosis of ADHD. Instead, the authors of DSM-5 recognize that, in practice, ASD and ADHD can co-exist, and that each requires targeted intervention. As we discuss in Chapter 5, psychiatric diagnoses resemble skirt lengths in their proneness to change; they vary according to changes in dominant thinking, in response to lobbying by stakeholder groups, and, yes, even in response to scientific advances. So who knows what changes DSM-5.1 will bring? Readers will easily locate detailed accounts of up-to-date diagnostic criteria and caveats online, so we will not feature them here.

Sluggish Cognitive Tempo (SCT), a diagnostic descriptor for children's attention and concentration difficulties that had its advent in the 1980s, is not in any edition of the DSM. Dr Stephen P. Becker of the Cincinnati Children's Hospital Medical Center, a key proponent of SCT as a separate entity from ADHD, says SCT is "…a cluster of sluggish, daydreamy, and apathetic behaviors and has historically been studied in tandem with attention-deficit/hyperactivity" (Becker, 2013, p. 1051). Barkley (2014, 2015) supports the idea of SCT as a distinct clinical entity, but argues that the label itself is undesirable at several levels, notably its pejorative overtones. He advocates instead for the term Concentration Deficit Disorder (CDD). Proponents of the SCT (or CDD) construct argue that it overlaps with inattentive forms of ADHD, yet is distinct from ADHD. As it is not included in any major diagnostic systems, and lacks clear-cut diagnostic criteria, we do not endorse its current clinical distinctiveness or its usefulness in informing discrete intervention approaches. Moves to widen the diagnostic net in this way should be viewed with caution, as the beneficiaries are not necessarily children and their families. We agree with Dr Allen Frances, an Emeritus Professor of Psychiatry at Duke University, that "We're seeing a fad in evolution: Just as A.D.H.D. has been the diagnosis du jour for 15 years or so, this is the beginning of another" (quoted in Schwarz, 2014).

ADHD is the most commonly-diagnosed child psychiatric disorder, with some estimates suggesting it is present in 5% of children, persisting into adulthood in around 50–60% of cases (Arns, Heinrich, & Strehl, 2014). ADHD is considered to be both familial and heritable – running in families for both biological and environmental reasons, and these factors have complex interactions with each other. Risk factors include male gender (4:1), and prenatal exposure to maternal smoking; while co-morbidities with other neurodevelopmental disorders (e.g., ASD, reading difficulties, language disorders, and conduct problems) are common (Thapar, Cooper, Eyre, & Langley, 2013). Environmental toxin exposure (pesticides, polychlorinated biphenyls, and lead) prenatally or in early life, has also been implicated as a factor contributing to the development of ADHD (Thapar et al., 2013). Diet and early family adversity also stand accused, but with little robust evidence to support causality (Thapar et al., 2013). In fact, these potential contributory factors are all works-in-progress in terms of their supporting evidence, and it is impossible in the case of a given child to definitively attribute their ADHD diagnosis to a particular factor or set of factors. We feel confident, however, in assuring you that your child's ADHD is *not* due to "Retained Reflex Syndrome" nor to its variant "Retained Neonatal Reflexes™", both spurious terms with *no formal standing in the medical or education literature*, as evidenced by a July 2016 search of four electronic library data-bases (Google Scholar, Ovid Medline, PsychINFO, and ERIC) that failed to return any peer-reviewed journal articles with either of them in their titles. Yes, healthy infants have certain so-called "primitive" reflexes that normally disappear over the first year, and yes, these are sometimes retained, but this occurs in the context of serious neuromuscular conditions such as cerebral palsy. These terms and their alleged relevance to developmental disorders such as ADHD and reading difficulties are, however, nonsensical.

That said, diagnostic controversies and inconsistencies, misinformation, half-truths and myths have been part of the ADHD landscape since it (or its past variants such as hyperkinetic impulse disorder) entered clinical use in the mid-twentieth century. An especially unhelpful myth is the prevalent notion of an "epidemic" of ADHD nowadays. Despite *perceptions* of a recent inexorable increase, a meta-analysis indicated that where standardized diagnostic processes are applied, an increase in the *actual* incidence of ADHD was not found over a three-decade period (Polanczyk, Willcutt, Salum, Kieling, & Rohde, 2014).

In addition to difficulty focusing and sustaining attention, children diagnosed with ADHD are often found to have reduced WM, although problems with WM are neither necessary nor sufficient for a diagnosis of ADHD (Willcutt, Doyle, Nigg, Faraone, & Pennington, 2005). Reduced ability to focus and sustain attention, combined with difficulty mentally manipulating information to perform set academic tasks, creates significant academic and social-emotional-behavioural issues. Therefore, copious research energy has gone into identifying treatments for ADHD in recent decades, and to a lesser but growing extent, WM. Lurking near the credible clinical and research laboratories are the usual quick-fix operators, who have manoeuvred lucrative niches for themselves in the still significant intervention gaps for this common and resource-hungry developmental disorder.

Can attentional and WM skills deficits be "remedied"?

Obviously (on the face of it at least), if deficits in attention and/or WM underlie many common neurodevelopmental disorders, then treatments designed to target these from "bottom up" should result in wide-ranging gains in cognition, learning, language, and behaviour. We wish. The search for a Holy Grail treatment for attentional and WM disorders has yielded a proliferation of approaches in recent decades. They range from the theoretically plausible according to current knowledge about the disorder, to the shameless parent-wallet-and-anxiety-targeting rip-offs that use parents' commitment to the best for their children as the obnoxious shoe-in-the-door.

Mainstream treatments for ADHD can be broadly classified as medication, behavioural interventions, neurofeedback, and cognitive training. Diets and dietary supplements, discussed in Chapter 10, are also advocated by some. We focus here on the first four, and then review some other popular "brain training" approaches and ideas for which evidence is weak or lacking, even though they flourish in the intervention marketplace and may also be adopted by schools.

Medication

There is some consensus in the literature that the current "gold standard" treatment for ADHD is a combination of behavioural management and medication (American Academy of Pediatrics, 2011; Sibley, Kuriyan, Evans, Waxmonsky, & Smith, 2014). Ideally, the initial focus is on behavioural approaches, which include parent and teacher training, particularly in the preschool years, with the addition and ongoing monitoring of medication if these do not deliver adequate improvements.

The stimulants dexamphetamine and methylphenidate (known by different trade names around the world) are the two main medications used to treat ADHD. These differ with respect to their underlying chemistry and effects, so individual children may benefit more from one than the other (Efron, Jarman, & Barker, 1997). Stimulants for ADHD may be prescribed in either short- or long-acting doses, with blood-levels of short-acting forms peaking after several hours, so they must be taken 2 or 3 times a day. The effects of long-acting (extended-release) stimulants last 8–12 hours, and so are usually taken once daily. Long-acting medications have the advantage of needing less vigilance than regular dosing across the day, and as children get older they may wish to avoid taking medication when peers are present.

Storebø et al. (2015) completed a Cochrane Review on methylphenidate use for children and adolescents diagnosed with ADHD, concluding that it may result in reduced teacher-reported ADHD symptoms, and improved teacher-reported general behaviour, and parent-reported quality of life. They also reported, however, that the low quality of the evidence in terms of methodological rigour means that the size (and, hence, clinical importance) of the reported effects was unclear. As well, they observed that the relative high frequency of side-effects, including sleep problems, headache, drowsiness, reduced appetite, weight loss, stomach pains, nausea and vomiting, and dry mouth is, of course, clinically important, *and* means that blinding of participants and assessors is difficult in research studies. Similarly, a Cochrane Review performed by Punja et al. (2016) showed that amphetamines reduced ADHD core symptoms according to parent, teacher and clinician ratings, but that the overall quality of the evidence ranged from low to very low, with high risk of study bias.

Sometimes, stimulants do not work well enough, and/or they cause unacceptable side-effects, and so less commonly-prescribed options may be considered. These include atypical antidepressants, such as atomoxetine and bupropion, and guanfacine and clonidine (high blood pressure medications). It is documented, however, that some of these drugs have side-effect profiles that are similar to stimulants, so may not be any better tolerated. Medication is generally not recommended for preschool children, and its long-term effects, positive and/or negative, are poorly understood. We recommend that you consult open-access practice guidelines in your country[1] to gain a broad understanding of the pros and cons of medication and then discuss options with your child's treating medical specialist.

---

1 In the United Kingdom, see: Attention Deficit Hyperactivity Disorder: Diagnosis and Management. NICE Guidelines. Available at: www.nice.org.uk/guidance/cg72/chapter/recommendations

In Australia, see: Clinical Practice Points on the Diagnosis, Assessment and Management of Attention Deficit Hyperactivity Disorder in Children and Adolescents. Available at: www.nhmrc.gov.au/guidelines-publications/mh26

In the USA, see: Attention-Deficit/Hyperactivity Disorder (ADHD). Available at: www.cdc.gov/ncbddd/adhd/guidelines.html

In Canada, see Canadian ADHD Practice Guidelines (CAP-Guidelines). Available at: www.caddra.ca/pdfs/caddraGuidelines2011.pdf

In New Zealand, see New Zealand Guidelines for the Assessment and Treatment of Attention-Deficit/Hyperactivity Disorder. Available at: www.health.govt.nz/publication/new-zealand-guidelines-assessment-and-treatment-attention-deficit-hyperactivity-disorder

In Europe, see Guidelines. Available at: www.adhd-institute.com/disease-management/guidelines/

Behavioural interventions

In addition to its relevance to academic learning, children's inattentiveness imposes significant tolls on social, emotional and behavioural development. This means that children diagnosed with ADHD will often, for all intents and purposes, present similarly to children with *pragmatic language impairments* (see Chapter 7), displaying difficulties with following conversations and instructions, inhibiting excessive talking, and waiting a turn, while frequently interrupting or intruding on others (Green, Johnson, & Bretherton, 2014), so a diagnosis of ADHD may accompany a diagnosis of language disorder and/or ASD. As we say repeatedly in *Making Sense of Interventions for Children with Developmental Disorders*, co-morbidity is the norm, and provides the backdrop against which interventions must be selected and trialled for each child. For children with attentional disorders, behavioural approaches are the mainstay, and involve training parents and teachers, as well as adjusting the environment to manage cognitive load and maximize successful attending, learning, and behaving, particularly when information and tasks are novel.

In Chapter 5, we briefly outline the theories underpinning behavioural interventions, and outline approaches that pertain to home and family life in some detail, so we focus here on behavioural approaches that are applicable in classrooms. The high prevalence rates of ADHD mean that one child in every classroom in America is so diagnosed (Fabiano et al., 2009), and behaviour management is a challenge for schools everywhere.

All behavioural interventions should be predicated on detailed *behavioural analysis*, conducted by an appropriately qualified clinician such as a psychologist or behaviour analyst, so that *antecedent events* and *reinforcers*[2] are identified, understood and, if necessary, addressed as first-line targets of any intervention. It is impossible to remove or modify every environmental factor influencing a child's behaviour; however, these do constitute the "low hanging fruit" and should always be considered first. We emphasize here, and in Chapter 5, that *behaviour is a form of communication*, and seeking to understand ways in which a child's behaviour can inform the practices and expectations of adults is a key goal of any behavioural analysis.

Modifiable environmental factors include classroom visual and auditory distractions that can sometimes be managed by teachers determining the

---

[2] *Antecedent events* occur *before* a behaviour and may be identified through behavioural analysis as predictable "triggers" of a particular behaviour (whether problematic or desired) for a child. *Reinforcers* are events that occur *after* the behaviour and influence the likelihood of the behaviour recurring in future similar circumstances.

nature, size and composition of small groups, the configuration of furniture and partitions, and manipulation of classroom seating arrangements (see Wheldall & Bradd, 2010). Just as the productivity and focus of adults vary as a function of their office-space configuration (De Been & Beijer, 2014), seating arrangements will impact on children's ability to display on-task behaviours. We agree with Wheldall and Bradd that, "Few adults would choose a social context in which to compose an important letter…and it amounts to little short of (albeit unwitting) cruelty to require individual work to be completed in seating contexts specifically geared towards interaction and conversation" (2010, p. 193).

While parents can find it difficult to influence their child's teacher or school regarding the approaches to behaviour management that are employed, we recommend that parents research school behaviour policies and the extent to which these guide actual classroom management and discipline approaches. Whole-school policies are increasingly required by education authorities, and dictate expectations concerning respectful behaviour, physical and emotional safety for all at school, and cyber-safety; such documents also define ways in which behaviour expectations may be contravened, e.g., through bullying, sexual harassment, and/or racial or religious vilification. Unfortunately, although many effective classroom behaviour management strategies have been identified through robust research, international studies show that these do not receive adequate coverage in teacher pre-service education, resulting in sub-optimal classroom practices and high levels of teacher stress (Dicke, Elling, Schmeck, & Leutner, 2015; Freeman, Simonsen, Briere, & MacSuga-Gage, 2014; O'Neill & Stephenson, 2014).

In their meta-analysis of what works to foster improved behaviour and academic achievement in classrooms, Marzano, Marzano, and Pickering (2003) identified four key factors: (1) predictable and known classroom rules and procedures; (2) the existence of clear and consistent disciplinary interventions; (3) the quality of teacher-student relationships; and (4) teachers' mental set (i.e., the teachers' willingness and ability to promptly identify and respond to problem behaviour, and to do so in a way that does not entail over-personalized responses). Similar findings were reported in Hattie's (2008) extensive review of what works in educational settings; this also identified the value of direct instruction over inquiry (problem-based) learning. This point goes to the heart of an ideological debate that is beyond the scope of this book; however, we are persuaded that children who either start from behind, or fall behind, at school often derive significant gains from

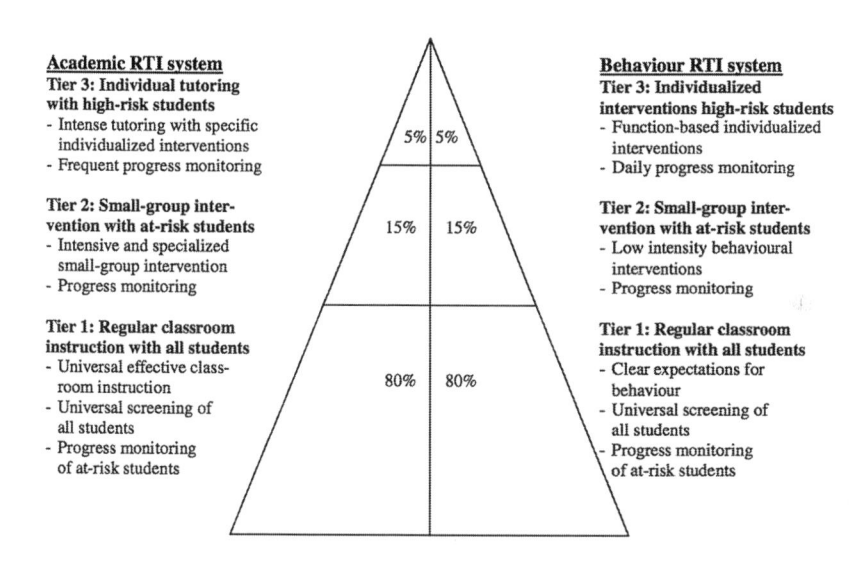

Academic RTI system			Behaviour RTI system
Tier 3: Individual tutoring with high-risk students - Intense tutoring with specific individualized interventions - Frequent progress monitoring	5%	5%	**Tier 3: Individualized interventions high-risk students** - Function-based individualized interventions - Daily progress monitoring
Tier 2: Small-group intervention with at-risk students - Intensive and specialized small-group intervention - Progress monitoring	15%	15%	**Tier 2: Small-group intervention with at-risk students** - Low intensity behavioural interventions - Progress monitoring
Tier 1: Regular classroom instruction with all students - Universal effective classroom instruction - Universal screening of all students - Progress monitoring of at-risk students	80%	80%	**Tier 1: Regular classroom instruction with all students** - Clear expectations for behaviour - Universal screening of all students - Progress monitoring of at-risk students

Figure 3.1 Three-tiered RTI approach in academic and behaviour domains. Source: Grosche & Volpe, 2013, p. 257; reproduced by permission

direct[3] (explicit) instruction, with its repeated opportunities for mastery, in order to make academic advances (Barnett, 2011; Stockard, 2010).

While not exclusively a behavioural issue, we note too that careful consideration should apply to the question of sleep quantity and quality. Sleep is important to the consolidation of new memories (Araújo & Almondes, 2014) and lack of it has been linked to inattention, behavioural deterioration, and increased accidental injuries in children and adolescents (Beebe, 2011). Sleep difficulties are more common in children with developmental disorders (Turnbull, Reid, & Morton, 2013), and should not be overlooked as a potentially modifiable factor (behaviourally and/or pharmacologically) that could influence classroom performance.

Response to intervention (RTI)

RTI is a three-tiered approach to assessing, monitoring, and responding to the behavioural and academic needs of children in mainstream and specialist

---

3 *Direct Instruction* (capitalized) is a specific teaching programme, where *direct instruction* (lower case) is a teaching method characterized by certain explicit instructional methods.

education classrooms that arose in part from USA legislative approaches, such as the *No Child Left Behind Act* (2001; www.k12.wa.us/esea/NCLB.aspx) and the *Individuals with Disabilities Education Act* (IDEA, 2004; http://idea.ed.gov), and is outlined in detail on the Center on Response to Intervention site: www.rti4success.org. As Figure 3.1 shows, its first (universal) tier refers to academic and behavioural approaches that are employed by teachers with all children in order to maximize behavioural and learning success. The overwhelming majority of children are expected to succeed, academically and behaviourally, as a result of Tier 1 classroom practices. In an RTI framework, teachers constantly use data derived from assessment tools and observational protocols to monitor student progress and determine whether additional supports are needed.

When children struggle to meet academic and/or behavioural expectations at Tier 1, they may be moved into Tier 2, with a small group of peers with similar support needs, to be provided with additional and/or more intensive instruction and behaviour support in order to "catch-up" with Tier 1 expectations. Ideally, such children return to Tier 1 when such goals are achieved, while a small proportion will need even more intensive and specialist 1:1 services, and these are offered at Tier 3. Again, the intention is that the provision of such supports should be time-limited, with students moving back down the tiers as they make up ground relative to their peers.

A strength of RTI is its focus on actual classroom practices. As Hempenstall (2012, p. 104) observed, it is assumed in an RTI framework that, "All students can learn and the learning is strongly influenced by the quality of instruction. In fact, it is argued that there is a predictable relationship between instructional quality and learning outcomes. It is expected that both general classroom programs and additional specific interventions will be evidence-based…". Although RTI has not been formally adopted outside the USA, we believe it has merit as a framework for considering and selecting educational and behaviour management approaches to the needs of all children, in a range of school settings. Our major caveat to this endorsement, however, lies in the quality of approaches employed at Tier 1. Unless optimal evidence-based approaches to academic instruction and classroom behaviour management are used at Tier 1, it is impossible to assert that Tier 2 and 3 services are actually reserved for children whose needs require specialized and intensive input. Grosche and Volpe (2013) underline that, because RTI is an American model, the only research on it is also American, so its applicability elsewhere is untested. Further, it is seen to have more utility as an intervention than a diagnostic framework, and has been applied more to remediating reading difficulties than to other developmental disorders that impact on classroom success.

Neurofeedback

The brain's neural activity involves *chemical* activity – the work of neurotransmitters such as dopamine and serotonin – and *electrical* activity. Neurofeedback, a form of biofeedback, relies on the fact that all kinds of brain activity (including sleep) result in electrical activity which can be detected and mapped using an electroencephalogram (EEG). During an EEG, multiple electrodes, applied to the scalp, transmit electrical signals via wires to a computer, which converts raw EEG data into frequency bands of interest so that comparisons between conditions (sleeping, reading, performing a mental task) and groups (e.g., children with/without ADHD), can be made to identify areas of the brain that appear to be active (or not) under particular conditions. These wave-forms have Greek letter-names: alpha, beta, delta, gamma, theta, and mu, categorized according to different levels of brain activity, developmental level, and some forms of brain pathology (e.g., epilepsy). Some studies have shown that the EEGs of children with ADHD differ from those of typically developing peers (e.g., Sonuga-Barke, Cortese, & Brandeis, 2013; Poil et al., 2014), while others suggest that there is no clear-cut distinction along clinical diagnosis lines, and that wide variability within an ADHD group can be expected (e.g., Buyck & Wiersema, 2014). Further, the stability of EEG changes over time in ADHD samples has been questioned (Holtmann et al., 2014). Nevertheless, the quest to harness EEG as a treatment modality has hurtled on relentlessly since the 1930s, and the advent of widely-accessible personal computers in the 1980s spawned a burgeoning industry. Unfortunately, rapid increases in the availability of technology have well outpaced science, with its characteristic caution and attention to detail in determining the efficacy of an approach. Neurofeedback has been defined as:

> *".... a theory-driven treatment based on operant learning strategies...The simultaneous and contingent feedback of neurophysiological signals is provided with the aim to learn to control the processes underlying these signals and thereby enhance (cognitive–emotional–behavioral) self-regulation. Changes in neurophysiological activity in the desired direction are reinforced by auditory and/or visual feedback. Feedback*

> *is usually presented in the form of simple computer games in which children can earn points (e.g., by moving objects on the screen)."*
> Gevensleben, Rothenberger, Moll, & Heinrich
> 2012, p. 448

What this boils down to is the presentation of computer games while the child is "wired to" EEG equipment that records and analyzes brain electrical data from the many electrodes placed on the scalp. The computer games are pitched at different developmental levels and are designed to be attractive and engaging to children and adolescents. Tasks might include striving to make a spaceship fly faster, which will only occur if a certain EEG condition is met and maintained. An aim of neurofeedback is to decrease *theta* waveform activity (associated with daydreaming or distraction), and increase *beta* activity which is associated with cognitive, emotional, and behavioural self-regulation (Arns et al., 2014; Baydala & Wikman, 2011; Gevensleben et al., 2012). The child receives real-time feedback about brain activity via EEG data, so knows if efforts at attending and focusing are meeting the criteria set by the clinician, as reflected in on-screen visual feedback. Neurofeedback thus incorporates principles of operant conditioning (see Chapter 5), whereby the aim is to change EEG activity through rewarding responses that display focused and/or sustained attention. Individual thresholds are adjusted across weeks of therapy, to gradually increase task complexity once initial gains are made.

Neurofeedback requires 30–40 sessions of around 45 minutes in duration, over 4–6 months, and is therefore associated with voluminous 1:1 therapist-child interaction. This poses an immediate methodological challenge to researchers, who rightly ask: to what extent are so-called "treatment effects" an artefact of therapeutic engagement and attention, rather than a reflection of some unique therapeutic benefits of the computer-based activity? (Arns et al., 2014). Systematic reviews and meta-analyses of neurofeedback and its effectiveness have highlighted this difficulty and a number of other methodological challenges, including questions as to the extent to which EEG changes correspond to meaningful behavioural changes detectable to adults who are "blind" (naïve) to the type of treatment received. Researchers also continue to tussle with finding appropriate placebo control conditions for comparison against neurofeedback – i.e., an equally engaging computer-based task that is not designed to have a therapeutic impact on learning. Importantly, too, few studies have examined whether apparent benefits achieved in the clinical setting transfer to tasks in the all-important real world where controlled feedback about EEG activity is not provided (Zuberer, Brandeis, & Drechsler, 2015). Further, there is evidence that neurofeedback is most effective in the context of effective parenting (Holtmann et al., 2014), which again calls into question the specificity of its effects. Recent systematic reviews (Arns et al., 2014; Cortese et al., 2016; Holtmann et al., 2014) conclude that, although research rigour has improved considerably in recent years, early optimism about neurofeedback's role in the treatment of ADHD may have been overstated. It is certainly the case that in some studies participants show gains (both on EEG and behavioural measures) in response to treatment, but it is too soon to be certain that behavioural gains reflect the treatment alone and are not simply an artefact of the study design (e.g., unblinded raters, meaning that observer expectancy biases results; or a positive effect of 1:1 adult attention in a calm, quiet room in treatment provided over 4–6 months). The jury is still out on neurofeedback.

Cogmed Working Memory Training (CWMT)

CWMT was developed at the Karolinksa Institute in Sweden by Klingberg, Forssberg and Westerberg (2002) and in 2010 was sold to Pearson Education where it is part of the Pearson Clinical Assessment Group. CWMT is a browser-based intervention, and App, that presents interactive games on a computer screen (overseen by a trained coach), requiring increasingly complex feats of concentration and memory in order to achieve successful outcomes. We found on the Cogmed website (www.cogmed.com), that 25×30–40-minute training sessions are completed online. The theoretical rationale for Cogmed training lies in the argument that WM is fundamental to attention and learning, and can be improved as a function of brain plasticity through specific and increasingly complex computer-delivered training exercises.

The evidence base for CWMT is *highly contested* and parents and researchers alike are forgiven for wondering whose earnest claims should carry most weight. Compare, for example, this from Söderqvist and Nutley (research directors at Pearson Clinical Assessment) who wrote in an undated (but presumably 2016) Pearson document:

> "As of March 2016, there are 80 original research studies examining the effects of CWMT published in peer-reviewed journals. The effects demonstrated in those are the basis for

> the claims that Cogmed currently makes. This document describes the policy underlying the formation of a Cogmed claim, as well as an elaboration of the evidence supporting each claim" (p. 1)

with this, from an independent academic review of CWMT against evidence-based criteria:

> "Given the state of the literature on CWMT, further investigation is needed before CWMT can be considered a clearly viable treatment for youth with ADHD." Chacko et al., 2013, p. 781

Two 2015 meta-analyses provide further examples of the mystifying evidence-status of Cogmed. One, conducted by Cortese and co-workers, concluded that although specific training on WM tasks results in improvements *on those tasks*, there was "…limited evidence for the clinical value of cognitive training for children with ADHD outside of the narrow confines of specific targeted neuropsychological processes" (Cortese et al., 2015, p. 173). Conversely, a meta-analysis co-authored by one of the developers of Cogmed (Spencer-Smith & Klingberg, 2015) reported clinically significant attention gains that generalize to improvements in everyday functioning. It is notable, however, that these authors initially identified 622 studies, with only 12 meeting inclusion criteria when filtered according to methodological rigour. This means that their conclusions are drawn from 2% of the studies, with 98% consigned to the metaphorical cutting-room floor. Hulme and Melby-Lervåg (2012) commented on the (then) current state of play with respect to WM training, pointing to an urgent need for more methodologically rigorous studies – larger sample sizes, random allocation to treatment arms, and multiple measures of key outcome variables (attention, learning, memory, behaviour). We would add the need for: careful blinding of raters (clinicians, parents, teachers), controlling the within-group variability (e.g., regarding age, clinical diagnoses, and co-morbidities), and identifying meticulous measures of skill transfer away from the computer screen towards the more complex and unpredictable demands of everyday life. This is exactly the kind of methodological rigour applied by Roberts et al. (2016) who examined academic outcomes two years after participation in Cogmed training in 452 children from 44 schools in Melbourne, Australia. Their open access paper records a failure of the intervention to produce measurable gains in reading, spelling, or maths, and in fact children in the Cogmed arm of the study recorded slightly lower scores on word reading and maths computation at the end of the intervention, leading the authors to conclude that "...our results raise questions regarding the potential for harm by taking children out of class on a regular basis for several weeks to provide an intervention such as this" (p. 8).

Much would be at stake, commercially and empirically, if computer-mediated training programs such as Cogmed could effect clinically meaningful, sustainable, generalizable gains across a range of social and academic demands in children's everyday lives. Perhaps unsurprisingly, then, this field has now reached the point where published *reviews of reviews* are materializing (e.g., Shinaver, Entwistle, & Söderqvist, 2014). Like Gathercole, Dunning, and Holmes (2012), Shinave et al. argue that some criteria used in meta-analyses and systematic reviews have been unduly strict. We see no compelling reasons, however, to make concessions on methodological rigour in this, or *any* approach to intervening for children with developmental needs, particularly given the diversion of time and financial resources that such approaches entail, and the ubiquitous opportunity cost. Cogmed has been (and is) the subject of intense research interest, so the contested, but increasingly negative nature of conclusions about its efficacy (see Roberts et al., 2016, above), by definition, means that we cannot endorse it as an evidence-based approach.

While Cogmed is the best-known computer-based approach to remediating attentional and WM difficulties, it has plenty of company in the marketplace. Variants include the Schuhfried (www.schuhfried.com) suite of programs, based on the exotic-sounding "Vienna Test System NEURO". The said Vienna System also has other streams: HR, TRAFFIC, and SPORT. Throughout *Making Sense of Interventions for Children's Developmental Disorders* we are critical of websites that have a dearth of peer-reviewed literature to which readers can refer. The Schuhfried site, including its CogniPlus page (www.schuhfried.com/trainings/cogniplus), is presented in a rather austere scientific-looking fashion, but fails to provide links to supporting research to back up the bold claims made about the programs' scientific bases, flexibility, and effectiveness across a wide range of neuropsychological disorders (everything, it seems, from ADHD in children to the rehabilitation of adults with acquired brain damage). Encouragingly, the NeuroMite page (www.neuromite.com.au) has a research tab, but clicking on it leads to an anticlimactic revelation: "The current study shows that there is strong evidence that cognitive (fluid) abilities underpin academic success. The capacity for students to perform well at school was strongly associated with divided attention, verbal memory, alertness, planning ability and sustained attention". Call the media. The "study" in question was only presented as a conference poster, so is worth pretty much the cardboard it may have been printed on as actual evidence. A series of polite but pointed emails to the Australian Schuhfried representative (a registered psychologist) requesting information about published evidence drew a blunderbuss[4] of neuropsychology references that bore no relevance to the CogniPlus or NeuroMite programs. Repeatedly pointing this out was starting to become embarrassing, so we eventually gave up.

It is worth noting here that "brain training" is big business, not just for children but also in the quest to prevent cognitive decline in adults. The *Lumosity* (www.lumosity.com) company produces desktop-, tablet- and smartphone Apps for brain training in English, French, German, Japanese, Korean, Portuguese, and Spanish, for a market that spans 182 countries. It recently took a hip-pocket hit from federal authorities in the US for deceptive claims about the capacity of its products to reduce cognitive decline, and for providing fraudulently obtained testimonials (Federal Trade Commission, 2016). History will tell whether the $US2 million fine will fuel more transparent, ethical practices. Nonetheless, the judgement stands as an admonition to providers in this space that consumers are entitled to scientifically-backed claims before they invest time, money, and hope in the next brainwave.

In addition to computer-based cognitive training, parents will encounter "low-tech" paper-and-pencil based interventions that make similar promises about their capacity to improve underlying cognitive, attention, and working memory skills. One such example is the Feuerstein Instrumental Enrichment (IE) program which, according to its website (http://acd.icelp.info) "...seeks to correct the deficiencies in fundamental thinking skills, provides students with the concepts, skills, strategies, operations and techniques necessary to function as independent learners, increase their motivation, develop metacognition – in short, to 'learn how to learn.'" A central thesis of IE seems to be that *intelligence* is modifiable, but we think that the more important focus for parents and teachers is children's *learning*, rather than their intelligence, in whatever way that might be measured (see pages 268–269). IE also has a strong narrative about the increased complexity of the modern world and children's need to think adaptively and respond flexibly to their environments. Similar rhetoric commonly turns up in modern education material, but does not necessarily translate into classroom practices that go beyond what teachers

---

4 A blunderbuss is a firearm with a flanged barrel to allow wide spray of shot and other projectiles. We think it apt here that its Wikipedia page describes it as having been "...effective at short ranges, but lacked accuracy for targets at long range" (https://en.wikipedia.org/wiki/Blunderbuss).

normally consider to be commonsense (e.g., repetition, salience, and novelty of information and materials), and we are aware of no evidence that repeated practice on isolated cognitive skills via paper-and-pencil activities improves academic performance any more than we could locate convincing evidence for computer-mediated approaches.

Brain Gym®

Highly visible globally, parents will likely encounter Brain Gym® (BG) via their child's school, in the mainstream or specialist education sector. BG was developed by Dr Paul Dennison who, according to the program's website (www.braingym.org): "In the 1960s, began the seminal research into reading achievement and its relation to brain development that would form the basis for the Brain Gym work—the remarkable movement-based learning program that has helped people of all ages turn their learning challenges into successes". You know us: "seminal research" saw us scurrying for peer-reviewed literature, particularly as Dr Dennison earned his PhD at the Faculty of Education at the University of Southern California. Investigations began in the 1960s, so there should be five decades' worth of peer-reviewed debate on BG. But no.

BG is based on an unscientific line of thinking that persists in some neurodevelopmental circles – that developments in gross and fine motor skill have direct relevance to aspects of cognitive, language, and memory development. Some clinicians recall with dismay the Doman-Delacato method, emanating from the Philadelphia-based Institute for the Achievement of Human Potential, founded in 1955. It is based on the idea (slated by the American Academy of Pediatrics in 1982) that developmental difficulties (whether due to verifiable brain damage such as cerebral palsy, or based solely on clinician assessment, such as ADHD) can be ameliorated through gross motor exercises ("pattern therapy" or "psychomotor patterning") aimed to boost neural pathways that somehow link gross motor skills with cognitive and language skills.

Undiscouraged by the lack of empirical support for such a notion, Dennison teamed up with his future wife Gail, an artist and movement director, and they co-created Educational Kinesiology – a conveniently authentic-sounding but nonetheless invented field. According to the BG website, "…the organization is committed to the principle that intentional movement is the door to optimal living and learning. Its mission is to support self-awareness and the ease of living and learning through safe, simple, and effective movement". Salient here is the liberal use of soft terminology: "ease of living", and "safe, simple and effective movement" – who argues that these are undesirable? Equally, who can define their presence or absence in an individual and, if present, the mechanism whereby they arose? Keeping it safe and simple at least attempts to respect the "first do no harm" dictum, but of course there is always harm in lost opportunity.

BG is now offered in more than 80 countries, via schools (predominantly) and businesses, and is built on 26 physical activities "…based upon empirical experience rather than neurological research". This disingenuous candour thinly camouflages BG's position, which we paraphrase as: "Instead of drawing on hard science, the approach is based on our own belief system". The 26 activities (e.g., The Elephant, The Cross-Crawl, The Double-Doodle, The Owl, The Energizer – described on the BG website) focus on balancing, re-patterning and multisensory stimulation. Sporting "cute" appealing names, they make equally "cute" and appealing claims, like improving confidence, stability, and self-expression, and reducing confusion and uncertainty. Such flat-feet-to-halitosis claims, we hope, set off alarm bells in consumers' minds.

There is little rigorous research about BG's efficacy in improving children's learning, either for those who are typically developing or for those who are experiencing difficulties. In the place of research rigour there are boundless testimonials, so while it is clear that BG creates a "feel good" glow, this is not the same as actually shifting the performance of *actual* children on *actual* skills that are important in the, well, *actual* world. We agree, therefore, with Spaulding, Mostert and Beam (2010, p. 26), who concluded that, "While these testimonials and anecdotal stories are persuasive, passionate, and compelling, they do *not* meet the established criteria for quality research in special education".

Reviewing BG raises the broader question of physical activity and cognitive functioning in children. In an era of sharp increases in childhood obesity levels in industrialized nations, few debate the face value of embedding physical activity into the school day. Physical activity is important in its own right for children's general health (cardiovascular function and body-mass index in particular) and in some cases results in opportunities to participate in team-based sports and outdoor projects that are intrinsically enjoyable and, some would say, character building. This notwithstanding, several reviews highlight the equivocality in evidence around the effects of physical activity on children's attentional and learning skills (Janssen, Toussaint, van Mechelen, & Verhagen, 2014; Rasberry et al., 2011; Singh, Uijtdewilligen, Twisk, Van Mechelen, & Chinapaw, 2012). The muddy state of "the science" is epitomized in this bet-each-way conclusion of a systematic review: "Results suggest physical activity is either positively related to academic performance or that there is not a demonstrated relationship between physical activity and academic performance" (Rasberry et al., 2011, p. S10). In part, the evidence is weak because methodological rigour was lacking in many of the studies conducted, so the question of links between physical activity and academic performance lingers.

Whole-brain/Brain-based learning

This extraordinary classroom approach is the brainchild (no pun intended) of California teacher Chris Biffle, and you can sample it via YouTube™ *ad nauseam*. Examples range from the first years of school to tertiary education, and follow highly scripted, prescriptive activities said to "activate the whole brain" in the learning process. It is difficult for us to do justice in text to what this approach looks like in action, but it can be summarized as class-based imitation and mimicry of set phrases and actions, that students must imitate immediately, using exactly the same intonation pattern as the teacher's. What *is* going on in those "*Teach!*" moments that create immediate, deafening classroom hubbub which would be overwhelming for children with ASD and/or attention and/or language processing, and/or emotional difficulties? How can the teacher monitor each pair of children who are supposedly "teaching" (repeating back) a piece of information that the teacher has just presented? To what extent do mimicry and compliance represent learning? How can higher-order concepts be taught (let alone learned) in this way? Normally, we would seek answers to such questions by consulting the academic literature for peer-reviewed papers that provide a theoretical rationale for an approach and examples of the way in which it has been trialled.

A rationale for an intervention needs to either align with current understanding of the workings of the brain, or provide a convincing argument as to why it deviates. In the case of Whole-brain/Brain-based learning, however, such searches return slim pickings indeed. Mostly, we find references to the Whole Brain Teaching website (www.wholebrainteaching.com), replete with glowing teacher testimonials, and the endless YouTube™ clips. Curiously, we found a link to "research" under a tab called "Goodies" (childish, we thought, for a site aimed at teachers), but when we clicked (via different browsers) we were transported to a blank page – a disarmingly honest representation of its evidence base. *Nowhere* on the website is any attempt to explain the underlying rationale of this approach, and a search of academic databases yielded only student "research" projects which are available online but not peer-reviewed and published in academic sources. The claims in one such paper (de Jager & du Toit, 2009) make for excruciating reading for anyone with even a modicum of neuroscience knowledge. With nary an ounce of supporting evidence, Whole Brain teaching techniques are explained with reference to the types of brain activation that are said to be occurring. For example, during the recitation of the *Five Classroom Rules* activity, "The limbic system engages the prefrontal cortex, Broca's area, Wernicke's area, the limbic system, hippocampus, visual cortex and the motor cortex" (de Jager & du Toit, 2009, p. 8). Dismissing the nonsensical circulatory nature of "the limbic system engaging the limbic system", this is nothing more than the stringing together of a list of brain regions to make unsubstantiated claims about what is happening during a classroom activity. You can find more of these neatly packaged "explanations" at www.wholebrainteaching.com. If teachers were taught neuroscience in their pre-service training they would be well-positioned to spot this kind of fakemelorum, but in its absence, are prey to multiple variants of neurononsense.

This approach is *at best* a crowd-control tactic, to gain students' attention and have them comply with military-style instructions of dubious learning value. That so many teachers buy into it, and that at least one education academic (located at Australia's Monash University) runs teacher professional development seminars on "Brain-Based Learning" (without having published research on the approach), leaves us greatly concerned about the exposure of teachers and children to time-wasting, atheoretical, non-evidence-based approaches, and associated woolly thinking. Claims that such approaches will assist teachers with "Getting the inside secrets of how to influence your student's brain chemistry" and provide "Brain-friendly tools and strategies for literacy instruction across all disciplines" (www.monash.edu/education/future-students/courses/short-courses/education-support/brain-based-teaching-strategies; accessed August 7, 2016) are both silly and grandiose. Teachers do not teach *brains*, they teach *children*, and the learning and behaviour of children is all they observe. They can neither observe nor measure their students' brain chemistry. This is pseudoscience writ large.

Laying some neuromyths to rest

Before closing this chapter, we consider other common neuromyths that permeate classrooms and parent chatrooms. First up, let's give the silly idea that *"we only use 10% of our brains"* a decent burial. You might believe it, and we couldn't possibly comment but suggest swinging the other 90% into action, right now, if you do. The brain is a complex, integrated organ, and we need it all. Yes, some people make amazing adaptations after stroke and other brain injuries, but 90% of the brain's real estate does not sit idle. Related to this is another ridiculous notion: the idea that the world divides into *"left brain" and "right brain" learners*. All human brains have a distinctive left and right hemisphere, evolved (in both evolutionary and individual developmental terms) to perform specialized functions. Broadly speaking, the left hemisphere is specialized for language and the right for visuospatial skills, but a massive bundle of neural fibres, the *corpus callosum* ("tough body"), links the hemispheres so that they work synergistically on all sensory, motor, cognitive, memory, language, spatial, and behavioural tasks that humans perform.

Learning styles

The belief that different learners have a natural preference for receiving new information via one sense (e.g., visual, auditory, or kinaesthetic/tactile, or "VAK") over the other, has been enormously influential in western education systems since the 1970s, and particularly since the publication of Dr David Kolb's *Learning Styles Inventory* in 1985. According to Learning Styles (LS) theory, teachers should provide instruction that optimizes learning for each child, by ensuring, for example, that visual learners have opportunities to *see* new information, auditory learners to *hear* it, and tactile-kinaesthetic learners to *touch and feel* curriculum materials (the latter being easier said than done as students climb up the grades). All of this follows, of course, a diagnostic process, in which the child's favoured LS is determined using a self-assessment tool. LS thinking spawned a decades-long, multinational industry of professional development materials and seminars for teachers and a plethora of tools for assessing students' preferences using the VAK framework.

Admittedly, the central thrust of LS thinking is reasonable, i.e., the idea that learners differ, bringing different background knowledge, interests, skills, and instructional preferences or requirements to the classroom. So far, so good, and most teachers would agree, we think, that a certain amount of "tailoring" is needed for individual learners in order to maximize their engagement and progress (notwithstanding that there are many common features among students that must be present for engagement and learning to occur). We think most teachers would also concur on the many shared elements in what makes for good learning, such as understanding the learner's starting point, explaining the aim of a learning task, breaking tasks down into manageable "chunks" so that small wins are readily accessible, and providing opportunities for repeated practice and consolidation of new knowledge and skills. However, the idea that all learners can be categorized into three groups (V, A, and K) flouts the basic learning principles that teachers apply in their classrooms every day, and has been roundly criticized and, in fact, dismissed in recent years (e.g., Howard-Jones, 2014; Pashler, McDaniel, Rohrer, & Bjork, 2008; Reiner & Willingham, 2010). In spite of these contemporary critical reviews, LS is one of the more resilient non-evidence-based contaminants to the education arena, having been credibly sold as robust and empirically-based to two generations of teachers. Dekker-Lee, Howard-Jones and Jolles (2012) reported that the LS neuromyth is embraced by over 90% of teachers so, along with other common forms of pseudoscience that have far too much prominence in modern education, we say it deserves to be obliterated from teacher pre-service and in-service education. Regrettably, this will take some time.

While Learning Stylists would have us believe that the world is cordoned off into three discrete sections to accommodate three different types of learner, there is an equally pernicious and silly polar extreme that holds that "all children learn differently". If there are more than 7 billion people in the world, that means that instead of three learning styles, there are actually, well, more than 7 billion, so a teacher's lot is not a happy one; happy one. In fact, there are more *similarities* than differences with respect to how children learn, and to the trained observer there are recognizable *patterns* associated with different developmental stages and with different developmental disorders. The purpose of assessment (whether by an SLP/SLT, psychologist, or other professional) is to identify those patterns and determine intervention priorities and approaches. The "all children learn differently" mantra, that chimes so sweetly with the truism, "everyone's an individual", is especially popular with purveyors of non-evidence-based nonsense.

Does screen exposure damage children's brains?

This is a question we are frequently asked by teachers who have heard, or read in popular media, about supposed harmful effects of screen[5] exposure ("screen-time") on children's brain development. There is an irony in this given the role of computers in modern education, and we suspect that, mostly, teachers are concerned about students' *non-academic* screen-time. That aside, some teachers' concerns are in response to the scientifically unsubstantiated

---

5 In this context, "screen" refers mainly to computers and mobile devices rather than to television.

claims made by British neuroscientist Baroness Susan Greenfield (2015). Dr Greenfield has a disappointing penchant for straying from the scientific method, favouring media limelight for popularist, invalid claims. In theatrical miscasting of correlation as causation, Dr Greenfield argues (2015) dramatically that much touted *alleged* recent increases in autism diagnoses (see page 68) are linked to the upsurge of screen exposure in young people's lives. Most worryingly of all for the scientific cause, Dr Greenfield makes these claims not in the peer-reviewed literature, where she knows they would require empirical evidence and be open to refute by scientific peers (and no, we do not necessarily refer here to barons, earls, and dukes), but in the context of an opinionated, populist book. There is no scientifically plausible evidence that screen exposure is "re-wiring" young peoples' brains in harmful ways, and claims to this effect should be dismissed as ill-founded hype (Bell, Bishop, & Przybylski, 2015; Mills, 2014). On the contrary, computer games in childhood can have beneficial effects on social and emotional development (Durkin & Barber, 2002) and there is emerging evidence of the psychosocial benefits of social media use by people with disabilities (e.g., Brunner, Hemsley, Palmer, Dann, & Togher, 2015). Given the wide popularity of videogames in childhood and adolescence, their use for enjoyment (if nothing else) by children with special developmental needs should be normalized, not stigmatized (Durkin, Boyle, Hunter, & Conti-Ramsden, 2013), with continuing scrutiny with respect to their educational and psychosocial pros and cons. We note here, though, that evidence is emerging to say that children's screen exposure should be minimized at night, as this may interfere with sleep (Hale & Guan, 2015; Hysing et al., 2015). There is also a small group of individuals with epilepsy who exhibit *photosensitive epilepsy*, a rare genetic epilepsy-variant in which seizure activity is associated with certain forms of light stimulation (Sadleir et al., 2015). It is said by some (e.g., www.epilepsy.org.au) that affected children may be more prone to seizure activity during screen exposure; however, we could locate no recent peer-reviewed literature that supports this assertion.

What is a Growth Mind-set and does your child need one?

For decades, interest has grown in the role of children's self-concept as learners, generating an enormous body of research on a range of self-related constructs, including self-esteem, and self-efficacy for learning (see Hattie, 2014). In more recent times, a topical "self" notion has entered the classroom in the form of "Growth vs Fixed Mind-set". This idea originates in particular from the work of Stanford University Professor Carol Dweck and her colleagues, and holds that children who have an implicit theory or belief that intelligence can be developed through effort and practice (i.e., those said to have a mastery, or *Growth Mind-set*), understand that "...struggle is an opportunity for growth, not a sign that a student is incapable of learning" (Paunesku et al., 2015, p. 785). By contrast, children who believe that their abilities are immovable, and hence experience academic challenges as a sign that they are "dumb", are said to have a helpless, or so-called *Fixed Mind-set* (Paunesku et al., 2015; Yeager & Dweck, 2012). According to proponents of this theory, a Fixed Mind-set is not only unhelpful for struggling learners, it is also problematic for high-achievers, who may initially attribute their success to innate ability and then neglect to apply adequate effort when tasks become harder, at which point unexpected failure occurs. In Mind-set theory, the kind of feedback and responses that students receive from teachers and parents (praise, encouragement, comfort, reassurance) can exert both helpful and unhelpful effects on Mind-set and on subsequent learning. Dweck (2007) argued that praise should focus on effort, processes, strategies, and perseverance, rather than the child's intelligence or talent, as the latter gives rise to a Fixed Mind-set.

Dr Dweck and colleagues have commercialized the Mind-set concept as MindsetMaker™, an online teacher professional development program and tools, and Brainology®, a blended learning curriculum (i.e., online and face-to-face delivery) for students, available at www.mindsetworks.com. Like many approaches that are enthusiastically promoted to parents, teachers, and schools, the Mindsetsworks site is heavily populated with testimonials, and even boasts the US Department of Education Institute of Education Sciences as a funding partner. We find this endorsement troubling, given that the document entitled "Evidence of Impact: Brainology® & Mindset Works® SchoolKit" hanging from the "Science" tab on the site, refers to four reports on Brainology®, none of which are published in the peer-reviewed literature. In an independent evaluation of Brainology, however, Donohoe, Topping and Hannah (2012) reported short-term changes in Mind-set that were not sustained at follow-up. There was also no significant difference in the academic performance of the two groups under study one year after the Brainology® intervention.

Growth Mind-set has new black status in education, which is another way of saying we fear it might be the new Learning Styles, or the new Multiple Intelligences: a smartly packaged piece of popular psychology that has some face validity but is translated into practice way ahead of the independent scientific analysis that establishes both its contribution and its limitations. *Of course* students need to have a level of belief in themselves as learners, and *of course* teachers must think carefully about how they craft and position feedback, in the process of supporting students' learning and helping them to persist in the face of difficulties. Both of these should be basic to any pre-service teacher education programme that covers learning theories. However, the message that all that is needed is a gritty shoulder-to-the-wheel mentality may be counterproductive for students with learning difficulties, who need more external support and repeated opportunities to achieve incremental mastery. We do not believe that diverting hours of staff professional development time and student class-time to promoting Growth Mind-sets is justified on the current science.

The monetization of ADHD

In this chapter we deal mainly with ADHD and its associated cognitive, behavioural and academic consequences. Because of the high prevalence of ADHD, and the wide-ranging daily challenges it creates for affected children, their parents, teachers, and society, its treatment is big business, avidly monetized by Big Pharma and, increasingly, Big IT with promises of browser and App-based treatments that will do Big Things in re-wiring and brain-training commerce. Their neuro-this and neuro-that buzzwords and scientific half-truths sound kind of plausible, but rarely bear up well under even gentle methodical inspection. In the ADHD marketplace, perhaps more than any other, disreputable snake-oil and pseudoscience merchants rake it in, monetizing a raft of supposed "underlying causes", and marketing aggressively to parents, individual teachers, whole schools, and school systems. Their cacophony and charisma can easily obscure the honest, plain-packaged offerings of legitimate behavioural approaches, honed by cognitive and educational psychology. Years of mixed-methods research is needed in this space; meanwhile, parents are advised to stay on the old black, and avoid the seductive new black and the off-road, wild terrain of big promises, big spends, big disappointments, and low returns.

4 Children with autism spectrum disorders

The initials "ASD" stand for autism (or autistic) spectrum disorders. The term refers to four lifelong conditions found under the heading of *neurodevelopmental disorders* in the DSM-5 (American Psychiatric Association, 2013). ASD encompasses the diagnoses of autism, Asperger syndrome (a separate diagnostic category prior to DSM-5), pervasive developmental disorder not otherwise specified (PDD-NOS), and childhood disintegrative disorder. ASDs are complex, and characterized by various combinations of: social interaction and communication deficits (unified in DSM-5 as "social communication" impairments); stereotyped or repetitive behaviours; sensitivities to sensory input; and, for about 38% of affected individuals, intellectual disability (ID), with a further 24% falling in the borderline IQ range (see pages 61, and 268–269). Parents, professionals, autism advocates, and people on the spectrum – some of whom prefer to be called "autistics" – muse and debate whether autism is a disorder, a disability, a cluster of deficits and symptoms to be treated, a neuro-divergent genetic variation or "neuro-minority" (Walker, 2012), or a way of being to be embraced as part of the diversity of the human condition.

No blood, cheek swab, hair, skin, urine tests, or brain scans can be run to diagnose ASD, and no ultrasound, amniocentesis or other form of crystal ball can be consulted prenatally. Instead, to identify ASD, an interdisciplinary team investigates a child's behaviour (the top predictor) and development, using evaluation tools that address the DSM-5 framework. This allows children diagnosed with ASD early in development, sometimes before they turn 3, to be described objectively relative to the severity of observed *social communication indicators* and *fixated or restricted behaviours or interests*, and the impact of any *associated features*: genetic disorders, and/or ID. To date, the suite of *early* predictors of ASD at 12–24 months, that correctly identifies just 30% of children on the spectrum, is a baby's response when their name is said, eye-contact, imitation, protodeclarative[1] pointing to show interest, and joint attention.

---

1 Pointing with an index finger to *request* an object is called protoimperative pointing, while pointing to draw attention to an object, to "comment" on it, or to share an interest in it is called protodeclarative pointing. The ability to use pointing to communicate typically develops by 12 months of age.

Social communication impairments vary in degree along a continuum (Gerber, Brice, Capone, Fujiki, & Timler, 2012; Norbury, 2014) and within and across individuals. Involvement ranges from the boys and girls who appear to occupy a private world, outwardly oblivious to others, to the so-called high-functioning (where "high functioning" does not equate to "highly intelligent") individuals who communicate awkwardly or reluctantly, miss or misread social cues and nuances, have odd "pragmatics" and good days (or moments) and bad days (or moments), with their communication skills that are strongly

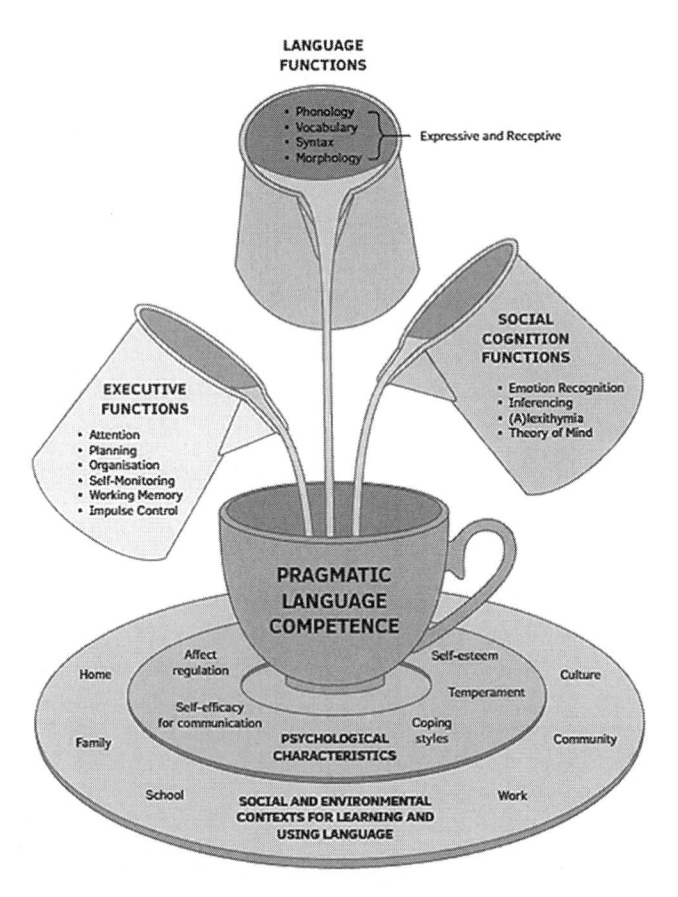

Figure 4.1 Pragmatic language competence.
Eloise Retallick: adapted from Snow & Douglas (2017)

impacted by social context (for expert first-person reflections see Sparrow Rose Jones and Morénike Giwa Onaiwu in Sutton, 2015). They constantly or intermittently lack the ability to *use* language in ways that are judged by others (unless the "others" happen to be autistic and/or inclusive in outlook) to be socially and contextually appropriate. For them, the interlinking contents and influencers of the pragmatic language competence "cup", displayed in Figure 4.1, are somehow "off". They may be valued, dismissed or belittled – and sometimes it is unclear which – as odd, original, eccentric, strange, geeky, or "a character"; or be embraced for their neurodiversity (Singer, 2016), as "naturally different" and not disordered or in need of remediation.

Genetics

Genetics research (De Rubeis, He, Goldberg, Poultney, Samocha, et al., 2014) led to the identification of mutations in 107 genes that may contribute to the probability of ASD. These findings, reported in *Nature*, bring a better understanding of the labyrinthine pathways involved in the disorder, and could eventually help in developing therapies. In an astounding prediction, the team foreshadowed that over 1000 genes might be implicated as ASD risk factors, but with many impacting modestly. Genetic disorders that can co-occur with ASD are: Angelman, Down, Fragile-X, Klinefelter, Landau-Kleffner, Prader-Willi, Rett, and Williams syndromes. When they co-occur, children exhibit the specific characteristics that define the particular syndrome *and* the ASD indicators. This partially explains the wide variability among individuals on the spectrum.

ASD and intellectual disability

Investigators at the Centers for Disease Control and Prevention (CDC) studied records from 2008, finding that 38% of children with ASD had ID (or an IQ below 70), 24% performed in the borderline range (71–85), and 38% had IQs in the average or above average range (above 85). They further found that significantly more females than males with ASD had ID, noting that ASD is 4–5 times more prevalent in males. In the period that the CDC has calculated prevalence rates of ASD and co-occurring ID, the rate of individuals with ASD who do *not* have ID has risen faster than the rate of individuals *with* ASD and ID. The overall rate of ASD was higher than in past US studies, at around 1 child in 68 children affected (earlier, it was 1:88).

Brain development and the environment

The prefix "neuro" in *neurodevelopmental, neurodiversity, neurotypical,* and *NeuroTribes* (Silberman, 2015) refers to the central nervous system (CNS) – the brain, brainstem, and spinal cord – which communicates via nerves with the organs of sensory perception responsible for hearing, taste, touch, smell, proprioception (the ability to sense where our body parts are in space without having to look), and vision. The CNS also communicates with muscles in organs such as the heart and stomach, and throughout the body to support both skilled (voluntary) and automatic (autonomous) movements. The brain functions of "neurotypical" or typically developing (TD) children grow predictably, in concert with *maturation* and *experience,* as youngsters learn from and adapt to consistent, changing, and new features of the *environment.* Environmental features are *internal* and *external.* This "neuro" development demands particular environmental inputs, and the relationships between brain development and experience with the environment are dynamic and interdependent.

Children with ASD experience their internal and external environments differently from neurotypical (NT) children, even when those around them are empathic, reassuring, bent on giving them "normal" input (message sent is not always message received), and are there to guide them with visual signposts: planners, Social Stories® (Gray & Garand, 1993) and routines-timetables. Figuratively, their nervous systems veer away from the everyday adaptations (e.g., responding positively to consolation, praise, reassurance or distraction) that generally help children deal with the changes and challenges of growing up.

For a child with ASD, life is largely shaped by incongruities between what their brain is equipped to handle in the moment and the behavioural, communicative, developmental, emotional and interpersonal challenges they are expected to conquer. The challenges may be as seemingly innocuous as the sound of a door slamming, cutlery set out differently from usual, or donning a new shirt with a tickly label; or as complex as being unable to calm down if one of these challenges becomes overwhelming, with the individual with ASD growing more anxious and agitated in the face of each kind and "comforting" intrusion.

Jack and the Weather King

Chatty, friendly, dog-loving, sensory-seeking, 8-year-old Jack, diagnosed with ASD, endured what his twin brother christened a "Jack Attack" in those exact door, cutlery, and shirt scenarios – which left him weeping inconsolably. Yet he was untroubled in some circumstances that a TD peer would probably see as risky. He was a confident runner and climber: recalling him shaking off his mother's protective grip and prancing through traffic, hands flapping, across a shopping street to befriend a surprised Jack Russell Terrier (which, in a rare use of possessive case, he called a "Jack's Russell") on the sidewalk opposite, is spine tingling.

Jack's climbing was concentrated on a desire to be "on top" of domestic appliances, preferably when they were operating. He would curl his wiry little body into a U-shape, hat pulled over his eyes, with his right ear glued to the surface of the appliance, evidently engrossed in the vibrations. "On top" of the washing machine and "on top" of the fridge were not too bad at home, a little tricky when visiting, but *nothing* compared with the 40°C/104°F afternoon when he climbed "on top" of his family's roof-mounted 1998 *Weather King* 10 SEER 5-ton heat pump unit, clad only in board shorts and a hat. His cries of "Jack needs to jump" (9 metres to the ground), and "Jack's on the roof" from a wee posse of pop-eyed small boys, alerted his father. Fingers trembling, he dialled 000, realising that Jack was stranded, barefooted, on the *Weather King*, powerless to cross the scorching metal roof in order to clamber down, and that jumping was seriously on the agenda. Fire and Rescue NSW arrived and acted quickly, without drama. His sweltering rescuers plucked him from his perch, preserving unruffled calm, while Jack wriggled and giggled, descending headfirst in a fireman's lift. He loved *that* level of stimulation.

Spellbound by the rescue crew and their paraphernalia, Jack's brother and his friends played "emergency rescue" for days. Did the incident spark an interest in Jack in Fire and Rescue, or stop his roof climbing; did he *learn* and *generalize* from the *experience*? No, no, and not really. Not once did he mention the incident. He never again climbed *his* roof, but rather than absorbing the idea that a rooftop is potentially dangerous, his fascination shifted from appliances generally, to *Weather Kings* only. With a dusty collection of 1990s *Weather King* brochures for reference – how his parents regretted squirrelling them away in the shed – Jack delivered regular soliloquies on their years of manufacture, features, model numbers and specifications, and climbed *other* roofs to find them. There was no telling him that their *Weather King*, imported by the family from the US, was unique in the district; Jack had to see for himself.

Autism news and reviews in print and electronic media

Imagine if Jack's story were reported as a case vignette in a research article in a quality journal. Chances are it would be picked up by a wire service, finding its way to the dwindling range of printed newspapers, or to electronic outlets like Medical Daily, RAND Health and Healthcare, or Science Direct, where it would likely acquire an overly-positive twist. Not so much, *"Boy Frightens Everyone, Learning Little"* as *"Spirited Lad's Rooftop Experience Paves Way for Autism Breakthrough"*, or something. In this vein, a real journal article, guardedly titled *"Nonmedical Interventions for Children with ASD: Recommended Guidelines and Further Research Needs"* was rejigged breezily by RAND as: *"What Evidence Says About How Best to Treat Children with Autism"*. TIME reports research under such headlines as: *"Behavior Therapy Normalizes Brains of Autistic Children"* and *"Autism Symptoms Disappeared with Behavioral Therapy in Babies"*; and the *New York Post* headlines a review of Levin (2015) with: *"The Miracle that Cured My Son's Autism was in Our Kitchen"*. This, even though Susan Levin states in her self-contradictory book (extolling a gluten-free diet, home-schooling, and the Son-Rise Program®): "Ben is now twelve years old. He has come a long way since he received his diagnosis. He is not cured of challenges, but he has shed many of his autistic characteristics." The reviewer may have missed that, drawn by: "Many people still don't believe recovery from autism is possible, but I know it is because of our experience with Ben".

Pity the family blasted with "the best way to treat" with "miracle cures" that "normalize brains" making "symptoms disappear", in reports that fail to say that while children with ASD *can* be helped in many ways, and research *is* forging ahead in its painstaking way, and all is *not* gloom, doom, heartbreak and melancholy, ASD is not *going* anywhere, specifically, not *away*.

> *"The studies that are reported with such fanfare in the media report outcomes that are measured exactly at the end of interventions that last for a matter of months. I believe that they help the children cope with the current challenge and they probably help the child and parent prepare for the next one coming up. How much hope they should offer for the longer-term future is questionable. For the parent participant I hope they show that if you can win one battle, you are likely to win the next one—as long as you can maintain your stamina there is hope there—but don't let down your guard because there be dragons ahead!"*
>
> Susan Rvachew, 2015
> www.developmentalphonologicaldisorders.wordpress.com

Dr Rvachew, a Canadian academic S-LP, highlights in her blog a study part-funded by Autism Speaks (www.autismspeaks.org): Szatmari, Georgiades, Duku, Bennett, and Bryson, et al. (2015) where a team of 14 investigators recognize the developmental (permanent) nature of ASD in reporting their research. They describe trajectories for children from diagnosis, between age 2 and 4 until age 6, tracking their autism symptoms (e.g., preoccupations, like Jack's interest in *Weather Kings*) and adaptive functioning (e.g., learning, or in Jack's case, not learning much, from internal and external experience). The research cautiously *suggests* that the predictors of outcomes for ASD symptoms (behaviour and development) *may* be biological (e.g., gender) whereas the predictors of outcomes for adaptive function *may* be environmental (e.g., early identification of ASD), and that autism symptoms and adaptive function are not coupled together.

> *"It is imperative that a flexible suite of interventions that target both autistic symptom severity and adaptive functioning be implemented and tailored to each child's strengths and difficulties."*
> Szatmari, Georgiades, Duku, Bennett, Bryson, et al. 2015,
> p. 283

Books about autism

Popular books on ASD abound, and many are far removed from the *"miracle that cured my son's autism was in our kitchen"*. It would be hard to find six books more different from each other than: *The Real Experts: Readings for Parents of Autistic Children* (Sutton, 2015), *Thinking Person's Guide to Autism* (Des Roches Rosa, Myers, Ditz, Willingham, & Greenburg, 2011), *In a Different Key: The Story of Autism* (Donvan & Zucker, 2016a), *Uniquely Human: A Different Way of Seeing Autism* (Prizant & Fields-Meyer, 2015), *Far from the Tree* (Solomon, 2012; 2013), and the critically acclaimed *Neurotribes: The Legacy of Autism and the Future of Neurodiversity* (Silberman, 2015).

Neurodiversity rights advocate Michelle Sutton (www.michellesuttonwrites.com) has capably compiled and edited 128 pages of illuminating essays and articles representing autistic voices: activists, parents, poets, students, teachers and writers. Her aim is to guide families in helping their autistic children to thrive, and she wrote it because she was unable to find the information she sought, as the mother of two autistic children. Described by Steve Silberman in an Amazon.com review as "a landmark book", *The Real Experts* is forthrightly pro-Facilitated Communication (FC) and anti-ABA (while we support neither position). It includes four essays by nonverbal and autistic FC user and advocate Amy Sequenzia, and a distaste for ABA (see pages 82–84) as abusive and damaging is evident throughout the book. It offers a unique insight into the rarely-heard opinions, perceptions and preferences of autistic adults across Australian and US settings.

Des Roches Rosa et al. (2011) brims with science, insights, informed opinions and sensible advice, largely written from parents' perspectives and by people on the spectrum. Key messages are that researchers and clinicians should express their findings in ways that are sympathetic to the dignity, self-esteem and needs of people with autism, and the importance of including them in conversations about ASD, as in *Nihil de nobis, sine nobis*: "nothing about us without us". The book, and associated website: www.thinkingautismguide.com, hold withering reviews of: the dangerous practice of chelation; the gluten-free, casein-free autism diet; FC and its stablemate the Rapid Prompting Method (while providing a November 2012 interview with Amy Sequenzia on her use of FC); the anti-vaccination lobby; biomed protocols; and Donvan and Zucker (2016a).

The unsettling *In a Different Key: The Story of Autism* (Donvan & Zucker, 2016a) leaves a bad aftertaste. Structured as a series of biographies, it focuses particularly on parents, parent-led autism organizations and autism in the media, in the tone of a deftly-edited TV news magazine with "up-next, dot, dot, dot" segues between chapters. Well-deserved potshots are aimed at particular techniques (e.g., FC), some people (e.g., FC devotee Douglas Biklen; and Andrew Wakefield, ill-famed for faking research that depicted the MMR vaccine as a "cause" of autism), and certain organizations. The founders of *Autism Speaks* (www.autismspeaks.org) Bob Wright and his wife Suzanne (b. 1946 d. 2016) sustain broadsides for lending unjustified legitimacy to Wakefield's anti-vaccination propaganda, later assuming neutrality, and finally disavowing a role for vaccines in ASD aetiology in 2015; while the Wrights' distasteful credo "children are lost to autism" is obliquely upheld by Donvan and Zucker.

Also among the huge cast of characters is Hans Asperger: kindly paediatrician doing his best in complex times, *saving* children from Nazi slaughter (the verdict of Silberman, 2015 in *NeuroTribes*), but likely a devious Nazi sympathizer, say Donvan and Zucker. Explaining their view, Donvan and Zucker cite the undocumented and shocking allegations of holocaust scholar Dr Herwig Czech in a talk at a 2010 conference held to honour Asperger.

Naturally, the speaker was pressed for evidence after the talk – *and* he received a series of requests over a period of years from Steve Silberman while he was backgrounding *NeuroTribes* – but to date, the elusive Dr Czech has not shared his findings with other scholars. We note, however, that Asperger's help in sending a child – Herta Schreiber – to a killing facility is regarded as a matter of historical record, and that this information is set to appear in future editions of Silberman's outstanding book.

Donvan and Zucker profile Bruno Bettelheim (villain and fraud), Raymond Babbitt (*Rain Man*), Temple Grandin, Alex Plank, and others as instruments of enlightenment; and Ivar Løvaas: antihero one minute, quirky hero the next. Dr Løvaas's atrocious misuse of the Skinnerian operant conditioning methods of shaping and aversives, including painful electric shocks[2] is puzzlingly condoned – along the lines that Løvaas felt it *necessary* to go to harsh extremes in order to "recover" autistic children and save them from self-harm.

Donvan and Zucker (2016a ; and see Donvan & Zucker, 2016b) fix grimly on bad science, bad practice, squabbling between autism advocacy heavyweights, and stomach-turning aspects of institutionalization. However, Ari Ne'eman[3] and other leaders of the neurodiversity movement are portrayed as divisive forces. Donvan and Zucker represent parents as hapless protagonists "dealing with", "living with" and "going home to" *autism* rather than *their children with autism*, and remain irritatingly coy about their own views. Instances of wrong reporting of scientific data by Donvan and Zucker are regrettable, as is their characterization of the murder of 13-year-old Dougie Gibson by his

---

2 Ruth Christ Sullivan PhD, elected in 1969 as the first president of the American Psychological Association (APA), mother of seven, including Joseph who is autistic, said that the APA accepted Løvaas using electric shocks on children. She is quoted in Feinstein (2010): "It was a way of getting their attention and getting them to talk…In the 1960s cattle prods were the only thing available. They were quicker. It might take two years to achieve what a cattle prod could achieve in a week. These days, no one should do it…".

3 Ari Ne'eman was Founding President of the Autistic Self-Advocacy Network (ASAN: www.autisticadvocacy.org) from 2006, announcing in 2016 a plan to step down. While endorsing evidence-based forms of AAC (see Chapter 6), we take issue with the supported typing and facilitated communication aspects of ASAN's Policy Statement which says, in part: "Many therapies and products for Autistic children and adults are helpful and should be made more widely available, such as physical therapy, speech therapy, occupational therapy, and augmentative and assistive communication technology (*including supported typing, facilitated communication* and other methodologies that support communications access). However, ASAN opposes the use of behavioral programs that focus on normalization rather than teaching useful skills". Current ASAN Board members include Morénike Giwa Onaiwu and FC user and advocate Amy Sequenzia, mentioned in this chapter.

clinically depressed father as a "mercy killing" – which is how an arresting police officer (inappropriately) termed it. In the authors' words: "Alec killed Dougie to put him out of a misery he believed to be inevitable" (p. 142). The lack of an index and reference list (which the 50-page "Notes" section does not offset) diminishes the book's appeal.

Strengths of Donvan and Zucker's 500-page history are the authors' flat rejection of Bettelheim's "refrigerator mother" meme, the interesting "Autism Timeline", the final chapter "A Happy Man" (Donald Triplett), and Parts VIII and IX, where the authors painstakingly describe the backdrop to the "autism epidemic" scare campaign from the 1990s through to 2010, propelled by Wakefield, *Autism Speaks* and, understandably (given the hype), frantic "autism parents". There is no ASD epidemic: but rather, diagnostic criteria are broader, identification more accurate, data collecting more sophisticated (e.g., controlling for effects of population growth), and the impact of diagnostic substitution (Bishop, Whitehouse, Watt, & Line, 2008) better accommodated.

Anyone excited by journalist Tom Fields-Meyer's 2011 *Following Ezra: What One Father Learned About Gumby, Otters, Autism, and Love from his Extraordinary Son*, will want to read *Uniquely Human: A Different way of Seeing Autism*, that Fields-Meyer co-wrote with Barry Prizant (www.barryprizant.com). If you *wanted* to see ASD as a litany of deficits to be blue-pencilled, Prizant and Fields-Meyer would disappoint. The authors, in Dr Prizant's voice, emphasize that the most effective approaches to autism do not set out to "fix" a person by expunging symptoms. Instead, they seek to: (1) understand the individual's internal and external experience, recognizing "behaviours" as adaptive strategies the person with ASD may call on when life is overwhelming; (2) seize openings to augment abilities and strengths; and (3) give support that will facilitate more appropriate behaviour and a better quality of life.

Professor of clinical psychology, Dr Andrew Solomon's (www.andrewsolomon.com) empathetic, eloquent *Far from the Tree* (Solomon, 2012 in the US; 2013 in the UK, differently subtitled) straddles popular and scholarly genres. Drawing on an immense data set derived from 300 interviews with parents of and people with "horizontal identities", Dr Solomon explores the personal and family impacts of ASD, child prodigy, criminality, deafness, disability, Down syndrome, dwarfism, rape-conceived children, schizophrenia, and transgenderism.

Families tend to value *vertical identities* or "*verticals*" – the characteristics we hope or anticipate our children will have, embodying what Dr Solomon calls "the onward march of our selfish genes". Verticals can include language, nationality, personality traits, race, religion and sexuality. An anticipated vertical identity is not necessarily either negative or positive. A family in which father, grandfather and certain uncles are considered to be hyperactive may readily assimilate a similarly inclined boy as "one of us", but have difficulty accommodating a little girl if she is the first female in the family to show ADHD characteristics. Similarly, reading problems are so usual in some families that parents see them as being vertical for their family, perceiving early signs and getting appropriate help quickly. We have no statistics, but our professional experience suggests that many families are ill-equipped to accommodate *horizontal identities* or *"horizontals"*, with their unexpected personas and needs that depart from the expected and wished for. Verticals are mostly respected while horizontals are often seen as defects.

A central theme of *Far from the Tree* is, "fixing is the illness model; acceptance is the identity model". Reading it, and it *is* a gripping read, we wished that the usually astute Dr Solomon were not so accepting of FC and of Douglas Biklen's brain development expertise. Describing nonverbal Ben, with ASD, whose mother has a PhD in special education and whose father was once an experimental psychologist, he writes (p. 247), "Some people who cannot produce oral words can communicate in writing, and some who don't have the muscle control for handwriting type instead, and some who don't even have the control for typing use other methods." To wit, Stephen Hawking and Martin Pistorius: so far so good. "Ben learned *facilitated communication,* or FC" (uh oh), "…a system in which someone helped him to use a keyboard by giving his arms nondirected physical support as he typed. There has been great debate about whether what is being expressed using FC is really the language of the disabled person or of the facilitator; Ben's parents are sure that he is controlling his FC utterances." Examples are given of "Ben's communication" via FC, including his exposing his aide, "an obese slovenly guy who always wore sweatpants" for raping him in a weight room, "while this other guy would watch". On page 758, Dr Solomon refers to Biklen (1993): "the seminal book on brain development in autism is Douglas Biklen's *Communication Unbound: How Facilitated Communication is Challenging Traditional Views of Autism and Ability/Disability*". We discuss FC in Chapter 6, so for now let us just say that we understand why Foxx and Mulick (2016; and see Todd, 2016) subtitled their Chapter 17, on FC: *The Ultimate Fad Treatment*.

ASD in children, and individualized, collaborative management

SLPs/SLTs work with children with ASD, their families, colleagues and the community in eight capacities:

1. ***Screening*** to detect children at risk for ASD, early, and to make appropriate referrals.

2. ***Assessment*** to establish aspects of social communication requiring intervention and support.

3. ***Diagnosis*** to ascertain, as members of transdisciplinary teams, the extent and impact of social communication indicators, and associated features, within the DSM-5 framework.

4. ***Intervention*** to help children with ASD with all facets of social communication, applying theoretically sound, evidence-based treatment.

5. ***Research*** to advance the knowledge base of the early identification and management of ASD.

6. ***Consultation and collaboration*** to work cooperatively with families, other SLPs/SLTs, education and health professionals to support goal setting and programme planning; and to provide broad input to policy makers, and agencies, to support service development.

7. ***Learning and teaching*** to extend or upgrade their own and others' knowledge and skills in working with those with ASD; and to provide student training and professional development.

8. ***Advocacy and political lobbying*** to contribute to bettering the quality of life and participation in society of individuals with ASD across the lifespan.

Beware the National Centre (or institute) for [insert a suitable title] (and acronym)

One of many things writing this book has reinforced in us, is to be careful not to assume that "white paper" and "national" in a document's title necessarily foreshadow authoritative, impartial information. Early in this chapter we cited research from the Centers for Disease Control and Prevention (www.cdc.gov), the foremost national public health institute in the US. Elsewhere, we cite the assuredly credible (Australian) National Health and Medical Research Council, the (US) National Reading Panel and the (Australian) National Inquiry into the Teaching of Literacy. On a roll with the "national" thing, we confidently approached the site, www.nationalautismcenter.org, of the conservative government-instrumentality-lookalike, National Autism Center (NAC). NAC is described as "May Institute's Center for the Promotion of Evidence-based Practice". In turn, May Institute is styled as a "national" nonprofit network (i.e., company) serving children and adults with ASD and other developmental and acquired disabilities, in over 150 US locations. The Center's "National" (are you getting the hang of this?) Standards Project's valuable 2015 report resulted from the collaboration of an expert panel, of whom 28/28 had doctorates, 9/28 were behaviour analysts, and 1/28 was an SLP: ASHA past President and 2016 Honoree of the Association, Patricia A. Prelock, PhD, CCC-SLP. Reviewing literature up to 2012, they classed interventions for ASD as "Established"[4], "Emerging"[5] or "Unestablished"[6]. Their report lists 14 **established interventions**[7] with evidence to show they are effective for children, adolescents, and young adults (under age 22) and one for adults over 22, with ASD (National Autism Center, 2015). Most of the 14 are from the behavioural literature (e.g., ABA, behavioural psychology, and positive behaviour supports). The panel notes that developmental psychology, special education, and SLP contributions to the autism literature are increasing, so that this (behavioural) trend may change in time.

NAC (2015) included the Picture Exchange Communication System PECS™ among the **emerging interventions**[8]. Those they deemed to be **unestablished interventions** are: Animal-assisted Intervention; Auditory Integration Training; Concept Mapping (Cognitive Orientation to Daily Occupational Performance: CO-OP); DIRFloortime®; Facilitated Communication; GFCF diet; Movement-based Intervention (e.g., the Alexander Technique, Feldenkrais, Pilates, Rolfing, and Trager); SENSE Theatre Intervention (preliminary support is available:

---

4 Established: Sufficient evidence is available to confidently determine that an intervention produces favourable outcomes for individuals on the autism spectrum, i.e., they are effective.

5 Emerging: One or more studies suggest that an intervention produces favourable outcomes for individuals with ASD; additional high-quality studies must consistently show this outcome before firm conclusions can be drawn about intervention effectiveness.

6 Unestablished: An intervention associated with no sound evidence.

7 Established interventions: Behavioural Interventions; Cognitive Behavioural Intervention Package; Comprehensive Behavioural Treatment for Young Children; Language Training (Production); Modelling; Natural Teaching Strategies; Parent Training; Peer Training Package; Pivotal Response Training; Schedules; Scripting; Self-Management; Social Skills Package; and, Story-based Intervention.

8 Emerging interventions: Augmentative and Alternative Communication Devices; Developmental Relationship-based Treatment; Exercise; Exposure Package; Functional Communication Training; Imitation-based Intervention; Initiation Training; Language Training (Production & Understanding); Massage Therapy; Multi-component Package; Music Therapy; Picture Exchange Communication System; Reductive Package; Sign Instruction; Social Communication Intervention; Structured Teaching; Technology-based Intervention; Theory of Mind Training.

Corbett et al., 2016); Sensory Intervention Package (preliminary support is available: Pfeiffer, Koenig, Kinnealey, Sheppard, & Henderson, 2011); Electro-Convulsive Therapy (ECT); Social Behavioral Learning Strategy, using Stop-Observe-Deliberate-Act (SODA); Social Cognition Intervention; and Social Thinking® intervention.

Individualized management in ASD

It goes against the grain, against common sense, and against professional ethics for SLPs/SLTs to endorse and implement one programme or intervention to the exclusion of all others. SLPs/SLTs possess the specialist skills and knowledge that are necessary to comprehensively assess and address the impairments of speech, language, and pragmatic language development (and eating in many instances) of individuals with ASD. In doing so, they have a duty to engage in E^{3}BP (Dollaghan, 2007), and to disclose to families the experimental (and hence unproven) nature of components of the treatment they offer, if they choose to include them. For any child referred to an SLP/SLT for help, individual, in-person assessment and management planning is necessary to determine the best fit between child-family-therapy-and-therapist. The intervention must then be fine-tuned relative to the child's responses and progress. Manualized, off-the-shelf/off-the-web packages delivered as supposed panaceas simply do not cut it (Travers et al., 2016).

No approach designed to address the core features of ASD has been identified as the *most* effective for *all* children with autism, and little is known about which children are most likely to respond best to each intervention, and the factors involved. For example, is progress governed more by the characteristics of the child and family, or by the characteristics of the treatment, or the skill of the clinician or team, or by some fortunate amalgamation of these? Optimal regimens will be evidence-based, delivered within naturally-occurring contexts and interactions that foster the development and generalization of skills that count for something in the "real world". They will include some combination of work on: *attention*; *behaviour and emotional regulation*: using communication to initiate and sustain social engagement and to request breaks and assistance; *cognitive skills and language abilities*: understanding and using nonverbal and verbal communication, symbolic play and executive functioning; and, *social reciprocation*: the pragmatic functions (see Figure 4.1) of initiating interactions, taking turns and providing contingent responses.

Roberts and Prior (2006) and Prior, Roberts, Rodger, Williams and

Sutherland (2011) looked at appropriate, autism-specific curriculum components for children up to age 7 that are relevant to guiding SLP/SLT practice. In the still-helpful 2006 document (see also Roberts & Williams, 2016), they highlight: "focusing on attention, compliance, imitation, language, and social skills; highly supportive teaching environments with a focus on generalisation and transition support; predictability and routine; a functional, communication-based approach to challenging behaviours; family involvement as part of collaborative partnerships with professionals; use of visual supports and augmentative and alternative communication" (p. 14).

Collaborative management in ASD

When behaviour analysts, OTs, psychologists, special educators, SLPs/SLTs and other professionals try to "go it alone" (and sometimes, in rural and remote settings, when money is tight, or when a family's belief system cannot incorporate multiple outside interventions, they have to go it alone), practice flies in the face of what the science tells us. E^3BP principles and the

Transdisciplinary Collaboration

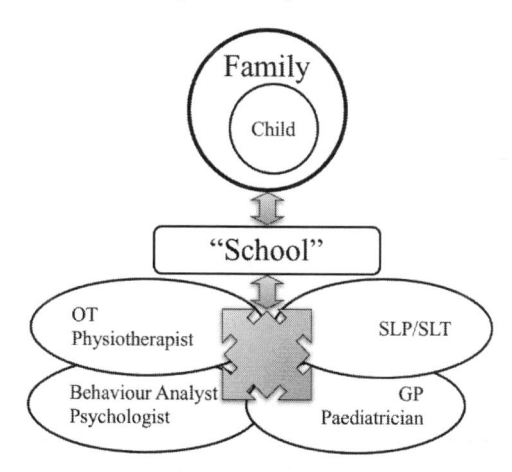

[Diagram: Family/Child circle connected to "School" box, connected to overlapping ovals containing: OT/Physiotherapist, SLP/SLT, Behaviour Analyst/Psychologist, GP/Paediatrician]

Figure 4.2 Transdisciplinary team showing interlocking lines of communication and collaboration.

ICF Framework[9] underpin a **transdisciplinary team** approach, where child and family are integral to the team. At a minimum, a team will involve the participants displayed in Figure 4.2.

Moore, 2013 (p. 1) defines transdisciplinary teamwork, as opposed to multidisciplinary[10] or interdisciplinary[11] teamwork, as involving "a team of professionals who work collaboratively, and share the responsibilities of evaluating, planning and implementing services to children and their families. Families are valued members of the team, and are involved in all aspects of intervention. One professional is chosen as the primary service provider for the family, and acts as the conduit for the expertise of the team. The full team remains involved, and the primary provider reports back to the team constantly".

Team members' ideals, preferences, knowledge and expertise are respected, shaping other members' actions, sometimes sustaining inherent pitfalls. For example, when a "strong" member embraces a fad, others may follow, as in the cases of, for example: an SLP/SLT using TalkTools® methods to work on speech, thereby encouraging an OT and special educator to use them too; a behaviour analyst's different approach to language intervention hindering SLP/SLT programming; and parents engaging in pseudoscientific hippotherapy, with a team respectfully (but reluctantly) acceding, even though it is absorbing time, money, and energy more beneficially spent elsewhere.

---

9 The International Classification of Functioning, Disability and Health for Children and Youth (ICF-CY) is a World Health Organization-approved, "derived" version of the International Classification of Functioning, Disability and Health (ICF, WHO, 2001) designed to record characteristics of the developing child and the influence of environments surrounding the child. Until October 2010 it was referenced separately as ICF-CY (2007). It has now merged back into the ICF and is referenced as such (WHO, 2016). Updates are available: www.who.int/classifications/icf/en/

10 Multidisciplinary teamwork: This model involves a group of professionals working independently with a family and having minimal interaction with one another. Each specialist conducts their own assessment, develops discipline-specific goals, and works directly with the child to remediate weaknesses identified in their assessments.

11 Interdisciplinary teamwork: This model involves a team of professionals that may conduct their own assessments and develop discipline-specific goals, but meet regularly to coordinate service planning. Actual service delivery is still done by the professionals separately, but as part of an overall plan.

Proprietary interventions

SLPs/SLTs, OTs, psychologists and special educators, and other professionals regularly undertake training to provide proprietary interventions for children with ASD and/or ID and complex communication needs. Such programmes include DIRFloortime®, the Hanen Programs®, Picture Exchange Communication System: PECS™, Prompts for Restructuring Oral Muscular Phonetic Targets: PROMPT©, Relationship Development Intervention® (RDI®), Responsive Teaching, and TalkTools®. Their certification or accreditation courses are for professionals who are *already* highly qualified at university level – and the standards required to gain such recognition are decided by the provider, who is rarely an educator.

Whereas an SLP/SLT, for example, might assess a novel therapy, looking at its research credentials and, if it stacks up, learning how to implement it through private study, reading journal articles, mentoring, peer supervision, or training (e.g., affordable CPD, CEE, CEU or Pro-D activities offered by ASHA, IASLT, NZSTA, RCSLT, SAC-OAC or SPA) – with these branded programmes "the knowledge" and "certification" are *only* available on the providers' terms. Required manuals, materials, and gadgetry usually come without research evidence, and are often *only* obtainable from providers and their agents, creating a fair bit of EFT activity.

SLP/SLT professional associations guide their members in this respect. Regarding ASD, Speech Pathology Australia (2009, p.12), cautions emphatically: "use only those interventions that are supported by research evidence, and in situations where they elect to deliver programs that are (a) commercial in nature, (b) in part or wholly outside the recognized scope of SLP/SLT practice, and/or (c) provided in a way that excludes the use of other empirically supported interventions, it is incumbent on the SLP/SLT to disclose these facts to their clients with ASD and their clients' families".

Fad, fashion, and science

In their outstanding *Controversial Therapies for Autism and Intellectual Disabilities: Fad, Fashion, and Science in Professional Practice*, veteran hogwash connoisseurs Foxx and Mulick (2016) provide descriptions and criticism of the good, the bad, and the ugly therapies in ASD and ID – but it is no spaghetti western[12] done on the cheap and biased towards a starring "good guy" and

---

12 Spaghetti western: a western film made cheaply in Europe by an Italian director.

amiable sidekicks. While Foxx and Mulick favour behavioural treatments, in selecting contributors they invited individuals who were among the "best suited by history and knowledge to write that chapter. Indeed, our collaborators break down into three general categories: behaviour analysts, those who would not describe themselves as behaviour analysts but who favour or are sympathetic to behavioural analytic approaches because of the strong science underlying them, and those who appreciate or acknowledge the empirical base of behaviour analyses but who would not identify with it professionally" (p. xv). The result is an Americentric (2 NZ, 2 UK and 41 US authors), forthright book, strong on historic and current manifestations of fads in ASD and ID, and why they persist. There are tales of the unexpected (e.g., their Chapter 7: Developmental disabilities and the paranormal, includes: a description of magnetic field deficiency syndrome – who knew?); fad classics like Sensory Integration Therapy; and a pleasing emphasis on empiricism, evidence and ethics. In the nicely executed Chapter 25, Dr Foxx explains (p. 428) that "ABA is not a fad, a pseudoscience, a dubious or controversial treatment, or politically correct" because it is supported by science, and its practitioners are subject to a code of ethics (Bailey & Burch, 2016). Never mincing words, he says (p. 426), "Pseudoscientific practices are perpetuated by professionals not staying current with the treatment literature."

The book has separate chapters on contentious practices in Special Education, and Speech-Language Pathology, but not in OT, Optometry or Psychology. Intriguingly for us, oral motor treatments are mentioned once in 568 pages, as a throwaway line on page 248 in the chapter on Sensory Integration Therapy – not in the SLP chapter by Cheryl D. Gunter and Mariele A. Koenig. The interventions Drs Gunter and Koenig deplore are (1) FC – it was sobering to see that of 11 mentions of Australia in the entire book, eight referred to FC, two to Therapeutic Touch Therapy and one to the dodgy Institutes for the Achievement of Human Potential. Then, (2) Fast ForWord™ (FFW), (3) Sensory Integration Therapy, (4) Whole Language (WL), and (5) Whole Language to Oral Language (WLOL), an acronym Norris and Damico (1990) adopted even though LOL[13] had already been coined. When we stopped ROFL, and discussing the abundant acronyms in SLP/SLT, we wondered how widespread the use of FFW and WL is among US SLPs working with children with ID and ASD.

---

13 LOL: Laughing Out Loud, was coined on a BBS (bulletin board system) called *Viewline* in Calgary, Canada, in the early-to-mid-1980s. ROFL: Rolling On the Floor Laughing.

> "We are particularly concerned about the failure of SLP to consistently promote and adopt the Scientist-Practitioner Model. Clearly, ASHA and academic programs in SLP advocate evidence-based treatment. However, in practice SLPs have traditionally assumed separate roles as researchers who study basic processes or as clinicians who provide a variety of clinical services. We believe that this division has led some clinicians to overlook the scientific dimensions of clinical work and it has led some researchers away from the experience of clinical practice. When science has taken a back seat to clinical practice, SLPs have tended to rely on a more intuitive form of clinical decision-making. While clinical intuition can be valuable when combined with science-based methods, it can result in vulnerability to fads and controversial practices without a scientific or theoretical balance. Clearly, sound clinical practice stems from multiple sources (Prizant & Rubin, 1999). However, 'an understanding and application of science must be a vital part of clinical practice in order to ensure that treatment methods are theoretically sound and empirically based with measurable, cost-effective outcomes' (Blischack & Cheek, 2001, p. 11)."
>
> Gunter and Koenig, 2016, p. 163

Intervention types

There are numerous interventions intended for children who have ASD. As team members, SLPs/SLTs find that some of the approaches, procedures and activities that they incorporate sit comfortably within their scope of practice, and some do not. The intervention-types include: augmentative and alternative communication (described in Chapter 6), and behavioural, developmental, relationship-based, communication-focused, and therapy-based interventions. The children involved in them may also be receiving biologically-based interventions, CAM, psychodynamic, and brain stimulation therapies.

Behavioural interventions include ABA, the Løvaas Method, and Learning Experiences-An Alternative Program for Preschoolers and Parents (LEAP). ABA, LEAP and Løvaas feature systematically applied operant learning techniques through the Discrete Trial Training (DTT) methodology. In DTT instruction, specific skills are broken down into small parts that are then taught, stepwise.

Developmental interventions (relationship based, or "normalized" interventions) centre on a child's ability to relate positively with others, and form "meaningful" relationships. They include, DIR®/DIRFloortime® and Relationship Development Intervention: RDI® (also styled RDI™ and RDIConnect™). There is modest independent research support for one aspect of DIRFloortime®, and none for RDI®.

Therapy based interventions comprise: Communication Focused, Sensory Motor, Combined, and Family Based interventions.

Communication Focused interventions may stand alone or they may be integrated within comprehensive programmes. Examples are the unethical and discredited Facilitated Communication (strategically rebadged as the Rapid Prompting Method (RPM), Soma® RPM, and Supported Typing) described in Chapter 6, as well as Functional Communication Training, the Picture Exchange Communication System: PECS™, Social Stories™, Social Thinking®, Speech Generating Devices (SGDs), visual strategies and visually cued instruction, and manual signing. There is no experimental support for **sensory motor interventions** such as Auditory Integration Treatments or for Sensory Integration Therapy. Among the **combined interventions** are LEAP, SCERTS®, TEACCH®, and the Early Start Denver Model (ESDM). **Family based interventions** aim to support and inform parents and teach them strategies. They include the National Autistic Society's (www.autism.org.uk) Autism Seminars for Families, EarlyBird and EarlyBird Plus programs; Positive Behaviour Support (PBS); and The Hanen Programs®. Affinity Therapy (www.lifeanimated.net), formerly Disney Therapy (Suskind, 2014), was developed by author and Pulitzer Prize winning journalist Ron Suskind, for his son Owen, with help from clinical psychologist and family therapist Dr Dan Griffin (www.drdangriffin.com). In his emotive book, Suskind (2014) tells how he and Owen began communicating verbally via Disney movie dialogue (see also www.ronsuskind.com): "A child disappeared into confusion, frustration, and silence. But deep inside his dark cave of isolation, he and his family began to dig for diamonds, working year by year, trial by trial, on a most improbable project: to find a way each of us can learn to animate our lives." Affinity Therapy is non-evidence based, draws on ideas and techniques from psychodynamic, neuroplasticity, and family systems theory, and according to its proponents is largely "family driven". It uses the "affinities" (special interests or preoccupations) of children with ASD reportedly to "provide a bridge" and "deepen the understanding" between parent and child. The affinities may be movie-or-video-related, or around media such as anime, maps, Minecraft, and Shining Time Station. Dr Griffin gives talks with titles such as *Disney & Life Animated: Families Using Affinities to Improve Social Skills and Beyond with Spectrum Kids*, and has written autism-related articles for his own website and for *The Huffington Post*. There is no information to be had regarding Affinity Therapy in the peer-reviewed literature.

Biologically-based interventions (prescribed, and other medicines) to "treat" the core features of ASD are not currently available. Still, children with ASD, preferably under the care of medical specialists[14] such as paediatricians or paediatric neurologists, may take prescribed medications to treat concomitant problems such as ADHD, anxiety, constipation, depression, sleep disorders, and seizures. Biologically based interventions such as hyperbaric oxygen chamber treatment; injections of EDTA for chelation, immunoglobulin, Lupron, secretin, and stem cells; the Miracle Mineral Solution (MMS); and the blood product Globulin component Macrophage Activating Factor (GcMAF) are not backed by science.

CAM interventions, which are non-evidence based, atheoretical, and biologically implausible, include acupuncture, anti-yeast therapy, chiropractic, craniosacral therapy, exclusion diets, homeopathy, naturopathy, osteopathy, and vitamin and mineral supplements. Chelation, GcMAF, MMS, homeopathic "vaccinations" for children, and withholding vaccination are potentially lethal.

Tinus Smits (www.tinussmits.com) offers "complete healing of autistic children" on his multilingual website (www.cease-therapy.com). The bio for its associated Twitter handle reads, "CEASE Therapy eliminates imprints of toxic substances like vaccines, antibiotics, anesthesia and other regular medication using homeopathy to reverse autism." CEASE Therapy combines isotherapy for "homeopathic detoxification" with orthomolecular support via

---

14 High-prevalence mental health problems (anxiety and depression) occur more commonly in children and adults with developmental disabilities, but symptoms are often either missed or misattributed as being "syndromal". Communication plays a central role in history taking, so it is vital that someone who knows the client's communication strengths and difficulties is present when medical specialist consultations occur.

Omega-3 fatty acid and vitamin C supplements to address "metallothonein deficiency" (purported to cause heavy metal poisoning); osteopathy if a child's birth was "difficult"; "classical" and "constitutional" homeopathy, and environmental adjustments such as adhering to the Specific Carbohydrate Diet, only drinking "pure water", having a child's (non-metal-containing) bed facing north or east, spurning microwaved foods, yeast and sugar, avoiding plastic containers, and refusing antibiotics. Parents are advised to, "Eliminate all electric appliances in the bedroom such as electric alarm clocks, TV, computers or audio equipment. Turn off Wi-Fi during the night (and day)". Training of homeopathic practitioners to become certified CEASE Therapists takes three to five "intensive" days, and the website includes links to certified practitioners' sites globally, where claims made for the curative powers of CEASE, for autism, ADHD, epilepsy, speech impairment, "and many modern chronic diseases" become even more farfetched. Dr Smits himself uses the fear and guilt cards unhesitatingly: "Autism is a serious disease that can be treated successfully, but even if I have given give [sic] you a lot of information about its treatment here and in my book *Autism Beyond Despair*, it needs professional help [from a CEASE Therapist]. Otherwise you will ultimately be disappointed and not get the results you hoped to achieve. Your child is too precious to treat yourself."

In a thoughtful review, two medical doctors (Levy & Hyman, 2015) discuss CAM treatments, like CEASE, that families may use or be tempted to use, to "treat" ASD. Covering natural products, mind-body practices, biological and biomedical treatments, they propose that in counselling families it is necessary to specify:

- the precise symptoms a particular CAM intervention is used to address
- the expected benefits, and potential side effects, of the CAM intervention
- how long it will be until the CAM intervention takes effect.

With these data they, and others, can establish the impact of a specific intervention, provided that interventions are introduced one at a time so that any effects can be correctly attributed.

Psychodynamic interventions rest on the unsupported assumption that ASD is caused by emotional problems the child has, due to impaired attachment or faulty bonding by parents, particularly the child's mother. Although there is unequivocal research evidence that ASD is a congenital, developmental, social communication disorder, and not an emotional "psychogenic" disorder arising from events in the interpersonal environment, psychodynamic therapies for ASD are widely applied in France. To their shame, this practice is ardently adopted and defended by prominent Freudian analysts (psychiatrists) located in France, and rightly opposed by those who value science in practice (Bishop, 2012).

Biomedical interventions in the form of **brain stimulation therapies** have been implemented to address ASD characteristics. They are non-evidence based, and potentially dangerous for children and young adults (and possibly others). They include electroconvulsive therapy: ECT (National Autism Center, 2015), and repetitive transcranial magnetic stimulation: rTMS or TMS (Oberman, Enticott, Casanova, Rotenberg, Pascual-Leone, & McCracken, 2015).

Intervention approaches

Here, we review interventions used by some SLPs/SLTs to support social communication progress in children with ASD: Løvaas Model and DTT, ABA, DIRFloortime®, Functional Communication Training, PECS™, Social Stories™, Social Thinking®, LEAP, SCERTS®, TEACCH®, family-based methods, and a residential community-based method, Camphill.

Behavioural interventions

The Løvaas Model and discrete trial training (DTT)

In the beginning, Norwegian-American clinical psychologist Ole Ivar Løvaas (b. 1927 d. 2010) established standardized teaching protocols for children with autism, based on behavioural principles, devoting a lifetime to advocacy, research and practice aimed at improving the lives of children and families impacted by autism. The Løvaas Model of Applied Behavior Analysis ("Løvaas Model": www.lovaas.com) is highly regimented and implemented for two to six years, relying heavily on discrete trial training (DTT) methods, for children aged 3 and upwards. DTT is used to reduce stereotypical ASD behaviours via extinction, and provision of "socially acceptable" substitutes for self-stimulatory ("stimming") and self-harming behaviours (for important insights, see Cynthia Kim's "Socially Inappropriate" and "The High Cost of Self-Censoring", and

Sparrow Rose Jones' "ABA—Applied Behaviour Analysis", in Sutton, 2015). The method evolved into Early Intensive Behavior Intervention (EIBI).

One of the first investigators to show that the behaviour of children with autism can be altered through teaching, Dr Løvaas was co-founder in 1965 of what is now the *Autism Society* charity (www.autism-society.org). Aspects of his work were contentious, such as: the frequency and intensity of treatment, time-money-and-emotional load on families, horrifying use of "aversives" to elicit compliance (smacking, shouting, electric shock, and withholding food, desired activities or wanted objects such as toys), claims of "recovery" from autism, and more (Silberman, 2015).

The Løvaas Model is delivered five days weekly, usually in the child's home, with sessions of five to seven hours' duration (35–40 hours weekly at over £20,000 annually). Sessions consist of "trials" with recurrent breaks. A trial ends if the "communicator" (the Løvaas practitioner, seated across a table from the child) considers that the child is becoming unfocused. Trials are composed of prompts (gestural, physical, tactile, verbal [e.g., in not-quite-pidgin and not-quite-English[15], *give me red, put in box, put on tin, show me soap*, etc.], and visual stimuli) delivered by the communicator, who aims to *shape* the child's behaviour so that they respond correctly to the prompts. If a child is unresponsive, makes an error, or is noncompliant, a "prompter", seated behind the child, provides either partial, or a full hand-over-hand help until the prompted response is completed. Correct responses are reinforced with some combination of praise, an "edible", treat, or playtime with a toy the child likes.

WWC reviewers (What Works Clearinghouse, 2010) considered 58 studies of the Løvaas Model. One met the WWC evidence standards; another met them with reservations; and the remaining 56 studies met neither their evidence standards nor eligibility screens. Based on the two studies that passed muster, the reviewers found potentially positive effects on cognitive development for children with disabilities, and *no discernible effects* on communication and language competencies, or social-emotional development, or behaviour, or functional abilities.

Applied Behaviour Analysis (ABA)

Whereas the Løvaas Model tends to be a one-size-fits-all arrangement, ABA

---

15 Reporting their comprehensive correlational meta-analysis, Sandbank and Yoder (2016) advise clinicians to reconsider intervention practices that prescribe shorter, grammatically incomplete utterances (e.g., "Pop bubbles", "Want ball?"), particularly when working with children with autism.

is always individualized. Although it comes in for a lot of flak from sections of the autism community (e.g., Sutton, 2015) and via the press, ABA is the ASD intervention associated with the strongest empirical evidence (Maul, Findley, & Nicolson Adams, 2015; Odom, Boyd, Hall, & Hume, 2010; Sallows & Graupner, 2005). Its detractors say that ABA is unethical, disrespectful and abusive because the success of ABA is defined as having a child behave like, or more like, a non-autistic person. Neurodiversity advocates stress that most people with autism want help with necessary life skills, but that they do not want their autism taken away. ABA's proponents describe it as an "applied natural science" as opposed to a social science, or as a "branch of psychology", or an "intensive education therapy".

ABA is a process in which assessment and interventions based on well-established learning theory are systematically **applied**, in order to improve socially significant **behaviour**, demonstrating through **analysis** that the interventions a practitioner (called a "behaviour analyst") employs with an individual are responsible for the improvement in the targeted behaviour.

> "ABA is a systematic approach for influencing socially important behavior through the identification of reliably related environmental variables and the production of behavior change techniques that make use of those findings. Practitioners of behavior analysis provide services consistent with the dimensions of ABA. Common services may include, but are not limited to, conducting behavioral assessments, analyzing data, writing and revising behavior-analytic treatment plans, training others to implement components of treatment plans, and overseeing the implementation of treatment plans."
>
> www.bacb.com Retrieved January 12, 2016

Contemporary ABA evolved from "behaviour modification", developed by B.F. Skinner (b. 1904 d. 1990) of Operant Conditioning and Verbal Behavior fame. "Behaviour modification" was displaced by "behaviour analysis", in a paradigm shift away from trying to change atypical behaviour to practitioners seeking to recognize the *function* of a behaviour, the antecedents and consequences promoting and maintaining it, and how it might be exchanged for "successful" behaviour. Practitioners' analysis is based on meticulous initial assessment of the function of a behaviour, and careful trialling and documentation of methods that produce quantifiable behavioural changes. Children as young as 2 years are seen, in interventions to support social communication and other skills, that: are naturalistic, follow the child's lead, use real-life teaching situations, mainly involve child-preferred activities, and encourage choice making. As Figure 4.2 shows, we see the appropriately qualified and ethical behaviour analyst (Bailey & Burch, 2016), and family as key players in the most basic of transdisciplinary ASD teams.

Developmental interventions

DIR® and DIRFloortime®

DIRFloortime® was devised by Stanley Greenspan (b. 1941 d. 2010), child psychiatrist (www.stanleygreenspan.com) and Serena Wieder, clinical psychologist. DIR® is an acronym for **Developmental Individual**-differences and **Relationship**-based model, an interdisciplinary framework designed to help clinicians, parents and educators do assessments and develop individualized educational or clinical programmes tailored to the needs of each child. DIRFloortime® is the practical application of the DIR® model, as a child-led, home-based, parent-implemented, relationship-centred, structured-play approach for infants and young children with ASD (Wieder & Greenspan, 2003). Its aim is to support children to achieve developmental milestones, thereby improving their ability to appropriately express emotion, engage reciprocally, connect socially, and grow intellectually.

Those wishing to train parents to deliver DIRFloortime® must undertake costly tuition provided by the Interdisciplinary Council of Developmental and Learning Disorders Inc. (ICDL): www.icdl.com. Training, open to *anybody*, leads to certification at five levels: DIR-Basic, DIR-Proficient, DIR-Advanced, DIR-Expert, and DIR-Expert/Trainer. It can be in-person, on videos and CDs, or through the ICDL portal (www.floortime.org).

Parents engaged in a DIRFloortime® programme dedicate countless hours to the endeavour. They work on the floor with their child, at least 20 hours per week at home, *and* in other settings, *plus* engaging in other therapies, *plus* 3 or 4 play dates a week for their child, with TD children. The DIRFloortime® philosophy is that all children must reach certain emotional and intellectual milestones, and that because children with ASD, *and those with other disabilities*, have difficulty reaching them, they need intense, individualized, eyeball-to-eyeball help, to "bring the child to a shared world". "Shared world", "emotional thinking", and similar descriptors of treatment goals and targets, are not operationalized – that is, the terms are not defined so that others can share the same frame of reference.

On the research page of the ICDL website, we found: "DIRFloortime® has the strongest research of any intervention to support its effectiveness in improving the core challenges of autism including relating, interacting, and communicating while decreasing caregiver stress and improving parent-child relationships". These ebullient claims are not supported by the literature, with the National Autism Center (2015), deeming DIRFloortime® "unestablished". Further, we could locate no studies of DIR® that explored "caregiver stress" or "parent-child relationships".

Some researchers (e.g., Dionne & Martini, 2011; Liao, Hwang, Chen, Lee, Chen, & Lin, 2014; Pajareya & Nopmaneejumruslers, 2011, 2012) offer modest evidence for DIRFloortime® as an effective parent-mediated treatment for improving social-emotional functioning of infants and children with ASD. The commitment in "parent hours", and estimated costs of $US2500 to $US3000 annually, per child (up to US$24,000 or £20,000), on top of fees for other interventions, will likely be prohibitive for many families.

Communication focused interventions

Functional Communication Training (FCT)

Based in ABA principles and well-established learning theory, FCT is a strategy for teaching behaviourally challenging individuals with ASD and/or ID to use more conventional, effective communication strategies with the overall aim of reducing their challenging behaviour (Hagopian, Fisher, Sullivan, Acquisto, & LeBlanc, 1998; Kurtz, Boelter, Jarmolowicz, Chin & Hagopian, 2011). Through functional assessment, the clinician identifies the purpose (e.g., wanting a snack) of the unwanted behaviour (e.g., thumping the pantry door). The child is taught how to ask for the snack more fittingly, using speech, signs, gestures or pictures (e.g., PECS™). The clinician does not set about eliminating the challenging behaviour until the child has learned the replacement one. The teaching steps are:

1. Identifying a more appropriate way for the child to communicate.

2. Systematically teaching the child the new communication skill.

3. Reinforcing (rewarding, e.g., through praise) the child's behaviour on the use of the skill.

4. Ignoring the challenging behaviour if it reappears.

5. Cueing or reminding the child to use the new skill when appropriate.

The clinician trains parents to implement the intervention at home, so that they can engage their child in 10–30-minute training sessions daily, and routinely reinforce the replacement behaviour when it occurs throughout the day. It is hard work for parents, but rewarding.

Mirenda (1997) performed a systematic review, reporting that FCT has the potential to result in an immediate, significant, and sustained reduction in challenging behaviour among individuals with autism. FCT is currently seen as best practice in addressing challenging behaviour in children with ASD. Furthermore, psychologists and SLPs/SLTs do not have to pursue expensive, "additional" training and certification! MUSEC Briefings – plain English reviews of pointless, and valuable education approaches alike – give it an unequivocal thumbs-up.

> *"FCT has a sound research evidence base and should be recommended as a primary intervention in a child's individual behaviour support plan."*
> Suzanne Cooke and Jennifer Stephenson
> MUSEC Briefing No. 29, 2011
> www.musec.mq.edu.au/community_outreach/musec_briefings

Picture Exchange Communication System: PECS™

Developed in 1985 by Andy Bondy and Lori Frost, the aim of PECS™ (www.pecs.com), trading as Pyramid Educational Consultants, Inc., is to apply behavioural principles to teach individuals with autism and/or ID to interact, and to make requests, by exchanging pictures, symbols, photos or objects for desired items. Instructors achieve this aim by pairing the "concept of expressive speech" with an object in repeated trials. Every session starts with a "preferred reinforcers survey" to gauge the best motivator for the child, at the time. No prerequisite skills (e.g., eye contact, pointing, and labelling), are required, and PECS™ begins with teaching a "social approach" to enable children to achieve concrete outcomes by getting items (e.g., toys), or doing activities (e.g., trampolining) they want.

PECS™ has six phases:

I. How to Communicate: Children are taught to exchange single pictures for highly desired items.

II. Distance and Persistence: Children use the single pictures to generalize skills learned in Phase I by exchanging them in different places, with different people and across distances, and are encouraged to be more persistent communicators.

III. Picture Discrimination: Children are taught to select from two or more pictures, in a communication book, to ask for favourite items or activities. A communication book is a ring binder with Velcro® strips enabling easy removal of pictures for communication.

IV. Sentence Structure: Children are taught to make "sentences" on a detachable sentence strip using an "I want" picture followed by a picture of the item being requested. The option to add adjectives, verbs and prepositions comes later for suitable children.

V. Answering Questions: Children are taught to use PECS™ to answer the question, "What do you want?"

VI. Commenting: Children are taught to "comment" (the term "comment" is used, not "answer" or "reply") in response to questions: "What do you see?" "What do you hear?" "What is it?" and to compose sentences starting with "I see—" "I hear—" "I feel—" "It is a—", etc.

There is limited well-controlled research into PECS™, with the results of several studies showing that *some* children with ASD benefit from its use, and that introducing PECS™ is linked with increased volubility (more talking) in some individuals. Its classroom use has been associated with better rates of communication initiations by students with ASD, and increases in the use of appropriate communication strategies by (typical) adult communication partners (Carr & Felce, 2007). So, PECS™ is an approach to watch with respect to future research outcomes.

Social Stories™

Carol Gray's Social Stories™ (Gray & Garand, 1993) go beyond social skills' training or how skills are "done". Practical and theoretically sound, they focus on teaching a child with ASD *how* to systematically evaluate why a person would use a particular social skill. They follow a 3-paragraph route, with age-appropriate pictures, intended to expose the behavioural *expectations* in a situation (paragraph 1: *When people are inside, they walk*), how people will think and feel if others do what is *expected* (paragraph 2: *Walking inside won't hurt me or other people*), and helping students focus on performing the *expected* behaviours (paragraph 3: *I will try to walk indoors. I can run when I am outside*).

Researchers at the University of Alberta, Karkhaneh and co-workers (2010) conducted a high-quality evidence-based systematic review of Social Stories™, concluding (p. 660) that their effects may be beneficial in terms of modifying target behaviours (social skills) among "high functioning children with ASD". The team noted, however, that "long-term maintenance, effectiveness of the intervention in other, less-controlled settings, and the optimal dose/frequency is unknown and requires further research". This is another intervention to watch in anticipation of further independent research.

Social Thinking®

Social Thinking® (Winner, 2000), is a product range and company developed by founder and CEO, Michelle Garcia Winner. The product, Social Thinking® (ST) was partly inspired by Social Stories®, and is for individuals with ASD who have good language skills and typical-range verbal IQs. The company, Social Thinking®, is approved in the US to provide CEUs for SLPs (ASHA members), social workers, psychologists, marriage and family therapists, counsellors, nurses, and teachers.

The aim of ST is to help students improve their "social cognition foundations" to interpret the intentions of others, and communicate more effectively through their own "social behavioural responses". There is some evidence that effects flow on, beyond social situations, to reading comprehension, narrative language for written expression, and academic undertakings (Winner & Crooke, 2009, 2014). Avoiding abstractions like *cooperate*, *negotiate*, and *respect*, ST has a vocabulary that is meant to make intentions and reactions in human communication explicit: e.g., *think with your eyes*, *keep your body/brain in the group*, *follow the plan*, be a *thinking of you kid* not a *just me kid*.

While Michelle Garcia Winner's work is favourably regarded by ST practitioners, and the ST methodology is grounded in research-based theoretical concepts that demonstrably underlie social communication (e.g., joint attention, inferencing, and theory of mind), we could locate no empirical evidence for it. We were surprised, therefore, to read that "Social Thinking® is the master key that unlocks all the other social doors" (Winner, 2013, p. 25). Still, we were interested to read Crooke and Olswang (2015). The first author, Dr Pamela J. Crooke, is the Social Thinking® Chief Officer of Research and Clinical Services, and Director of Social Thinking Training and Speakers Collaborative.

Crooke and Olswang argue for approaching research from more than one perspective, exploring practice-based research (PBR) (Dollaghan, 2007, pp. 133–135). They illustrate PBR, without demonstrating cause and effect, by reporting part of a retrospective study (albeit preliminary and thus limited in scope), examining three ST strategies: *thinking with eyes*, corresponding to the theoretical concept of joint attention; *expected/unexpected*, corresponding to the concept of inferencing/theory of mind; and *whole-body listening*, corresponding to the theoretical concept of executive functioning for self-regulation.

> *"If we wish to reduce the research–practice gap and promote a form of research–practice integration, then we must embrace a variety of research perspectives, in particular those that value the practitioner in the process. The traditional research pipeline, along with its valued internal validity, is absolutely necessary for discovering mechanisms of change and documenting the efficacy and effectiveness of our assessment and treatment protocols. PBR is not meant as a replacement but rather a complement to assist in closing the research–practice gap. What PBR brings to the discovery process is the valued input of practitioners."*
> Crooke and Olswang, 2015, pp. S1880–S1881

In their review paper, an outraged Leaf et al. (2016) do not refer to Crooke and Olswang (2015) in concluding that "Social Thinking®, to date, cannot be considered evidence based, empirically supported, or a scientific approach" (p. 1). They concluded their barbed critique with heated advice that, "Social Thinking® should be a lesson to all behaviorists that the field of ASD treatment is still saturated with pseudoscientific and antiscientific approaches; professionals in the field of ABA must do a better job of educating the public while promoting the field of ABA so that all individuals with ASD receive the most effective interventions" (p. 6).

On the Social Thinking® homepage (www.socialthinking.com, accessed July 12, 2016), it says, "At our conferences we share our latest frameworks, lessons, and strategies for teaching social thinking and related social skills to people aged 4 years old through adulthood. We offer 15+ full-day courses, each offering unique concepts and strategies regarding a particular theme or age group. All information presented can be used immediately in the classroom, home, community, and workplace!" Nearby, is a "What people are saying" section where SLPs, a school psychologist, and others are quoted. There is this, from an SLP: "I love how realistic the approach is, and doable!! Based on real clinical experience, adaptable to individual needs/strengths. Great that all the vocabulary is simple, easy to understand, and not full of professional 'shop talk'". The psychologist says: "Social Thinking is the philosophy that I ascribe (sic) to professionally. It serves as my guide through assessment and intervention." Another SLP enthuses: "OMG you are my hero ☺ and I use just about everything you publish!"

The existence of the testimonials worries us; as do the "latest frameworks" and "unique concepts and strategies" rather than frameworks, concepts, and strategies that *build* on the *existing* evidence base, and are backed by peer reviewed, published evidence of the effects and effectiveness of Social Thinking® – sans hype.

Combined interventions

Learning Experiences – An Alternative Program for Preschoolers and Parents (LEAP)

Children engaged in LEAP work to a rigorously applied individualized education plan that combines a mainstream curriculum, classroom adaptations and teacher instruction; with aspects of ABA (chiefly EIBI), peer-mediated instruction, incidental teaching, self-management training, prompting strategies, and systematic parent training. Among the techniques employed are errorless learning, time delay, pivotal response training, PECS™, and positive behaviour support. Its wellspring is that children with ASD will learn better in integrated settings alongside TD age-peers, if those peers have been taught (trained specifically) to help them. Intervention targets are ambitious, encompassing, *with appropriate support*: social and emotional growth, language and communication abilities, independence, choice making, coping with transitions, behaviour, and overall improvements in cognition and physical abilities.

Strain and Bovey (2011) performed a well-designed randomized controlled trial with preschoolers and their teachers. They found positive impacts after two years of the *full* LEAP training and support model, with statistically significant and substantively important effect sizes on the average classroom-level measures, across four domains: behaviour, communication, intellectual, and social. In the study, Strain and Bovey examined whether (1) a two-year LEAP training, that included a support module for teachers, yielded better outcomes for preschoolers with ASD, than (2) a limited LEAP model with no teacher development support. In the "teachers in" condition, "classrooms" received 23 days of LEAP training and coaching over 24 months, incorporating presentations, discussions, and demonstrations by LEAP trainers; onsite training and support including practice sessions, observations, and feedback; maintenance checks; and LEAP materials and manuals. Their positive findings relate strictly to the training with "teachers in" and not to the diluted version delivered to the comparison group.

SCERTS®

Many SLPs/SLTs consider the SCERTS® Model (www.scerts.com) (Prizant et al., 2006) to be an exemplary ASD intervention. Developed by three SLPs and an OT, it is a team-based educational and treatment framework combining **S**ocial Communication, **E**motional **R**egulation, and **T**ransactional **S**upport. The authors state, without explaining *their* interpretation of team structures, that a transdisciplinary or multidisciplinary team best implements SCERTS®, in partnership with the child's family. It affords systematic assessment and programme planning for children and adults with ASD and related disabilities, and their families, across wide ranges of age and ability. It helps families, educators, therapists and nonprofessional staff to work in a well-coordinated fashion, thereby maximizing progress. SCERTS® is a service provision model rather than a specific programme. Implementing it does not mean excluding other practices or approaches, as it has the flexibility to integrate practices from various methodologies. To date, there is no research regarding the *overall* effectiveness of SCERTS®, but its components are built on well-established research so it warrants ongoing research and clinical interest.

Treatment & Education of Autistic & Communication related handicapped Children TEACCH®

World famous, "Division TEACCH" was established in 1966 in the Department of Psychiatry of the School of Medicine at the University of North Carolina (UNC). In 1972, the North Carolina General Assembly passed groundbreaking legislation enabling TEACCH to become the first state-wide community-based programme of services for individuals with ASD and other developmental disorders. Today, as the UNC TEACCH® Program (www.teacch.com), it serves individuals with ASD across the lifespan, conducts multidisciplinary training, and does research. It has two certification levels, Practitioner and Advanced Consultant. The main ideas behind the intervention model, "Structured TEACCHing" are: the need to grasp the learning characteristics of individuals with ASD, and the importance of visual supports to promote meaning and independence. The "Culture of Autism" idea, as a way conceptualizing the patterns of thinking and behaviour seen in individuals with ASD, is central to TEACCH®. It includes: relative strengths in processing visual information; attention to details but difficulty grasping how those details fit together as a whole; trouble combining ideas; difficulty organizing ideas, materials, and activities; difficulties with attention; difficulty with time concepts, including moving too quickly or too slowly and problems perceiving the beginning, middle, or end of an activity; communication problems that always include pragmatic impairments; a tendency to become over-attached to routines; very strong interests and impulses; and marked sensory preferences and dislikes.

The principles of Structured TEACCHing are: understanding the culture of autism; developing an individualized person- and family-centered plan for each client or student rather than a standard curriculum; structuring the physical environment, with physical boundaries between different tasks, workstations and clear schedules of daily activities; and using visual supports to make the sequence of daily activities predictable and understandable.

University of Auckland researchers, Virues-Ortega, Julio and Pastor (2013) performed a meta-analysis of 14 TEACCH® intervention studies. They reported that TEACCH® had: small effects on perceptual, motor, verbal, and cognitive skills; and negligible to small effects on communication, activities of daily living, and motor function. Gains in social and maladaptive behaviour were larger, but need replication. Virues-Ortega et al. cautioned that their analysis should be considered to be exploratory, as only limited data were available.

The Early Start Denver Model (ESDM)

The Early Start Denver Model (Rogers & Dawson, 2010), initiated in 1981 by Dr Sally Rogers of the University of California MIND Institute (www.ucdmc.ucdavis.edu/mindinstitute), broadly resembles TEACCH® in that it is based around a personalized, family-centered plan that fosters parents' use of a child-centered responsive interaction style. By embedding recurrent teaching opportunities into play (Rogers et al., 2012), in naturalistic settings, it aims to augment existing gains in children aged 12–48 months. Parents meet quarterly with their child's treatment team to discuss goals, objectives, activities and instructional plans across situations (home, daycare, preschool). ESDM incorporates the shaping of natural, and then conventional gestures; and teaching motor-imitation skills related to language, and the meaning and importance of speech. It employs aspects of functional behavioural analysis: communication training; reinforcing alternative (more conventional) behaviours; and "redirection" to alternative behaviours children can use to achieve goals. Online workshops, to become an ESDM certified therapist, are available via the MIND Institute link above. In Australia, the Autism Specific Early Learning and Care Centre (www.latrobe.edu.au/child/services/aselcc) offers ESDM non-certification training for parents, professionals and para-professionals in the Asia-Pacific region.

Widely embraced, and heralded as "evidence-based", according to reviews by Weitlauf et al. (2014) and Roberts and Williams (2016) the current *level* of evidence for ESDM is low, especially in terms of long-term effectiveness, so it does not yet achieve the Foxx and Mulick (2016, p. 216) seal of approval. We note, however, that Dr Rogers and others (Dawson et al., 2010) conducted a randomized controlled trial, demonstrating that, over a two-year period, a group of children diagnosed with autism who received the ESDM treatment showed greater gains in adaptive behaviour than a matched group who were engaged in intervention with community-providers. Furthermore, the children in the ESDM group were more likely to be reclassified from having autism to having PDD-NOS. Subsequently, Fulton, Eapen, Črnčec, Walter, and Rogers (2014) provided somewhat encouraging support for ESDM, when delivered in a community setting with "relatively minimal" (p. 8) one-to-one intensive therapy, as having the potential to reduce children's maladaptive behaviours. We await with interest further independent research into this long-running combined intervention.

Family-based interventions

Family support and education programmes that show promise but which require further evaluation in the form of large-scale independent studies, are Autism Seminars for Families (previously The Help! Program) and the EarlyBird and EarlyBird Plus programmes, all developed and operated by the National Autistic Society in the UK. Others are Positive Behaviour Support (PBS) and The Hanen Programs®, notably More Than Words.

The Camphill movement

The Camphill movement comprises over 100 residential communities in 20 countries. Inspired by the work of Rudolf Steiner (b. 1861 d. 1925), it was started in 1939 in Scotland by Dr Karl Koenig (b. 1902 d. 1966), an Austrian paediatrician and educator, and his colleagues. Following a Waldorf/Rudolf Steiner curriculum, it provides educational intervention, craftwork instruction, practical training in workplace and life-skills, and therapies to schoolchildren, young people, and adults with learning disabilities (ID), ASD, mental health problems and other special needs. Teachers and other carers live with the students in households that simulate extended families. The Camphill philosophy, *anthroposophy*[16], is that irrespective of an individual's apparent disability, that individual's spirit – the fundamental core that makes us all human – remains "unbroken". Hence, all people warrant equal respect and comparable chances in life, in order to realize their potential. Many Waldorf/Rudolf Steiner schools, with no nearby Camphill communities, pursue the Camphill methods, which aim to foster natural abilities and support development in all areas. The effects and efficacy of the method await evaluation.

ASD in children, and pseudoscience

We discuss ASD relative to: Sensory Integration in Chapter 5, Facilitated Communication in Chapter 6; Auditory Integration Training/Treatments in Chapter 8; chelation, diet and biomedical interventions (biomed protocols) in Chapter 10. Here, we look at ASD and animal-assisted intervention, psychological astrology, CAM, GemIIni™, Relationship Development Intervention®, and the Son-Rise Program®.

Animal-assisted intervention

Human interaction with animals has demonstrable psychosocial benefits (O'Haire, 2010). Animal-assisted intervention (AAI) is a broad term used to describe diverse ways of involving animals in activities of daily living,

---

16 Anthroposophic (Anthroposophical) medicine is a form of CAM devised by Rudolf Steiner and Ita Wegman (b. 1876 d. 1943) in the 1920s. It is based on occult (esoteric and paranormal) conceptions and Dr Steiner's spiritual philosophy, anthroposophy. Its practitioners use various interventions, including massage, exercise, counselling, and substances akin to homeopathic dilutions. Some Anthroposophic doctors oppose childhood vaccination.

rehabilitation, social care, education and therapy for adults and children. The weak (albeit largely positive) evidence base for AAI may be partly attributable to methodological constraints, including difficulties in study design. Animal ethics preclude researchers from randomly assigning animals to people who may or may not want them, and it is impossible for investigators and participants to be "blinded" to an animal's presence.

AAI exists in numerous forms, and may take place in people's own homes, in hospital, care, and custodial settings, on care farms, in schools, and as a function of organizations (e.g., Riding for the Disabled[17]: www.rda.org.uk). Animals are used to provide assistance to people with ASD, behaviour problems, chronic mental illnesses, diabetes, epilepsy, generalized anxiety disorder, ID, post-traumatic stress disorder, sensory impairments, and more.

Assistance animals (or *service animals*) are animals that live with, and provide specific support for, an individual with an impairment; and *therapy animals* are used in animal-assisted therapy (AAT). AAT is defined by the International Association of Animal-Human Interactions Organizations (IAHAIO) as "a goal oriented, planned and structured therapeutic intervention directed and/or delivered by health, education and human service professionals. Intervention progress is measured and included in professional documentation. AAT is delivered and/or directed by a formally trained (with active licensure, degree or equivalent) professional with expertise within the scope of the professionals' practice. AAT focuses on enhancing physical, cognitive, behavioral and/or socio-emotional functioning of the particular human recipient" (Jegatheesan, Beetz, Ormerod, Johnson, Fine, Yamazaki, Dudzik, Garcia, & Choi, 2014, p. 4). Representing the views of the IAHAIO, Jegatheesan et al. note (p. 7) that while observation and contemplation of animals in the natural world and in wildlife sanctuaries is acceptable, wild species (e.g., dolphins, elephants, capuchin monkeys, prairie dogs, arthropods and reptiles), even if they are tame, should not be involved in AAT interactions.

Companion animals stay with their charges full time, or for long or short periods. The animals are of almost any variety, from birds, caged or visiting outdoor feeders (e.g., for patients in bed to observe through a window or in courtyards and gardens), to resident cats, dogs, fish, guinea pigs, hamsters, rabbits, and sheep in schools and at home. Companion animals are not

---

17 "Riding for the disabled" as an activity is not necessarily a component of an intervention/therapy/rehabilitation. One of its roles is simply to provide the necessary environmental supports and assistance to a person with a disability to ride a horse: for purpose of learning to ride, or for the experience, enjoyment or challenge of riding, or to instruct other riders.

assistance/service animals like, for example: guide dogs that help visually impaired people move about safely; capuchin "organ grinder" monkeys, taught to help people with severe mobility limitations by operating lights and picking up dropped objects; hearing dogs, trained to alert their human partners to the sounds of daily life, such as a baby waking, smoke alarms, faxes and phones; or assistance animals that may signal to an owner with diabetes that a potentially fatal drop in blood sugar levels is occurring, or warn an owner with epilepsy of an impending seizure.

Saving the day

In children's books and media, there is a recurrent theme of animals as saviours. Recall Aesop's *Androcles and the Lion* of mythic Greece, Paul Gallico's *Snow Goose* at Dunkirk, and dozens of heartwarming tales of resolute cats, gentle St Bernards, and *Croix de Guerre* awardee Cher Ami and other gallant carrier pigeons liberating people from imminent death. Not to be outdone, *Lassie* (The Wonder Dog) saved lost brothers who were dying in the snow; *Skippy* (The Bush Kangaroo) in episode upon episode spared Sonny from a sticky end, and Anna Sewell's 1877 *Black Beauty* (the eponymous horse) narrates, in the first person, how he prevented his groom at Squire Gordon's, Mr John Manly, from descending to a watery grave.

It is a charming *idée fixe*, rich in anthropomorphism, sentimentality and drama, appealing to many authors and readers. Similarly, AAI or "pet therapy" for children with ASD (for which there *is* a nascent evidence base: see O'Haire, 2013) piques imaginations as the foci of books, movies, documentaries, and commercial ventures (e.g., www.eagala.org for Equine Assisted Psychotherapy and Equine Assisted Learning). They range from the elitist – who can afford a month traversing Mongolia by horse with a 5-year-old (Isaacson, 2009) – to the emotional, evangelical, and enticing for parents willing to try anything to help their children with ASD.

For one example, the book, *The Horse Boy: A Father's Quest to Heal His Son* (Isaacson, 2009), has become a documentary film (*The Horse Boy Movie*, 2009), a global business, Horse Boy World (www.horseboyworld.com, home of Brain Building and Kinetic Learning) and a topic in the 2015 ITV 2-part "factual series" *Man and Beast* with Martin Clunes. The publicity blurb (www.itv.com/presscentre/ep2week21/man-beast-martin-clunes) for the second episode of *Man and Beast* reads, "Martin learns how horses are being used for helping autistic children. Rupert Isaacson has devised the Horseboy Method, from which hundreds of autistic children have benefitted from the therapeutic powers of horses". If the respectful actor has his doubts during this encounter, he does not let on – which is *not* the response Clunes fans have come to anticipate from his brusque alter ego, the EBP-fixated, duly sceptical Doc Martin.

> **Pseudoscience alert**
>
> *"The term hippotherapy refers to how occupational therapy, physical therapy, and speech-language pathology professionals use evidence-based practice and clinical reasoning in the purposeful manipulation of equine movement to engage sensory, neuromotor, and cognitive systems to achieve functional outcomes. In conjunction with the affordances of the equine environment and other treatment strategies, hippotherapy is part of a patient's integrated plan of care."*
> www.americanhippotherapyassociation.org
> January 19, 2016

O'Haire (2013) performed a systematic review of empirical research on AAI for ASD, that utilized dogs, dolphins, guinea pigs, horses, llamas, and rabbits, noting that the presentation of AAI varied greatly across the 14 studies reviewed, and that most had "many methodological weaknesses". Reported outcomes (universally positive) included gains in social communication and decreased problem behaviours, autistic severity, and stress. O'Haire concluded that there is preliminary "proof of concept" of AAI for ASD, and she called for rigorous research.

Dolphins: Wild animals as therapy props

Dolphin-assisted intervention can consist of having the child swim with dolphins, touch them, or be given the impression that they are taking care of them, and that in response the dolphin loves the child. Alternatively, it can be a structured, bespoke for each child, Dolphin Assisted Therapy (DAT). In DAT, the child is encouraged to complete pre-set tasks such as placing a ring or peg in a certain spot on request, or verbalizing on command. Being permitted to interact with the dolphin then rewards the child who touches it, kisses it, or "rides" it, holding its fin. There is no evidence to support either form. In a position statement, the Whale and Dolphin Conservation Society says that DAT is unlikely to meet the psychological or physical welfare needs of either human participants or dolphins (Brakes & Williamson, 2007, p. 18), concluding: "it is highly recommended that the practice of dolphin assisted therapy be terminated".

Hutchins (2016) begins her ASHA Leader feature: *Communing with Dolphins*, with: "A dolphin jumps high into the air—and a new neural pathway is emblazoned in the brain of a child struggling to speak". The article celebrates the work of Janet Flowers (Certified Autism Communication Navigator), who integrates dolphins, sea lions, tropical birds, ducks, and other animals into short-term intensive treatment for children aged 3–13, from around the world, with significant communication disorders or delays including ASD, CAS, and Down syndrome. Dr Flowers has her own protocol, and has reportedly distanced herself from DAT (see Editorial comment on Ray, 2016), though it is unclear how the dolphin aspect of her menagerie methodology, "Short-Term Intensive Treatment", differs substantively from it. Hutchins quotes Flowers: "The emotional center of the brain can also send skills and knowledge to long-term memory…Seeing a dolphin perform immediately after achieving a goal generates memories through the brain's amygdala. This path differs from the traditional way of learning new skills, which involves activating the hippocampus. In other words, if you're teaching a skill at the time you're having a dolphin jump for a child, they'll likely remember it!".

Seeking explanations for these improbable neural mechanisms and their "likely" effects on memory and learning, we perused Dr Flowers' website (www.drjfi.org), where she logs being "recognized for her decades of achievements in the speech-language pathology community for her therapeutic approach, philosophy and research". Unable to locate research reports, we connected by email with Dr Flowers in April 2016, and requested a copy of the oft self-cited Flowers (2003) or any of her publications on marine mammals in therapy, to be informed that the 2003 work was her doctoral dissertation, which was not available on request. Meanwhile, the response to the Hutchins (2016) article from Ray (2016, p. 5) raises key ethical issues around mistreatment of wild animals, while also stating that "the exploitation of the families that are taken in by it should be considered unethical, not glorified".

Psychological astrology

There was a wave of irate incredulity among SLPs/SLTs in blogs and social media, and waspish responses from us, coupled with concerns for potential victims, when Hill (2015) posted to her *Smart Talkers* speech and language therapy blog (www.smarttalkersblog.com), a guest entry by Staffordshire Hi-Tech Astrologer and Personal Coach, Alison Chester-Lambert (with a master's degree in Cultural Astronomy and Astrology). As our horoscopes foretold, teleporting through the celestial taradiddle on Ms Chester-Lambert's galactic websites was a stellar chore. There was, for instance, a claim that: "Psychological Astrology can help us to understand the inner world of those who cannot communicate. This is because the birth chart can describe the basic motivations, likes, dislikes and desires of the person. And it can describe these things better than we can describe ourselves in most cases…it will describe the inner world of your child down to a tee".

Before pressing on to Castor and Pollux we read www.midlandsschoolofastrology.co.uk and www.alisonchesterlambert.com, and, predictably for anyone who knows how thorough (a scientifically established characteristic of Sagittarians and Arians) we can be, the websites of kindred Psychoastrological spirits, divining not one whit of evidence. Our analysis is displayed in Figure 4.3.

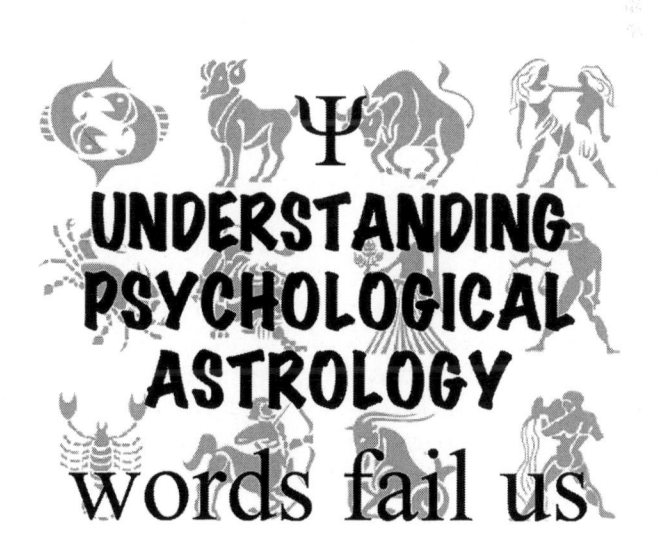

Figure 4.3 Ψ Understanding Psychological Astrology.

GemIIni™

"Video modelling" is a promising, but somewhat divisive, evidence-based teaching technique that uses video recording and display equipment to provide a visual model of a targeted behaviour or skill (Bellini & Akullian, 2007; Morlock, Reynolds, Fisher, & Comer, 2015; Shukla-Mehta, Miller, & Callahan, 2010). It has been the topic of much research (e.g., Rayner, Denholm, & Sigafoos, 2009; Wilson, 2013).

Overall, results of a systematic review of 19 studies (Delano, 2007) indicated positive gains in social communication, "functional skill", perspective-taking, and difficult behaviour. Delano signalled, however, that: "A small pool of studies was reviewed, and treatment effects were not measured. Consequently, it is unclear at this time whether video modelling is more or less effective than other models of instruction for learners with autism, and too soon to make detailed recommendations for practitioners" (p. 41).

Enter founder and owner of GemIIni™ Systems, Inc. (www.gemIIni.org), and instigator of the term "discrete video modelling", Laura Marie Kasbar. GemIIni™ is described as "a specific form of video modelling based on the discrete trial method of applied behavior analysis [that] was developed and documented by Laura Kasbar in 2000 as a way to teach children who do not respond well to other kinds of therapy, including traditional applied behavior analysis (ABA)."

Mrs Kasbar says of GemIIni™, "With more than three decades of research and studies conducted with hundreds of thousands of people, science has proven that video modeling is one of the most effective ways to teach speech and reading skills. In addition, research shows that GemIIni's discrete video modeling is more effective than standard video modeling."

> **Pseudoscience alert**
> *"We are seeing all aspects of behaviors associated with autism improve. There is a neurological basis for these improvements which academics and neurologists believe may have to do with teaching to the basal ganglia and encouraging the transfer of information from the default network to the active network in the brain...People with very advanced language skills, even NT students who are advanced for their age, can use GemIIni. There doesn't appear to be an age or ability level. It is working with toddlers and 65-year-old stroke victims."*
> Laura Kasbar, 7 June 2015
> www.quora.com

It takes moments to sign up, create an account, and add one or many "students' " names – no questions asked, and with no permissions from parents or guardians if the "students" are not your own children – and proceed to purchasing a membership, and "treating" a child, or children, without the inconvenience of an assessment of *any* kind. The claims on the site are farcical. There is *no* independent research into GemIIni™. The "neurology" that underpins it is laughable: "On a neurological level, the brains of people with autism are larger than the typical person, making it possible for them to learn and store tremendous amounts of information, but much less capable of using that information." The interpretations of juried research into video modelling as an entity (e.g., Morlock et al., 2015 who used GemIIni™ videos, but who did not evaluate the efficacy of "discrete video modelling"), implying that they provide support for the GemIIni™ product, are blatant misrepresentations. The "sell" is inexorable, and we should all steer clear.

Back from the brink: Relationship Development Intervention® (RDI™)

Styled as a "cognitive developmental model", RDI™ was created by an entrepreneurial psychologist, Steven Gutstein, to be delivered at home, by parents. It is popular with teachers, "behavioural therapists", and RDI™ Certified Consultants in Australia, Canada, China, India, Italy, Japan, Malaysia, Mexico, New Zealand, Singapore, Switzerland, the UK and the US, and aspects of it are delivered in classrooms around the world. Its RDIconnect™ Internet presence (www.rdiconnect.com) is a website wonderland of wearying word pairs, intended to mesmerize and engage: "balanced learning", "cognitive apprentice", "dynamic intelligence", "experience anchor", and "neural underconnectivity" (whatever *those* might be). On the site, you can arrange to do an online parent course, "Join the RDI Learning Community Today to Get the Help Your Family Deserves", and "Gain the confidence and tools to pull your family back from the brink so that you can go on doing what you do best—being a family".

The basis for the intervention is that the "neural underconnectivity" in people with ASD leads to a rigid and fixed worldview. Being averse to both change and novel information, people with ASD do not develop "dynamic intelligence": the ability to think flexibly and take different perspectives, process different sorts of information simultaneously (e.g., listen and see at the same time) or make decisions. The intervention's six objectives, relate to emotional referencing, social coordination, declarative language, flexible thinking, relational information processing, and foresight and hindsight.

One of Dr Gutstein's maxims is, "With mental illness, you're fixing broken minds; with autism, you're creating a mind". While such apothegms do nothing for us, it is clear that he has a way with words, as evidenced by his many books and "professional posts and articles" online. This gift does not, however, extend to conducting and publishing research. We could not unearth evidence-based practice guidelines, systematic reviews, or independent empirical evidence of the efficacy of RDI™. Any "evidence" we found was anecdotal, testimonial, in-house, advertorial, and located on the RDIconnect™ website.

The Son-Rise Program® (Options Method)

In 1974, Barry (Bears) Neil Kaufman and Samahria Lyte Kaufman started The Son-Rise Program® (SRP®) for their son, Raun (b. 1973), who was diagnosed with autism. Its associated company, the Autism Treatment Center of America™ (www.autismtreatmentcenter.org), was founded in 1983 as "the worldwide teaching center for The Son-Rise Program®, a powerful and effective treatment for children and adults challenged by Autism…The treatment and educational model has changed the way children with Autism are helped worldwide."

At the core of the SRP® is the belief that children on the autism spectrum have difficulty forming relationships, but can be helped to do so through playful interaction with an adult, in a specially set-up room in the family home. The adult follows the child's lead, and does not set an agenda. This includes "joining" children in their behaviour, rather than trying to stop or modify it. So, if the child is lining up cars, eyeballing a tiny detail on the wallpaper, throwing blocks, flapping and bouncing, or wrecking the joint, the adult follows suit. This imitation is said to help build trust, showing the child love and acceptance, without judgement. This in turn is said to make it easier to build a relationship. Ultimately, with a good bond established, the child is motivated to learn new skills within activities of interest. Simple.

As a consequence of the Son-Rise Program®, administered by his parents, Ruan was, we are told, cured of his autism over a three-year period, from 18 months of age. His IQ rose from less than 30 to whatever it takes to graduate with honours from high school, earn a degree in Biomedical Ethics from Brown University, and become the Director of Global Outreach for The Son-Rise Program® at the Autism Treatment Center of America™. From his parents' and his own reports, Ruan Kaufman has done well; but the Son-Rise Program®, not so much. In over four decades of its existence, there has been one peer reviewed, but methodologically flawed, study of the SRP (Houghton, Schuchard, Lewis, & Thompson, 2013). In two words: stay away.

Be prepared

We have mentioned four books, presenting disparate viewpoints, that help to inform, inspire, challenge and bring guidance, comfort and necessary tools to prepare for the next step, to those travelling the ASD journey as parents: Des Roches Rosa, et al., 2011; Prizant and Fields-Meyer, 2015; Solomon (2012; 2013); and Sutton, 2015. Here is one more book. Like any parent, if you are the mother, father or grandparent of a child, young person or adult who is on the spectrum, you will think at times – probably a lot of the time, if truth be told – about your "child's" adult life. If you are an adult with ASD, then you will inevitably think often about the quality of your life: what you have accomplished, how you participate in society, and what is still to come; how you are or will be as a parent; and how the world sees you, and you see it. If you are so placed, the exhilarating, respectful *NeuroTribes: The Legacy of Autism and the Future of Neurodiversity* (Silberman, 2015) may be for you. Science journalist and social justice advocate, "raised to be sensitive to the rights of the oppressed", Steve Silberman proposes a model for acceptance, understanding, and full participation in society for people who think differently. This optimistic, game changing book, illuminated with ideas, is for people with ASD, and *all* concerned for them.

> *"Be prepared to overturn all prior knowledge you had about autism. With meticulous research, Steve Silberman has unearthed the surprising truths about the history of autism, uncovering the roots of the lie of the autism "epidemic". Be prepared to share the deeply compassionate understanding that the author bestows on the many different individuals we now include in the autism spectrum. His empathy touches even the villains of the story, and this is both moving and apt when he advises us all to embrace diversity. This gripping and heroic tale is a brilliant addition to the history of autism."*
>
> Uta Frith
> Emeritus Professor of Cognitive Development,
> University College London

Whatever you read, we hope it helps you to be prepared. If you recognize that there are no easy fixes, and if you routinely do your homework (see our 7-point safety check in on pages 292–298), request and weigh the evidence behind interventions, and check practitioners' credentials, you are set to become a critical consumer of information, research, and services. If you are open to changing your mind, if necessary, on the basis of your own digging, then you are an educated consumer, and potentially, a consumer advocate. If you can resist the hype, the hard sell, and the allure of the magical panacea – and can spot pseudoscience in a single bound – then, in our books, you are a superhero[18]!

---

18 "In modern popular fiction, a superhero is a type of heroic character possessing extraordinary talents, supernatural phenomena, or superhuman powers and is dedicated to a moral goal or protecting the public." Wikipedia

5 Behaving, Feeling, and Getting Along with Others

One sure-fire method for humans to draw attention to themselves is to behave in ways that deviate from the expected social norm. This "norm" is highly variable, depending on age, prevailing social customs, cultural, ethnic and religious mores, and immediate context, making it difficult for parents to teach, and for children to master, the spoken and unspoken niceties of social behaviour. Why is conduct that is greeted cheerily in one situation deplored in another?

Social disapproval and ostracism are generally unpleasant for humans, and we are socialized to avoid them, so it is no surprise to see evidence suggesting that our brains experience social exclusion through physical pain pathways (Eisenberger, 2012). Curiously, we are socialized to play *against* our emotions in many situations, simply to maintain a semblance of social harmony. Imagine the mayhem if everyone said just what they felt when jammed into Economy seats on a long-haul flight. Bolshie remarks about caterwauling babies, rowdy toddlers, she-bagging and manspreading passengers hogging space in fully reclined seats would soon spark aerial pandemonium. So, before considering the relative merits of behavioural interventions for children and adolescents with developmental disorders, we examine behavioural self-regulation itself. We stress that for children and many adults, *behaving* is the outward manifestation of *feeling*. If we forget this, we will misinterpret and/or miss important diagnostic and management information.

Behavioural self-regulation

The ability to self-monitor and self-regulate behaviour, in ways that are responsive to the social and emotional requirements of a situation, is a challenging and later developing human skill. As any new parent knows, newborns have no concept of self-regulation. For them, it is all about having biological needs met: *now*. We understand, and accept, that the only tool at infants' disposal is crying, and if crying fails to meet their needs, they cry louder and longer. Becoming accustomed to having their distress acknowledged, babies gradually learn that the nearby sound of parents' voices signals that comfort is imminent, and they begin to quieten, prior to being fed. This takes time and repetition, assisted by the processes of bonding and attachment, in which infants and their caregivers become attuned to each other's needs and emotional signals. The early emergence of *self*-soothing starts in toddlerhood, to be followed by years of practice. Significant physical or emotional challenges will provoke setbacks, so that soothing by a trusted adult (e.g., a parent, grandparent, or childcare worker) will be needed for the little one to regain equilibrium.

Alongside self-soothing behaviour, children develop empathy for others' emotional states, and the ability to curb strong, socially undesirable interpersonal and behavioural responses. Two toddlers, playing in parallel or cooperatively, will inevitably clash, usually over a toy both covet, irrespective of who actually owns it. Neither has empathy for the feelings of an aggrieved playmate, robbed of the use or control of a toy, and both aim to win at all costs (even if that means biting). Such skirmishes are the focus of much early parenting, resulting in teachable moments about sharing, and (hopefully) developmentally appropriate disciplinary approaches such as distraction, a firm "no" and short-term time-out, as opposed to smacking, bargaining, shouting, or demonstrating how

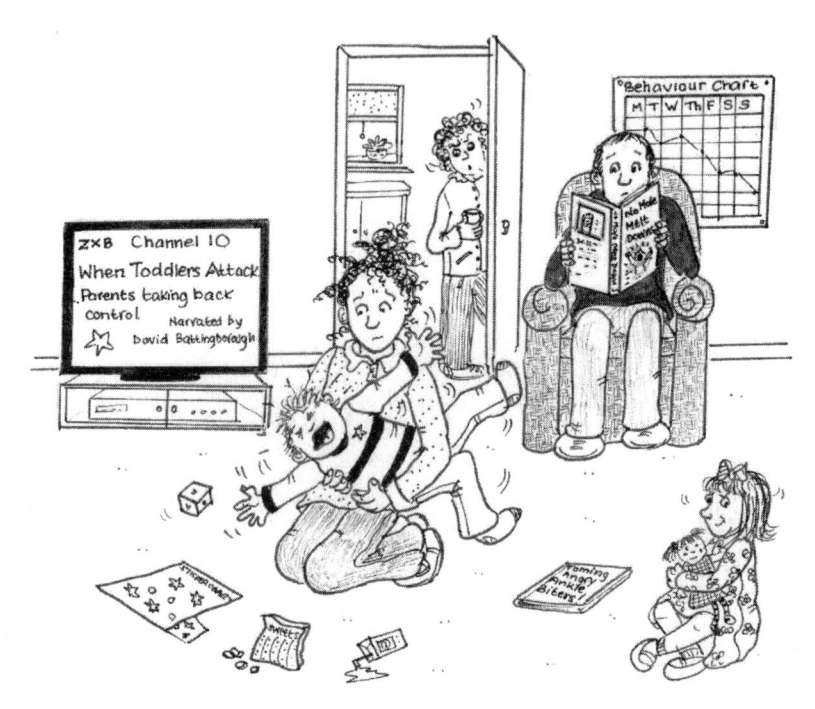

Helen Rippon

biting "feels". Eventually, parents' roles as external regulators (of emotional states and behaviour) must yield to internal control.

Newborns and toddlers are not expected to display internal self-regulation, but we do expect such capacities to begin appearing by roughly age 5, as part of the "school readiness" package. In the preschool years, therefore, children are typically exposed to games and activities that promote turn-taking, reciprocity, sharing, cooperation, and waiting. These skills do not come naturally to most preschoolers, so must be learned through direct explanation, modelling, shaping, and reinforcement. For information about these processes, and the work of influential 20th-century social learning theorists like Albert Bandura, see www.learning-theories.com. Children vary in how readily they acquire and refine self-regulation skills, and setbacks are common, e.g., in emotionally charged circumstances, or when they are tired or sick. Concurrent developments, in cognition, memory, sensory perception and language, support the development of behavioural self-regulation, and difficulties in one or more of these domains can compound delayed or problematic behavioural development.

Behavioural and emotional self-regulation relies on optimal functioning of several cortical and subcortical brain-regions. Subcortically, there is the limbic system (see Figure 5.1), a neural circuit deep within the cerebral cortex, comprised of structures that include the hippocampus, amygdala, and mammillary bodies. The limbic system is essential in regulating affective (emotional) states and, because of its role in memory, can trigger pre-conscious responses, e.g., in people who were exposed to early trauma, and who are then re-exposed to a person, place, sound, smell or object associated with the prior traumatic experience (see pages 117–118 for more on classical conditioning). Limbic structures are also central in activating the fight-flight-or-freeze response in circumstances of extreme physical or emotional threat. There is a huge, recent literature on the long shadow cast by early maltreatment (abuse and/or neglect) with respect to brain development and children's capacity to fully engage academically and socially at school. This work is beyond our scope, so interested readers are referred to investigations by Dr Bruce Perry, via the Child Trauma Academy in the US (www.childtraumaacademy.com), where there are links to openly accessible research and practice papers of relevance to parents, teachers, and clinicians. We also recommend the open access Australian publications: *Creating Calmer Classrooms* from the Commissioner for Children and Young People (2007), and the Australian Childhood Foundation's *Making Space for Learning* (2010). Trauma-informed practice shows promise as a means of making classrooms feel safer, more predictable, and less stressful for *all* children, particularly those who have been, or are, exposed to high levels of stress in at home. Distress is sometimes masked by children in ways that can easily and understandably (although often incorrectly) be re-attributed by adults, including teachers. Teaching dysregulated, unpredictable, distressed children is unquestionably stressful for teachers, feeding teacher burn-out and attrition from the profession (Ross, Romer, & Horner, 2012). We therefore endorse recent initiatives by some teacher pre-service programs to cover trauma-informed practice in their curricula.

The cortical regions most commonly associated with learned and conscious behavioural self-regulation are the frontal lobes, especially the prefrontal regions located just behind the forehead. The prefrontal regions are responsible for "higher-order" executive skills such as planning, self-regulating, curbing impulses, focusing attention selectively and screening-out distractions, thinking in the abstract, and taking the cognitive and emotional perspectives of another person.

"Thinking in the abstract" means being able to consider concepts and ideas that are intangible or invisible, e.g., phenomena like trustworthiness and respect. Given the range and complexity of these cognitive skills, it follows that the prefrontal regions are among the latest to mature, with final maturation

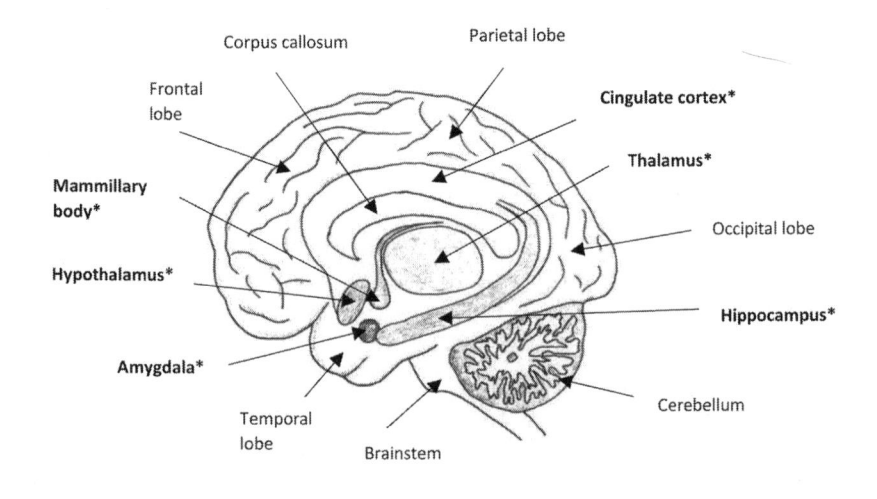

LIMBIC SYSTEM*

Figure 5.1 The limbic system. Emina McLean

occurring well into the 20s (Blakemore & Choudhury, 2006). This progress involves two key processes: *myelination*: the formation of an insulating sheath around neurons to assist them to conduct electrical messages more efficiently; and *neuronal pruning*: the removal of inefficient pathways, so as to consolidate neural circuitry that efficiently supports new and emerging skills. This late maturation of the prefrontal regions (plus the hormonal surges associated with adolescence) is largely responsible for the regrettable predicaments that can accompany late adolescence and early adulthood: involvement in road trauma (particularly in the company of peers), unplanned or regretted sexual activity (resulting in pregnancy and/or sexually transmitted infections), detrimental alcohol and other drug consumption, and over-representation in interpersonal violence statistics. Sometimes, more than one of these risks is present at one time, exacerbating the perils of immature prefrontal regions.

Behaviour problems are serious mental health concerns

It is vital to remember that behaviour problems are *serious mental health concerns*; something that is easy for parents, teachers, and clinicians to overlook. Consciously keeping this principle uppermost invites us to (1) understand what lies behind behaviour, thereby sidestepping lazy, judgemental assumptions, and (2) identify contributory factors to adverse patterns of behaviour. It is also important to know that mental health problems (emotional and behavioural) are significantly more common in people with developmental disabilities (Einfeld & Tonge, 1996; White, Chant, Edwards, Townsend, & Waghorn, 2005). In some cases, this echoes features of the underlying disorder, but a medical diagnosis cannot singlehandedly account for the behavioural profile of a given individual with a neurodisability. Furthermore, the presence of a neurodevelopmental disorder does not remove the importance of *temperament* (e.g., children's personal qualities of extroversion, adaptiveness to new situations, and perseverance with long, challenging, or unpleasant tasks), nor the influence of *culture*. Behaviours (e.g., noisy interjections while in company; avoiding eye-contact with authority figures; laughing when you make a mistake) judged improper and embarrassing in one culture, may be well-tolerated and even encouraged in another. In addition, there are obvious family-to-family variations within cultures with respect to behavioural regulation of children.

Rather than being categorically distinct, children's emotional and behavioural difficulties will sit somewhere along a continuum, from *internalizing* to *externalizing* disorders, with substantial masking of one by the other.

Regrettably, internalizing and externalizing disorders, where behaviour problems and emotional difficulties intersect, are often conceived as separate and even mutually exclusive, which they are not. The internalizing and externalizing disorders interface is well summarized by Caroline Miller, of the (US) Child Mind Institute (nd):

> "A child who appears to be oppositional or aggressive may be reacting to anxiety—anxiety he may, depending on his age, not be able to articulate effectively, or not even fully recognize that he's feeling...... It's not uncommon for children with serious undiagnosed anxiety to be disruptive at school, where demands and expectations put pressure on them that they can't handle. And it can be very confusing to teachers and other staff members to "read" that behavior, which can seem to come out of nowhere".

Internalizing disorders predominantly encompass anxiety and depression. Anxiety, in turn, is characterized by excessive worry, and can be accompanied by social and other phobias (disproportionate fears), as well as panic disorders and post-traumatic stress disorder. In children, common signs of anxiety include bed-wetting, school-refusal, and difficult-to-pinpoint somatic (bodily) symptoms such as tummy pains and nausea. Less commonly, selective mutism can occur where a child only speaks to certain people (e.g., parents) in few situations (e.g., only at home). The overriding feature of depression is low mood, generally for periods of two weeks or more, accompanied by loss of pleasure in activities that are normally enjoyed, together with pessimism about self, others, and the world in general. When depression is severe and/or unremitting, it can negatively impact cognition (e.g., by impairing concentration and memory). Unfortunately, anxiety and depression often co-occur, though one may become evident first and be more obvious than the other. Both respond well to intervention, whether pharmacologically- or psychologically-based, although psychologically-based "talk therapies" such as Cognitive Behaviour Therapy (CBT) rest on the ability to "think about one's own thinking" which holds challenges for children and adolescents with developmental disabilities but is not necessarily beyond their reach with appropriate scaffolding (see page 138 for an example of scaffolding in the context of circle time). The benefits of pharmacological treatment can be marked, particularly in moderate-to-severe cases, and may facilitate successful use of psychological therapies. Unfortunately, medicines can also have adverse side-effects (Masand & Gupta,

2002), and their benefits typically wane when treatment ends. It may be helpful to pair psychotherapy and drug treatment (Clarke et al., 2005); however, there is a dearth of research on this question in children and adolescents with developmental disorders, so families and clinicians need to work together as scientist-practitioners to evaluate effectiveness in individual cases.

While internalizing disorders like anxiety and depression may be misdiagnosed, have their severity trivialized, or go undiagnosed, externalizing disorders are just that, "external" and unmissable by those around the child, because they are disruptive, particularly to parents and teachers. Miller's words illustrate that <u>behaviour is the observable tip of the emotional iceberg;</u> it does not convey what is happening under the surface, where visibility is poor.

Although most diagnostic systems present internalizing and externalizing disorders in separate categories, they are really co-occurring disorders, which are not always recognized as such. According to the Diagnostic and Statistical Manual of the American Psychiatric Association (DSM-5; 2013) the main forms of externalizing disorder are ADHD, oppositional defiant disorder (ODD) and conduct disorder (CD). We cover ADHD in Chapter 3, focusing here on ODD and CD. The features of these disorders are well-summarized on the American Academy of Child and Adolescent Psychiatry website (www.aacap.org).

True to its name, ODD refers to behaviours such as defiance and lack of cooperation in circumstances where cooperation can be reasonably expected on social and developmental grounds. Typical ODD behaviours include frequent temper tantrums, challenging of rules, excessive arguing with adults, non-compliance with reasonable requests, deliberate actions that annoy or upset others, apparent spitefulness, and eagerness to exact revenge when aggrieved. Some children with ODD may eventually, in adolescence, be diagnosed with CD, because they exhibit several of the following behaviours: physical and/or verbal aggression towards people and animals (including cruelty to animals), threatening and intimidating behaviour, use of weapons (e.g., knives), stealing, lying, damaging others' property, and frequent truancy. While oppositional and challenging behaviours are normal aspects of children's development, ODD and CD are not developmentally normal. They signal to parents, teachers, clinicians, police, and children's courts that the young person needs careful psychological assessment, to identify (and hopefully address) underlying predisposing and perpetuating factors, within the child, within the environment, or within both.

We cannot rely on children and adolescents to tell us in words that they feel distressed, or to say why. There is good evidence that children with severe behaviour disturbances are at high risk for unidentified language impairments (e.g., Snow & Powell, 2011), and behaviour, not words, may be the only way some children can signal distress. Behaviour can also be used to communicate skill-deficits. A student who misbehaves rather than completing set-work may be trying to tell the adults that, "I don't understand what you want me to do here". The co-occurrence of learning and behaviour difficulties in the primary school years is always a red flag for unrecognized language difficulties, and SLP/SLT assessment, in consultation with the teacher and educational and developmental psychologist, is advised in such situations (see Cross, 2011 for further detail).

Diagnostic processes and terminology for behaviour disturbances

Like all sub-specialties pertaining to people with disabilities, psychiatry has in-house terminology to describe and differentiate disorders. Unlike some other branches of medicine, however, these terms do not describe disorders that are diagnosed through laboratory-based or radiological tests. Instead, they are derived from detailed histories, skilled observation, discussion with a range of interviewees, and use of behavioural scales and structured questionnaires. As a profession, psychiatry continues to strive to adopt more rigorous diagnostic classification systems, but most practitioners will probably agree that significant subjectivity and loose interpretation lingers. This, combined with the usual co-morbidities, means that an individual patient will have different labels applied by different practitioners at different times. Each revision of the DSM and the International Classification of Diseases (ICD) sees off some labels and introduces new ones, in efforts to reflect scientific advances. The changes are inevitably swayed by interest groups' lobbyists, and satisfying all stakeholders is impossible. Ironically, as the severity of disability *increases*, the feasibility of applying conventional, useful, diagnostic labels for behavioural and emotional difficulties *decreases*, so that clinical skill and strong interdisciplinary teamwork are needed to manage knowledge gaps and diagnostic uncertainties.

Developmental disorders and mental health problems

There are many reasons why children and adolescents with developmental disorders are more prone to behavioural and emotional difficulties than their typically-developing (TD) peers. Nonetheless, we caution vigorously against sloppy attribution of behavioural patterns to a child's biomedical diagnosis, as in "*it's syndromal*". Parents tire of hearing that their child with Down syndrome (Ds) must have "a lovely nature", when really, some children and adolescents with Ds display, every day, defiant, oppositional, unpredictable behaviour. A syndrome is but one *part* of who a child is, and a range of bio-psycho-social factors must be considered to understand their behaviour and, moreover, to understand and respond when their customary behaviour *changes*.

Taking a bio-psycho-social perspective on behaviour

Using a bio-psycho-social framework means considering the biological basis of a condition (e.g., whether the disorder is syndromal, metabolic, traumatic or idiopathic), the individual's psychological characteristics (e.g., temperament, coping styles, and self-concept), and the child's and family's social, cultural, and environmental circumstances. In days gone by, the medical model of disability was dominant, but in recent times it has been augmented by conceptual models that are informed by psychosocial aspects of living with disability and we applaud the introduction of this wider lens. Meanwhile, it is important to *understand* the biomedical aspects of a condition in order to fully appreciate the challenges that the young person may face, and to ensure that necessary medical and surgical treatments are provided. Ds, for example, is associated with cardiac anomalies, and an elevated risk later in life of developing Alzheimer's Disease (Wiseman, Alford, Tybulewicz, & Fisher, 2009). Acquired brain injury carries heightened risk of post-traumatic epilepsy (Liesemer, Bratton, Zebrack, Brockmeyer, & Statler, 2011) and children with cerebral palsy may require surgery to relieve joint contractures (Aisen, 2011). Two children with the same biomedical diagnosis will have different profiles of strengths and needs. Understanding an individual's psychological characteristics, together with sensitivity to social and cultural contexts, supports better tailoring of educational and therapeutic responses. Conversely, focusing unduly on one or two dimensions while ignoring others will almost certainly constrain a child's progress. A bio-psycho-social response relies on careful, thorough history-taking and also on the involvement of the whole interdisciplinary team, with the family as essential participants.

Sitting alongside the bio-psycho-social approach are the "Four Ps" – the predisposing, precipitating, perpetuating and protective factors associated with mental health problems, whether emotional or behavioural (or both) in nature. The Four Ps, mapped over the bio-psycho-social framework, aid our

Table 5.1 Four Ps Grid: Abbie.

Four Ps	Bio	Psycho	Social
Predisposing	Abbie has a developmental disability, so this increases her risk of MH problems under stress. At age 15, she is displaying pubertal body changes and some moodiness that might have occurred irrespective of the recent school change.	Abbie has had limited experience of dealing with major life changes, so cannot call on previous examples of situations that have been emotionally difficult for a while, but have then become easier.	
Precipitating		A teacher aide reports that Abbie was teased by another student on her first day because she did not know where to place her belongings. This was distressing for Abbie and she withdrew socially from her peers.	A recent house move and change of school has disrupted Abbie's sense of connectedness and routine within a broader social network.
Perpetuating		Abbie believes that she will never like her new school as much as she did her old one.	Refusal to go to school means Abbie is not making new friends.
Protective	Abbie is in good physical health and enjoys sport. Getting her involved in school sport may be beneficial.	Abbie does not have a history of anxiety or depression.	Abbie's parents are supportive and eager to know how best to support her. They trust the staff at the new school to work towards solutions for Abbie. Abbie has strong relationships with two cousins who live near her new house.

understanding of behavioural difficulties, particularly when they co-occur with a communication impairment that complicates or even prevents history taking. This framework is also helpful in determining the focus of an intervention. The kinds of information that can arise from this way of thinking are exemplified in Abbie's Four P's Grid, in Table 5.1.

Abbie is 15 and has Ds. Until lately, her behaviour and mental health (MH) have been unremarkable, but since changing schools after a house move, she has been withdrawn, refusing to attend school most days. Unable to resolve the current impasse, and realizing that this is more than teenage angst, Abbie's increasingly worried parents turn to the school psychologist, who carefully collects history information from Abbie, her parents, teachers, classroom aides, and clinicians, producing a summary of her current status.

Using this framework, the team sees with greater clarity Abbie's pattern of strengths and difficulties, and opportunities for focused support are identified. They decide that Abbie may benefit from reassuring psychoeducation about handling change, allowing her to accumulate concepts and words to help her understand this confusing experience. Psychoeducation is also important for Abbie's parents, who seek guidance on how much to intervene and how much to "step back", but be available should Abbie seek their support. They ask teaching staff how she can participate in school sport, and an enthusiastic buddy is assigned to help her to assimilate socially. Her cousins are also urged to spend time with Abbie away from school, now that she lives nearby, so that she can enjoy positive social and emotional experiences, separate from school and from the immediate family. Close monitoring of Abbie's psychological wellbeing shows that she is not clinically depressed, so that it is not appropriate or necessary to initiate medication. Her reluctance to attend school abates, and she makes two friends.

Behaviour change in the context of severe communication impairment

When children and adolescents have severe and complex communication impairments, it is imperative to recognize that negative changes in behaviour may signal undiagnosed medical conditions and/or psychosocial distress. Medical conditions such as urinary tract infections, gastro-oesophageal reflux, upper respiratory tract infections, middle ear infections, appendicitis, undiagnosed tendonitis and fractures, and menstrual/gynaecological disorders can all cause severe, sometimes sudden-onset discomfort that may initially manifest as behaviour change. It is critical, therefore, that behaviour change is recognized as a *form of communication*. The tricky task for parents, teachers, clinicians, and carers is to determine *what* is being communicated. Uncharacteristic and unexplained distress, irritability, and withdrawal are all red flags for possible medical issues that require assessment and management, or signals that the young person is being mistreated, e.g., by carers or inadequately supervised fellow residents in a residential facility. We wish that mistreatment were not a consideration, but as discussed in Chapter 6, it is unfortunately true that suboptimal care, and even criminal acts, are sometimes perpetrated on people with disabilities. Bad, unsafe "care", or abuse by housemates can result in distress, exhibited behaviourally, e.g., as retreat, anxiety, irritability, or belligerence, so having a reliable means of communication (if possible) and a trusted advocate is critical.

When children or adults have severe physical disabilities and associated medical problems, they may come under the overlapping care of many medical specialists. In addition to the family general practitioner (GP), neurologists manage epilepsy, gastroenterologists look after disorders of the digestive system such as reflux, diarrhoea and constipation, orthopaedic surgeons operate on fractures and contracted limbs, psychiatrists manage disorders of mental state and attention, ophthalmologists address impaired vision, ENT specialists assist with disorders of hearing, swallowing, and nasal function, respiratory physicians deal with lung disorders, gynaecologists treat menstrual disorders...the list goes on *and on*, to include dermatologists, endocrinologists, paediatricians, rheumatologists, and more. These practitioners have specialized knowledge and can contribute in important ways to support everyday functioning and independence. A troublesome downside of having several specialists involved is that there may be little or no communication between them, with an associated high risk of polypharmacy. The (Australian) National Prescribing Service (2000) says,

> *"Polypharmacy is the concurrent use of multiple medications. It can be associated with the prescription and use of too many or unnecessary medicines at dosages or frequencies higher than therapeutically essential. However, multiple medications are often necessary and can constitute best care for patients."*

Polypharmacy poses serious risks because of potential drug interactions that can create confusion, drowsiness, muscle weakness, memory problems, agitation and nausea. These are unpleasant in themselves, and can increase the probability of injury. If unrecognized or misdiagnosed, they may also contribute to well-intended but inadvisable decisions to stop or increase medications, and may contribute to poor compliance with medications in general. In addition, many people (disabled or not), use over-the-counter medications (e.g., proprietary analgesics, antihistamines, sleep preparations, slimming aids, dietary supplements, and CAM "remedies"), often without mentioning them to medical practitioners, fearing disapproval, or thinking them "harmless" and so not needing consideration in the broader medications profile (see pages 273–274). It may be helpful, therefore, for a pharmacist to periodically review medications to identify those that might reasonably be discontinued or reduced, and to determine whether the initial indications for their use persist. Polypharmacy must be considered where behaviour and/or cognitive function decline, and is best prevented through clear communication between practitioners. Families can be the best conduits for this communication, as they may be the only ones who know the exact extent of the care team.

Behavioural principles and interventions

The pioneering 19th- and 29th-century work of behavioural scientists Ivan Pavlov (b. 1849 d. 1936) and B.F. Skinner (b. 1904 d. 1990) left enduring influence on developmental psychology generally, and teaching specifically. Through his celebrated experiments with bells and salivating dogs, Dr Pavlov identified that two previously unrelated events or phenomena can become linked in ways that influence future emotional and behavioural responses. Childhood sexual abuse victims often recount how an aroma, e.g., the scent of an aftershave, can have a life-long aversive effect, regardless of the circumstances in which they later smell it. This is because two previously unrelated (unconditioned) events have become involuntarily paired for the affected individual; this is called *classical conditioning*. Dr Skinner, in slightly later work, examined ways in which responses that are under voluntary control can be shaped by consequences (positive or negative), resulting in a description of *operant conditioning*. Operant conditioning occurs when parents and teachers reward a desired behaviour (positive reinforcement), when they withdraw a reward following undesired behaviour (negative punishment), when they punish undesired behaviour (positive[1] punishment), and less commonly (thankfully) when they remove something unpleasant (an "aversive") in response to desirable behaviour (negative reinforcement).

A working grasp of classical and operant conditioning, and social learning theory (see page 107) can be helpful with many aspects of parenting, teaching, and therapy, as adults spend innumerable hours trying to teach children new

---

[1] Operant conditioning is easier to understand if you remember that, in this context, "positive" means adding something and "negative" means taking something away.

knowledge and skills. The mechanisms whereby classical conditioning has influenced a child's responses in a particular situation may be somewhat obscure; for example, how is a teacher expected to know that 6-year-old Pattie has learned to associate suddenly loud adult voices with imminent violence? Pattie is always neatly dressed, and there are no outward signs of neglect. However, things are volatile and unpredictable at home, where she has (unconsciously) learned that the sound of grown-ups unexpectedly talking loudly signals a need for hyper-vigilance to threat (resulting in difficulty concentrating in class). By contrast, the mechanisms by which operant conditioning influences children's behaviour are more obvious, particularly to trained observers. Many children enjoy (if not seek) adults' attention, but if the only reliable way of achieving this is to play up, then it should surprise no-one if misbehaviour becomes an issue in the home or the classroom. If, on the other hand, adults provide *contingent praise*, i.e., positive comments/affirmations in response to *specific* desirable behaviours (e.g., being well-mannered, sitting quietly, staying on task, and taking turns), then that behaviour has been positively reinforced, and will likely occur again.

Specific descendants of behaviour theory include time out on the spot (TOOTS), applied behaviour analysis (ABA) (see Chapter 4), a contemporary version of "behaviour modification", and cognitive behaviour therapy (CBT) discussed below. TOOTS acts as an effective circuit-breaker in response to an undesirable behaviour, and can involve physical removal of the child to a safe and observable location that is not intrinsically rewarding in some way (think "naughty corner"), or it can simply involve the removal of social attention, as occurs when eye-contact, smiling, and other forms of engagement are temporarily withdrawn.

Behavioural interventions to manage infant sleep

Anyone who has experienced parenthood knows the stock-standard questions to expect, along with the endless flow of unsolicited and free advice (typically worth exactly what you paid for it). Those stock-standard questions begin with the baby's gender and weight, and rapidly segue to sleep. If you think the Olympic Games are tough, try psyching up for interrogation sessions at extended family gatherings, where folkloric "evidence" on infant crying and sleep flows like water, and pious tut-tutting, exchanged knowing glances, and smug self-satisfaction are just the beginning.

Sleep "problems" are common, being identified by adults caring for some

20–30% of infants and toddlers (Mindell et al., 2006), and may be even more common and/or persistent in children with developmental disorders such as ASD (Richdale & Schreck, 2009) and ID (Richdale, Francis, Gavidia-Payne, & Cotton 2000). So sleep is an area of early challenge in many families. In part, this problem is of our own making in industrialized nations, where value judgements about "good" babies (who sleep through or for longish stretches) and "difficult babies" (who wake frequently at night) abound. How inconsistent it is that the same infant behaviour that attracts sweet-voiced comfort and reassurance by day, can result in isolation and abandonment, and sleepy growls from the big bed, at night. How perplexing it would be for the infants themselves, if they had any sense of day and night, which of course they do not, until sometime around the middle of the first year.

Sleeping has unique status among developmental milestones. Do new parents workshop ways to get their typically-developing infants to roll over? To sit unassisted? To hold a rattle? Of course not. Parents know that babies progress at different rates in different areas of development. Yet this sensible logic seems not to apply to sleeping. There is no evidence that babies "should" sleep through the night by magical Week-X of life. This is a milestone like any other, occurring with enormous variability.

Because humans are a contact species, close mother-to-infant proximity is imperative, allowing easily accessed comfort and suckling via breast or bottle. Attachment theory was developed by British psychiatrist John Bowlby (b. 1907 d. 1990) in the second half of the 20th century, and has been extensively studied and elaborated, retaining a strong, respected place in contemporary developmental mental health theory and practice (see Cohen, 2001). The essence of attachment theory is that infants are innately driven to maintain closeness to their primary caregiver. Experiences from 0–2 of being responded to in warm, reliable, and timely ways by caregivers constitute the basis of the child's internal working model of how relationships work. Secure early attachment is a building block of resilience and of future self-soothing behaviour; hence parental responses that foster secure attachment *promote*, rather than threaten, these important later developments.

There are many things an infant cannot do: ride a bike, resolve a quadratic equation, and self-soothe. Self-soothing is as complex and sophisticated as the first two. Somehow, many parents and hovering family elders allow themselves to be blind to this, setting the scene for struggle, frustration, and a sense of failure. Still under-developed at birth, the human brain cannot support high-level processes like emotional self-regulation, so infants are not ready for the massive task of self-soothing and the experience of being abandoned to cry creates enormous physiological stress and emotional distress. Measurement of blood levels of the stress hormone cortisol has been used to gauge infants' physiological stress in response to "sleep training" approaches like controlled crying and cry it out. While babies may reduce their crying over a few days, their cortisol levels can stay high, indicating that they may still feel stress even though their crying has reduced (see Blunden, Thompson, & Dawson, 2011). This means, sadly, that a quiet baby is not necessarily a calm baby. Professor Helen Ball, of Durham University explains:

> *"It's not part of a baby's evolved biology or behavioural repertoire to be sleep trained anyway, therefore it's completely normal for a baby to resist such a process — however gradually it's done. The fact that it's possible to sleep train babies doesn't mean it is an appropriate thing to do. We have no idea of the consequences."*
> www.bellybelly.com.au/baby-sleep/cry-it-out

This is a controversial and often emotive topic, with infant mental health experts arguing against behavioural management of sleeping difficulties because of their potential for long-term harm to emotional development, most particularly, early secure attachment (e.g., Blunden et al., 2011). Other child health researchers, (e.g., Price, Wake, Ukoumunne, & Hiscock, 2012) present evidence of no demonstrable emotional or behavioural harms in 5-year-olds whose sleep difficulties in infancy were managed via a "behavioural sleep intervention". It is significant (and obvious) that "remediation" of infant sleep and crying difficulties has important implications for parental wellbeing (Hiscock, Bayer, Hampton, Ukoumunne, & Wake 2008). What remains unclear, however, is the extent to which parent distress arises from their perception that their baby "should" be sleeping longer and waking less. We do not doubt the scientific rigour of the randomized controlled studies like the one cited above, but note the possibility that such approaches are unsuitable for some subgroups of children, and that children with special needs may be in such subgroups. We also note that a recent systematic review of behavioural approaches to infants' crying (Douglas & Hill, 2013) concluded that "An evidence-based approach to sleep problems in the first 6 months avoids behavioral interventions, including extinction and graduated extinction" (p. 505).

On balance, we concur with the Australian Association for Infant Mental Health (AAIMH), which states: "Controlled crying is not appropriate for use before the baby has a real understanding of the meaning of the parent's words; the infant or toddler needs to know that the parent will return and needs to feel safe when the parent is absent" (AAIMH, 2013). We recommend that parents of all children, typically developing or not (and the latter is not always evident in infancy) establish realistic expectations of what infants can and cannot do with respect to sleeping and self-soothing, particularly in the first year of life. We also recommend against the use of non-evidence-based approaches to infant sleep such as cranial osteopathy, aka craniosacral therapy – the manipulation of an infant's skull bones and/or spine in order to "correct" so-called misalignment associated with the birth process. Here, we look no further than the words of Emeritus Professor Edzard Ernst: "wild assumptions, flimsy science and wrong conclusions" (www.edzardernst.com).

Some parents deal with daytime sleep difficulties by using baby-carriers that provide soothing proximity and physical contact, allowing the parent to complete at least some routine tasks. Although long discouraged (and often actively disapproved) in western societies, co-sleeping can happen safely, reducing the burden of night-waking, if not its frequency (Bartick & Smith, 2014). Important caveats are that co-sleeping should not occur on sofas or in vehicles, and risks are reduced through breast-feeding, avoidance of smoking, putting babies down to sleep on their backs, and ensuring that where they sleep is not over-heated (Bartick & Smith, 2014; Blunden et al., 2011). Establishing regular bedtime routines can also help to some extent (Mindell, Telofski, Wiegand, & Kurtz, 2009). Sleep deprivation is no fun, but it is especially punishing when it is accompanied by a pervasive, guilty sense of failure as a parent. Sleeping through is a milestone like any other, and children will get there when they are good and ready.

Smacking (slapping)

On the sunniest of days and in the best of circumstances, parenting is an inherently challenging and unpredictable task. Parents cannot (nor should they) devote 100% of their time and energy to their children. There are household jobs to be done, schedules to adhere to, and myriads of competing demands such as jobs, eldercare, health, (physical and mental), study and financial stressors (and the outside possibility of some personally focused down-time!). It is little wonder, then, that the sometimes uncooperative, recalcitrant, rude, destructive and disrespectful behaviour of children pushes parents' coping skills to the point of frustration overload and they find themselves mid-smack. What's "wrong" with that?

While smacking opens an immediate release valve for parents' frustrations, it does so by allowing the parent to exploit their superior size and strength over the child. A smack will generally stop the problematic behaviour, but it does not necessarily teach the child better self-control and internal reasoning processes for future consideration of what is "right" and what is "wrong". Rather than "teaching a child a good lesson", evidence indicates that children who are regularly smacked (particularly when this is associated with hostile parenting) are at greater risk of developing oppositional and aggressive behaviour (Gershoff & Bitensky, 2007). A curiosity associated with this aspect of parenting is that "smack" is a euphemism for what in other circumstances would be called assault. A parent who hits their troublesome 2-year-old in the name of discipline would, if they repeated this act against a troublesome adult, risk criminal offence charges. Most parents who smack do so (a) acknowledging that they themselves were smacked as children (the "*it didn't do me any harm*" argument), (b) believing that smacking is a reasonable and logical way of responding to undesirable behaviour, and/or (c) perceiving that corporal punishment and discipline are one and the same. Yet there is no clear line between what one parent calls "reasonable discipline" and what another (or indeed the law) might call abuse. Sweden led the world in banning corporal punishment of children by their parents in 1979, and a further 36 countries have followed. Interestingly, only one of these (New Zealand) is primarily English-speaking. In Australia, for example, controversy surrounds the extension of corporal punishment bans that currently exist in most schools, childcare centres, and youth detention facilities, to NT government schools, SA and QLD private schools, and to the home. If you doubt that this is an issue heavily steeped in politics and culture, consider that at the time of writing, there are 19 US states that still permit corporal punishment in schools (http://ocrdata.ed.gov).

It is not our mission in *Making Sense of Interventions for Children's Developmental Disorders* to stigmatize certain practices or the parents who employ them. Rather, we seek to present reasoned arguments based on empirical evidence to guide families, particularly those who are raising children with developmental disorders. Jones et al. (2012) reported on a systematic review and meta-analysis concerning children with developmental disabilities, identifying that they face an elevated risk of experiencing all forms of maltreatment – i.e., physical and emotional neglect, violence (including sexual assault), and emotional abuse. The reasons for this are multifactorial, ranging from inadequate understanding on the part of carers (whether families, foster-parents, or residential care workers) about the basis of behavioural problems in developmental disability, social stigma, and inadequate family support and respite services (see Snow, 2009 for further elaboration). And the good news? There is ample evidence that healthy, well-adjusted, self-regulating children can be raised without recourse to physical punishment. Some strategies to achieve this are listed on pages 128–131. Raising a child who has a developmental disorder is fundamentally more psychologically challenging for parents than raising TD children, hence the suggestions made in this chapter will inevitably yield mixed results. Nevertheless, we can confidently state that there are *no reputable sources* that advocate the use of corporal punishment to promote cooperation and/or reduce undesirable behaviours in children with developmental disorders. On the other hand, it is sometimes advocated that restraint in various forms must be employed, and that requires separate consideration.

Restraint (physical and/or chemical)

The United Nations Declaration of the Rights of Disabled Persons (UNDRDP; United Nations Human Rights, Office of the High Commissioner, 1975) has been ratified by some 190 member states and so guides disability policy and law in western nations such as the UK (see www.disabilityrightsuk.org), Australia (www.humanrights.gov.au), Canada (www.ccdonline.ca), New Zealand (www.hrc.co.nz), and the USA (http://usicd.org/index.cfm/crpd), though it must be noted that some states have ratified the convention with reservations, which can be viewed on the UN Treaty Collection site (https://treaties.un.org). Several articles in this convention are intended to guide equitable, respectful and minimally restrictive approaches to the provision of services (whether medical, educational, vocational, and/or independent living). The behaviour of children and adolescents with developmental disabilities can be such that their own or others' safety is threatened, and/or they are unable to participate in a range of community settings because their behaviour is considered socially inappropriate (e.g., undressing, urinating or masturbating publicly). In such cases, physical or chemical restraint, may be considered. Such restraint might include restrictive clothing (e.g., garments fastened at the back that are difficult to remove unassisted), psychotropic medication to reduce agitated behaviour, and, as has recently been (controversially) reported via the media in some Victorian schools (e.g., Cook, 2015), cages to physically contain students whose classroom behaviour is difficult to manage. While we acknowledge that there are circumstances where the least restrictive environment is, in fact, quite restrictive, we caution that restraint should only be employed under the supervision of appropriately qualified specialists (e.g., psychiatrists, clinical and/or educational and developmental psychologists), and should emanate from careful behavioural analysis to identify potential antecedent events (internal, social, or environmental triggers). Sometimes these can be successfully addressed, minimizing or reducing recourse to more restrictive approaches that do not address underlying causes, but merely act as "Band-Aids", with potential adverse side-effects. We also support interventions that better equip teachers, health, and residential care workers with behaviour-management knowledge and skills. We have yet to meet a member of such groups who describes this aspect of their pre-service training as adequate.

School suspensions and exclusions

Schools have always been places where rules are rules and consequences exist for those who flout them: so don't slouch, and tuck your shirt in. Sometimes, a student's behaviour in school is considered so disruptive and/or harmful to the wellbeing of fellow students or staff that their removal is deemed necessary, so they are suspended, or expelled. In their cross-national study of the use of suspensions and expulsions in the USA and Australia, Hemphill, Toumbourou, Herrenkohl, McMorris and Catalano (2006) reported that such practices may backfire, *increasing* the likelihood of antisocial behaviour, particularly in boys who are academic under-achievers and who hang out with antisocial peers. This finding was corroborated in a study of 100 youth offenders completing custodial sentences in Australia, in which 87 participants had experienced suspensions and/or exclusions from school (Snow, Woodward, Mathis, & Powell, 2015). The fact that *all* of these young people were ultimately sentenced to custodial youth detention-centre terms suggests that their risk trajectories were not favourably altered by these sanctions. Judicious use of suspensions in particular may be helpful in circumstances where there are more protective factors than risk factors in a child's life. Parents can be "protective factors" when they are emotionally attuned and responsive to their child's needs, and willing and able to work in concert with their school to reinforce shared values and goals with respect to behavioural expectations. School administrators have a challenging task in ensuring that schools are safe work places and learning environments for all. In our view, rather than simple recourse to suspensions and exclusions, it would be preferable to see school staff better equipped and professionally supported to analyze and respond to problematic behaviour in ways that promote continued participation by vulnerable students. Suspensions can constitute a perverse reward for students who dislike school, and expulsion basically makes the student someone else's problem until such time as he or she is the whole community's problem by virtue of contact with the criminal justice system, mental health agencies, and/or public housing services.

Boot camp for adolescents

Every so often, an intervention comes along that looks (at least to readers and viewers of sensationalist media and the writers who produce their copy) like a quick-fix for a complex problem, while simultaneously fuelling armchair social commentators' view that all that is needed is some old-fashioned common sense and a swift kick up the backside. Boot camp for misbehaving adolescents is right up there in this category. While the term "boot camp" does not have one narrowly-defined and commonly accepted meaning, it is generally taken to refer to stints of short-term, residential, intensive and compulsory discipline regimens. Teenage boot camps, run along military lines, emerged in the USA in the 1980s in an effort to force disruptive teenagers to behave in ways that are judged as acceptable by adults. Strictly imposed schedules, demanding physical activities, and harsh, confrontational punishment and humiliation for non-compliance are all hallmarks of this approach. Like fashion, boot camps come and go as policy approaches. One was trialled and abandoned in 2015 in Queensland, Australia when an independent review failed to support its continuation (Queensland Government, 2015).

Boot camps do not address the underlying causes of disruptive behaviour (which in the case of young people in contact with the law can often be traced to psychological trauma associated with long periods of parental neglect and/or abuse), instead adopting a one-size-fits-all recipe-book approach. In 2005, Wilson, MacKenzie and Mitchell conducted a systematic review of studies examining the effectiveness of military-style boot camps, concluding that they are not effective in reducing offending, and actually have similarly low success rates to incarceration. We do not advocate the use of this approach, given its weak theoretical rationale and evidence base. Bergin (2013) further critiques its limitations, and poor cost-effectiveness.

Sensory Integration Therapy

Some interventions, like Sensory Integration Therapy (SIT), for children with developmental disorders become popular with mainstream practitioners before contemporary principles of evidence-based practice are established, occupying comfortable and stoutly evidence-proof niches in some clinicians' armouries. SIT was developed in California in the 1960s and 1970s by A. Jean Ayres, becoming a revered go-to therapy among many OTs worldwide. Dr Ayres (b.1920 d. 1988) argued that children with certain developmental disorders (e.g., cerebral palsy, specific learning disability, and autism) had difficulty synthesizing incoming sensory information (e.g., via the organs of vision, olfaction, hearing, touch and proprioception) at a cortical level. This poor synthesis (or "integration") caused learning and/or behaviour difficulties, which she termed sensory integrative dysfunction – symptoms of which Dr Ayres said she had in childhood – for which the treatment is (da-da!): Sensory Integration Therapy (SIT: Ayres & Robbins, 2005[2]). There is a critical distinction between (a) what Dr Ayres rightly observed regarding the sensory sensitivities and preferences of children with ASD, and those with some forms of ID, and (b) appropriate ways of responding to them therapeutically. Sensory-based therapies delivered by OTs use a variety of standard-issue equipment, such as balls, weighted vests, and swings, while more entrepreneurial practitioners offer 21st-century props with fun names like "Miracle Belts", "Disc'o sit", "Movin'sit", "Steamroller" and "Steamroller Deluxe", "Starfish Cushions", "Rainbow Parachutes" and "Air Pressure Squease Vest - like a hug" (promoted at www.calmingkids.com.au). They may be fun for some children to experience, in which case they should be employed for their enjoyment as reinforcers, but not necessarily with an expectation of therapeutic gains or transfer of new skills to other contexts. Further, some children may find these activities and approaches aversive, so at a minimum, we recommend an assessment by an OT who is a specialist in the area of developmental disorders.

The American Academy of Pediatrics (2012) does not recommend the use of diagnostic labels such as "sensory integration (or processing) disorder", advising instead that signs and symptoms of sensory deficits should be subsumed and managed within a broader, mainstream diagnosis such as ASD. We think it is important that sensory difficulties be recognized, assessed, and carefully managed on a case-by-case basis after appropriate behavioural analysis, noting that systematic reviews (e.g., Barton, Reichow, Schnitz, Smith, & Sherlock, 2015; Lang et al., 2012) failed to establish robust evidence for the efficacy of SIT for children with ASD. This is all the more noteworthy for the enormous research effort into both "sensory integration disorder" and SIT over fifty years. Studies are available that appear to show benefits of some forms of SIT

---

2 Dr Ayres died in 1988, and her co-workers continue to release revised editions of this text.

for some samples, but, or should we say *big* but, study designs are typically weak and suffer from common methodological flaws such as lack of follow-up post-intervention. SIT has a modicum of face validity, probably yields some benefits for some children, has professional buy-in from *some* OTs, and historical standing in certain circles that is difficult to shift. We agree in part with the bottom-line articulated by online health and wellness writer, Erica Patino that:

> *"There's no harm in having your child try sensory integration therapy. But be aware that there may be more effective ways to help your child with sensory issues."*

Our caveat is that all non- (or soft-) evidence-based interventions carry with them an opportunity cost, that is, the lost time that can never be regained but that could have been spent in ways that carry a better probability of producing meaningful gains.

Bizarre bazaar

So far, we have dealt with interventions that have had a foothold in mainstream practice for decades, some of which look a little jaded now in the light of progress and scientific scrutiny. Before discussing practices for which we think the evidence base is at least somewhat established, we will detour along the more bizarre alleyways of the behaviour bazaar. Some of the approaches that follow will not be given unwarranted coverage here because of their loopy-index, but we do want to convey a sense of the silliness that abounds. Complementary and Alternative Medicine (CAM) approaches, such as chiropractic, homeopathy, kinesiology, naturopathy, neurolinguistic programming (NLP) and cranial osteopathy, are easily accessible, make grandiose and often attractively-packaged claims, but (our editor probably will not permit another *big but*) as they have *no plausible scientific arguments* (nor evidence) they have no role in any child's treatment regimen. CAM practitioners' testimonials and advertorials do not constitute an evidence-base, and their legitimacy cannot be established anyway. Be smart, and keep walking.

Living in a 24/7 socially networked world may have advantages, but ready access to a global audience and market for self-styled experts is not one of them (unless you are one, and are making money out of it). Take, for example, Josh Shipp, a US 30-something former "foster kid" (his term) turned "the teen whisperer" (more Shippspeak) whose Twitter bio (based on his study sample size of 1 adolescent at-risk) reads, "Every kid is ONE caring adult away from being a success story". How admirable that Mr Shipp has triumphed over adversity, but how disquieting that he finesses and spreads a message to parents and teens, struggling with *any* behavioural issues, that all that is lacking is a caring adult. Mr Shipp's trump card is that he has "appeared" on Good Morning America, Oprah, 20/20, MTV, and CNN, but we are unamused. While personal experience is powerful, achieving adulthood via the school of hard knocks is an insufficient basis for declaring expertise on matters as vital and as complex as emotional and behavioural adjustment in adolescence. Charisma is no substitute for evidence; which brings us to daytime TV, and Dr Phil (see also pages 267–268). With promos like "*I Sleep With A Gun Because I Am Terrified My 19-Year-Old Son Will Kill Me*" and "*My Daughter Is A Lazy, Lying Mooch Who Neglects Her Kids*", what could possibly go wrong? As you know, and we *know* you know, platforms that function to entertain and profit from people's misery and shame will not light the way to intervening effectively and humanely for young people with emotional and behavioural difficulties. Quizzes, arbitrary "dos and don'ts" lists, shocking statistics, and "warning signs" are all, well…warning signs. Watch for entertainment, and a sense of schadenfreude if you must, but that is all.

Approaches supported by least some good evidence

There is a truism that parenting is simultaneously the most important and challenging job on Earth, and the one for which people feel least prepared. Parenting style is influenced by many factors, including culture, personality (parent and child), and parents' experiences of how they themselves were reared. To be clear: there is no one "right" child-rearing "method". Instead, there are parenting approaches (plural) and behaviours (plural) that increase the probability of raising a child who displays generally cooperative, self-regulated behaviour by late childhood. They apply irrespective of the presence of developmental disability, and are summarized below.

- Be emotionally available to your child at his or her developmental level.

- Avoid harsh, coercive, and/or erratic parenting responses. By the same token, avoid being overly permissive, as children need boundaries and limits. They also need parents who are *parents*, not "friends" or "mates".

- Comment favourably on desirable behaviours your child displays, avoiding unwarranted praise that is not contingent on an actual behaviour.
- Circumvent power-struggles that do not really matter (aka "pick your battles").
- Reflect on your parenting skills and style; discuss these with trusted friends and family members and consult written material from reliable sources.
- Without underestimating your child, have realistic expectations of what he or she can achieve cognitively, linguistically, socially, and behaviourally at a given age.
- Accept that sharing does not come naturally to toddlers and preschoolers, and continues to be challenging into the early primary-school years. Sharing needs to be modelled and taught, and children need support to deal with the difficult emotions this important skill can arouse.
- Flag transitions and expectations. If you want your child to get ready to come to the meal table, make this known 5–10 minutes in advance, so that an enjoyable activity is not sharply terminated, causing inevitable distress and potential conflict.
- Gain your child's attention before making a request. Children's attentional and memory skills are under construction, so they can easily agree to do something without fully processing what is required, or the expected timeframe.
- Know that young children's distractibility can be an asset to parents when things are getting out of hand. Rather than engaging in a power-struggle, direct your child's attention elsewhere to head-off a tantrum. It works sometimes.
- Give your child choices, where possible, so they can make decisions and exert some control, e.g., over whether they have a bath before or after dinner.
- Remember that behaviour can be a window on emotions. Ask yourself what might be "driving" a particular response. Not all behaviour is about seeking attention; sometimes it reflects avoidance or sensory self-stimulation.

- Have clear expectations, but do not impose unrelenting high standards across all developmental domains.
- Expect ups-and-downs and plateaus in children's development and remember that different children acquire knowledge and skills at different rates.
- Apply consequences that are proportional to the misdemeanour, without delaying them (or the child may miss the connection between behaviour and outcome).
- Acknowledge your, and your child's progress, even if it is slow and incremental.
- Allow cooling-down time after an outburst of challenging behaviour has been managed. This allows both you and your child to "re-set" emotionally before trying to discuss what happened.
- Help your child to learn words for emotions. This helps to create order out of internal and external chaos.
- Bear in mind that younger children and children with language difficulties cannot give good verbal accounts of their actions or the feelings underlying them. Behaviour is communication.
- Develop family routines around getting ready for the day, mealtimes, and bedtime. These will need to vary sometimes, but predictability helps everyone know what comes next and what is expected of them.
- Turn off screens and electronic devices at mealtimes. Get together for the evening meal so that family conversation and engagement is fostered. Build up positive interactions, for emotional capital to draw on in more difficult times.
- Guard against shouting at or ridiculing your child, and name-calling, as they build emotional barriers between you making communication generally more difficult.
- Take it as a "given" that tantrums are developmentally normal for young children and may persist in children with developmental difficulties. Children's tantrums generally mean they are emotionally and cognitively overwhelmed and for the moment are unable to verbalize/manage their wants or feelings in a better way.

- Maintain calm, if you can, when facing emotional outbursts such as tantrums. Losing *your* cool will surely escalate emotions, turning a spot-fire into a raging bush-fire.
- Resist the urge to smack. Perfectly good citizens can be raised without corporal punishment.
- Work with school staff when they impose reasonable consequences for unacceptable behaviour.
- Retain your sense of humour.
- Remind yourself that you are the grown-up. This means that whether or not you intend to, you are modelling emotions and behaviour to your children every day. Children are great imitators, so it is not fair to punish them for reproducing emotional responses and behaviours they observe in their parents or other adults.
- Model behaviour you would like to see and hear. If you don't want bad language, avoid calling your child "a little @$%!" or your fellow motorist "a stupid #@!%".
- When things go pear-shaped and you swear, argue with your partner, or behave in other ways that later cause you shame and embarrassment, come clean with your child. Modelling self-reflection and the taking of responsibility will engender respect, affirming for your child that lapses are not fatal errors and can be learning opportunities.
- Give yourself (and your partner, if you have one) regular pats on the back. This is hard work.

Sometimes parents need extra support with childrearing, and may consider enrolling in a parenting programme. Some parenting programmes focus on children's *behavioural regulation*, and others emphasize *emotional attunement* between parents and their children. These emphases are neither separate nor mutually exclusive, and there are evidence-based approaches for both. We suggest, however, consultation with a psychologist or other counsellor to determine which focus best suits an individual case. We cannot review the many parenting programmes here, but focus on two that come from slightly different theoretical angles, and that are the subject of considerable published research: Triple-P and Tuning into Kids.

The Triple P – Positive Parenting Program® (Triple-P)

Triple-P is an example of a parenting programme that has a predominantly behavioural focus and is widely considered to be evidence-based. It was developed in Australia by Dr Matt Sanders, a professor of Clinical Psychology at the University of Queensland. According to its website, Triple-P (or PPP) is "…a parenting and family support system designed to prevent—as well as treat—behavioural and emotional problems in children and teenagers" (see www.triplep.net (nd)). Triple-P targets families that are in some way vulnerable, e.g., because of parental mental health problems, or the presence of developmental disability in a child. Ideally, it aims to *prevent* problems in the family, school and community but is often sought by families in distress because of behaviour management difficulties that have already arisen. Triple-P strongly emphasizes parents' *self-efficacy*, that is, their belief and confidence that they can be effective and successful as parents. It operates across five key developmental levels until age 12, with specialized programmes for parents of adolescents (Teen Triple-P), parents of children with disabilities (Stepping Stones), parents navigating separation or divorce (Family Transitions), indigenous parents (Indigenous), and parents of children who are overweight (Lifestyle).

Through Triple-P, parents learn to self-assess their parenting, "own" the problem, set goals, determine a plan of action, and then implement and evaluate it. Triple-P is adaptable to the relevant social and cultural contexts of families, and has been adjusted for use in over 20 countries. Parents learn skills around boundary-setting, creating positive and safe learning environments, giving instructions/making requests in ways that promote cooperation and success, and considering the underlying function of a child's behaviour (Sanders, Turner, & Markie-Dadds, 2002). Triple-P operates across five levels (universal, selected, primary care, standard, and enhanced), depending on the intervention intensity and focus required. Treatment intensity and duration are therefore variable, but standard Triple-P normally requires about 10 hours over 8–10 sessions (Sanders, Mazzucchelli, & Studman, 2004).

As the subject of exhaustive peer-reviewed research, Triple-P enjoys enormous popularity and respectability across academic, government, and media platforms. In Australia, it has received millions of taxpayer dollars to support broad-based community roll-outs. It may even be that Triple-P is the topic of more peer-reviewed literature than any other intervention described in this chapter, so there is no shortage of studies on which to weigh up effectiveness. That said, there is a conspicuous dearth of Triple-P studies conducted independently, by impartial researchers. For example, Scottish researchers did a systematic review and meta-analysis of 33 studies evaluating outcomes of Triple-P programmes, finding that in 32/33, the authors had conflicts of interest (Wilson et al., 2012). Other criticisms of Triple-P research (see Coyne & Kwakkenbos, 2013) include limited follow-up periods (to monitor retention of gains) and the lack of no-treatment control groups (as opposed to using wait-list controls). This means that the general effects of attention and support that would be present in *any* parenting programme (to wit, something is usually better than nothing) are not adequately controlled for. Coyne and Kwakkenbos also highlight over-reliance on mothers' reports of progress (with an absence of views sought from fathers), selective reporting of outcome measures, and a general failure of pre-registration[3] of research trials. Overall, Wilson et al. reported a "lack of convincing evidence" (p. 13) concerning the effectiveness of Triple-P at a population[4] level, though their analysis suggested it may have a place for families of children with more severe problems. Triple-P's theoretical rationale has merit, but these reviews indicate that caution should be exercised by parents, teachers, and clinicians regarding expectations of long-term gains. Parents and their children may derive benefits from Triple-P, but its effectiveness may not be as dramatic and broad-based as its website enthusiastically proclaims. It is important that parents know this, so that they (a) have realistic expectations of what participation in the programme might achieve, and (b) do not blame themselves or their child if gains do not mirror the dramatic progress portrayed in its advertising.

With its focus on parents of children with disabilities, Triple-P's Stepping Stones (Sanders et al., 2004) is well within our remit. Its rationale lies in the more frequent co-occurrence of behavioural and emotional difficulties in children with developmental disorders, and the resulting psychological burden for parents and siblings. Sanders et al. correctly note that this co-morbidity generates a double disadvantage for children: it is difficult for them to understand and learn what is required of them, simultaneously resulting in exclusion from community settings where appropriate behaviour is role-modelled by others (most particularly, schools). Irritable and fractious adult responses to

---

3 Pre-registration of a clinical trial offers some protection against the non-reporting of results that are either not significant or go against the hoped-for outcome. When a trial is pre-registered, the researchers are committing to seek publication in a peer-reviewed journal, irrespective of the findings. This means that, over time, the published literature should contain a more balanced view of the state of play concerning a particular intervention and its evidence-base.

4 Population-level interventions shift the distribution of health risks through policies and practices that influence underlying social, environmental, and economic inequalities (Hawe & Potvin 2009).

challenging behaviour are understandable, but can serve to exacerbate, rather than ease, difficult interactions. Like Triple-P, Stepping Stones is based in social learning and behaviour theory, and emphasizes the two-way influence that parents and children exert on each other's responses. According to Sanders et al. (2004), Stepping Stones aims to strengthen parents' skills in managing common behaviour problems associated with developmental disabilities, while reducing their use of harsh and punitive discipline. It further seeks to develop parents' personal coping skills (to reduce parental stress), while enhancing their abilities to discuss parenting issues and to develop their own problem-solving strategies. Focusing on children's communication skills is central to Stepping Stones, meaning that SLP/SLT involvement in its design and implementation will be necessary for many children.

There is some promising evidence concerning the effectiveness of Stepping Stones for improving parenting efficacy and reducing the stress some families experience as a consequence of a child's developmental disability. For example, Whittingham, Sofronoff, Sheffield and Sanders (2009) described a small RCT in which parent-report of behavioural difficulties in (predominantly) verbal children with ASD improved as a group, though not in all cases. In fact, some of the significant changes were evident in only one-third of the group. As the treatment group comprised only 29 families, this equates to improvements on important measures for only ten families. Where gains happened, some were maintained six months after the programme ended, but again, it is notable that these researchers used a wait-list control group rather than comparing Stepping Stones with another intervention. We can safely assume that "something is better than nothing", so the lack of a comparison with another intervention makes it difficult to assess the extent to which a *general* benefit of an intensive parent-support and behaviour-oriented programme was observed, as opposed to a benefit associated with Stepping Stones *specifically*. In a subsequent study, Sofronoff, Jahnel and Sanders (2011) examined the impact of delivering the key components of Stepping Stones in two 90-minute seminars. Improvements were reported, and were maintained at a three-month follow-up, but their sample-size was again small and undoubtedly biased towards women in stable marital relationships, where mental health issues did not predominate. As one of the arresting features of developmental disability is its heterogeneity, studies with larger, more representative samples are needed in order to determine the impact of approaches such as Stepping Stones, whether delivered directly or via seminars.

Tuning into Kids (TIK)

TIK also originated in Australia, from the work of Dr Sophie Havighurst and her colleagues at the University of Melbourne and the Royal Children's Hospital. TIK arose in part from concerns that it may be inappropriate to emphasize behavioural management of children when significant emotional factors and family stressors impede parents' ability to bond with their child. Hence, where Triple-P has a significant focus on parents' self-efficacy for and goal-setting around parenting at a *behavioural level*, TIK emphasizes parents' *emotional attunement* with and *responsiveness* to their children. Like Triple-P, TIK is delivered across 8 sessions, employing role-plays, video-based materials and psycho-education. It draws on the evidence-based emotion coaching work of American relationship therapists John and Julie Gottman (www.gottman.com). The five basic elements of emotion coaching are summarized by their website staff writer Ellie Lisitsa (2012), and are listed below.

1. *Empathy*: "When children show their parents vulnerabilities, they want their parents to be their allies".

2. *Seeing your child's expressions of emotion as opportunities for teaching and intimacy*: "Rather than seeing negative expressions of emotion as a problem that needs to be 'dealt with' or 'fixed,' or even as the result of some kind of parental incompetence, the realization that such moments can be used to teach your child may come as a huge relief".

3. *Treating a child's feelings with empathetic listening and validation*: "Rather than asking a child how they feel, observe them—their facial expressions, body language, gestures, and the tone of their voice. If your toddler is crying, she probably doesn't know why. Asking her won't help".

4. *Helping your child to find words for their emotions*: "Providing words [to describe the problem] can help children transform an amorphous, scary, uncomfortable feeling into something definable, something that has boundaries and is a normal part of life… [something that] everybody has and everybody can handle".

5. *Set limits while helping your child to problem solve*: Here, the Gottmans refer to the importance of parental limit-setting and rule-making, while giving children opportunities to make choices and do some things for themselves.

According to its website (www.tuningintokids.org.au), TIK has a specific focus on helping parents to become aware of and regulate their own emotions, as a basis for gaining improved awareness and understanding of their child's emotions and subsequent behaviour. Emulating the Gottman emotion coaching principles outlined above, TIK emphasizes assisting children to identify, label and understand their emotions, and strengthen their problem-solving capacities when faced with emotionally challenging experiences. This reflects the view that, "Parental attempts to change children's behavior without responding to underlying emotions might miss addressing the meaning or function which that behavior holds" (Havighurst et al., 2013, p. 249). Like Triple-P, TIK (and to a lesser extent its derivatives, Tuning into Teens and Tuning into Tots) has been subjected to peer-reviewed research since its development a decade ago, and there are indications that it produces clinically significant gains for parents and children. We do note, however, that some of the same criticisms directed at Triple-P apply to TIK also, e.g., reliance on waiting-list controls, relatively small samples, a tendency to exclude children with developmental disorders that might be more resistant to intervention, and a preponderance of mothers as the participants/informants. It is also true that (like Triple-P) the bulk of research on TIK has been conducted by investigators involved in its development. Interestingly, though, a study by TIK investigators (Duncombe et al., 2014) compared Triple-P and TIK and a waiting-list control-group for children in the first four years of school who, on the basis of assessment on validated measures, were at-risk for behaviour disturbances. Duncombe et al. reported that Triple-P and TIK were both superior to the waiting-list control condition and were *equally effective* at producing meaningful gains that were detected by teacher-observers who were blind to (random) group allocation. These workers concluded therefore that "The finding that both TIK and PPP are effective in an early intervention setting can provide greater choice and flexibility for practitioners involved in helping children with emerging conduct disorder" (p. 13).

Parenting programmes in summary

According to a review of 17 controlled trials of nine intervention approaches, "Parenting program components that are consistently associated with the largest effects include increasing positive parent–child interactions and communication skills, teaching parents to use time out and consistent discipline strategies, and providing parents opportunities to practice new skills with their children in training sessions" (Petrenko, 2013, p. 655). Parents of children with developmental disorders should all, therefore, have access to evidence-based parenting interventions that contain *psychoeducation* components (information that explains the underlying basis of behaviour and its effects on everyday functioning and relationships), *skills* components to increase the effectiveness of communication and discipline approaches, and *self-care* components to reduce the effects of cumulative stress on parents' mental health and wider family functioning. There is also some consensus that *multisystemic* interventions (targeting parents, teachers and the child) are superior to those with a single target (e.g., just the home, or just at school), as children need to experience consistency across the settings in which they interact every day.

The benefits of these interventions will vary between approaches and between families; however, there is sufficient evidence from generally well-conducted studies to indicate that, as a general rule, participating families should expect to achieve improved understanding of the basis of challenging behaviour, and skills that lead to observable gains in behaviour and overall emotional functioning. Parents and clinicians who are curious to understand the basis of and evidence for a particular parenting programme can consult the California Evidence-Based Clearinghouse for Child Welfare (www.cebc4cw.org), funded by the California Department of Social Services, which provides good guidance on selecting and critiquing available programmes.

Circle time and restorative conferencing

Modern classroom practices strongly emphasize the worth of strong self-esteem, behaving appropriately, sharing, being respectful and welcoming to others, and taking responsibility for wrong-doings by apologising and engaging in approaches aimed at restoring respect and equilibrium. Broadly, such practices are in the remit of two related approaches: circle time and restorative practice.

Circle time is often a component of a whole-school strategy for promoting positive behaviour, managing behavioural difficulties and helping children to discuss and resolve conflict or other distressing experiences that can occur during the school day. Circle time can be used to share everyday reflections, feelings, and experiences, or responses to specific occurrences of bullying, exclusion, physical or verbal aggression, interference with belongings or property, and other common behavioural violations in the classroom and school-yard. In its implementation, children sit in a circle, and a discussion is led by the teacher, who seeks to promote effective verbal communication (expression and comprehension) skills, eye-contact, turn-taking, and empathy. Lead-in phrases such as "I feel happy when…" or "I feel afraid when…" might be used to facilitate younger children's participation, and turn-taking can be taught by having the speaker hold a particular object that signals that it is their turn to talk. Circle time is undoubtedly preferable to confrontational, disciplinarian approaches that create "winners and losers", as it aspires to a level playing field where everyone can have a say, be heard and respected, and listen. Circle time is, however, highly verbal, and may be intensely challenging for children with developmental disorders, in the sense that its cognitive, linguistic, pragmatic, and behavioural demands are quite high (paying attention, sitting still, following and remembering what has been said, responding appropriately, and so on). In the hands of a skilled teacher, clinician, or classroom aide, however, circle time might provide the verbal and emotional "scaffolding" needed by vulnerable children in order to fully engage. Over twenty years ago, Housego and Burns (1994, p. 29) reflected on circle time and concluded that:

> *"If circle time is to be of real value to the children we teach, we need to be as rigorous in scrutinising our practice here as we are in other areas of the curriculum. We may need to give much more thought to the way it is conducted. We may even begin to question whether its aims are not more effectively carried out in other ways."*

Unfortunately, as subsequently outlined in a review by Lown (2000), circle time lacks a clear definition, theoretical rationale, and consistent procedures, so its evidence base is poor. Leach and Lewis (2013) have also cautioned that circle time can have the unintended consequence of making some children feel lonely, isolated, and bullied. It is pleasing to see the emergence of rigorous research of this widely used, but under-studied approach (e.g., Cefai, Ferrario, Cavioni, Carter, & Grech, 2014), but at the moment it is difficult for us to endorse a practice that probably varies widely from school to school in all aspects of its implementation.

As children progress into secondary school, they may be asked to participate in a restorative conference, if they are the victims or perpetrators of wrong-doings. Restorative conferences about a particular incident should be facilitated by a trained convener in order to maintain a focus on the wrong-doing and how it can be redressed by those present. Common questions posed in such conferences may include:

- What happened?
- What were you thinking at the time?
- What have you thought about since?
- What is the impact on other people?
- What do you think needs to be done to make this right?

When young people have a diagnosed and recognized developmental disorder, allowances can be made by all parties for their reduced comprehension skills, slow responses, and need for repetitions and extra time. Many students, however, do not have observable or diagnosed difficulties in these areas, and may struggle in the context of a restorative conference, particularly if this is high-stakes in terms of possible disciplinary consequences. Restorative conferences tax individuals' narrative language skills (while "telling their story"), and also require them to identify emotional states in others (e.g., sadness, confusion, embarrassment, anger), and respond appropriately (i.e., in ways the other party deems acceptable). We cautiously endorse the use of restorative conferencing, with the caveat that staff must be formally trained in its facilitation and, most particularly, they need to understand the often hidden communication disabilities experienced by children with developmental disorders. As noted above, such difficulties can sometimes manifest behaviourally, and can trigger unhelpful responses by adults (e.g., criticism, shaming, and exclusion). Further information about the use of restorative practices with special needs populations can be found in a text by Burnett and Thorsborne (2015). The need for careful preparation for the verbal demands of restorative conferences, particularly where these are part of a legal process, is outlined by Hayes and Snow (2013).

Early intensive behaviour interventions in autism

Contemporary thinking supports a sustained and largely successful push, by both clinicians and researchers, to enable identification of ASD at the earliest possible age, ideally before 2 years, so that intensive multidisciplinary early intervention can commence (Barbaro & Dissanayake, 2009). Typically, early identification begins when developmental concerns are raised (e.g., regarding socialisation or early talking), perhaps by a parent or grandparent, and then discussed with a health professional such as a family doctor or a maternal and child health nurse. As there is no laboratory test (e.g., based on a blood sample) that can definitively diagnose or exclude ASD, what should follow is a comprehensive multidisciplinary assessment, using structured interviews and observational protocols, such as the Autism Diagnostic Observation Schedule (ADOS; Lord et al., 2000), Autism Diagnostic Interview – Revised (ADI-R; Lord, Rutter, & Le Couteur, 1994) and the Diagnostic Interview for Social and Communication Disorders (DISCO; Leekam, 2013).

Autism assessment teams vary in their composition, but typically include a child psychologist or psychiatrist, a SLP/SLT, and an OT. In early intervention (EI) transdisciplinary intervention teams will comprise the child's family, and the professionals discussed in the previous chapter and shown in Figure 4.2. Early identification and EI are designed to go together, in order to minimize and ideally prevent behavioural, learning, and social adaptation symptomatology. The impetus for earlier identification also reflects the fact that, historically, by the time many children have been formally diagnosed with an ASD (3–5 years), the achievement gap between them and their peers is already quite wide, and they are about to commence school, where social and academic demands will increase dramatically. Additional benefits of early identification include the red flag created in the case of younger siblings, who face an elevated risk for diagnosis for ASD (Bradshaw, Steiner, Gengoux, & Koegel, 2015), and the opportunity for a detailed developmental assessment by a paediatrician to identify co-morbid medical conditions (e.g., epilepsy) that may require medical management.

The actual form of early intervention on offer can vary widely, ranging across highly structured approaches such as Applied Behaviour Analysis (ABA), SLP/SLT services, sensory integration therapy (pages 125–127), diet (see Chapter 10), and/or medication (see pages 37–38). The other dimension on which these approaches show wide variation is their evidence base, so extravagant claims and enthusiastic testimonials flag the usual cautions.

The US National Research Council (2001) recommends that:

> *"Based on a set of individualized, specialized objectives and plans that are systematically implemented, educational services should begin as soon as a child is suspected of having an autistic spectrum disorder"* (p. 220).

> *"Educational services should include a minimum of 25 hours a week, 12 months a year, in which the child is engaged in systematically planned, developmentally appropriate*

educational activity aimed toward identified objectives" (p. 220).

"Lack of objectively documentable progress over a 3-month period should be taken to indicate a need to increase intensity by lowering student/teacher ratios, increasing programming time, reformulating curricula, or providing additional training and consultation" (pp. 220–221).

The US National Research Council further recommends that early intervention has a focus on the following six domains and processes: functional spontaneous communication, social instruction, the teaching of peer-oriented play skills, cognitive development, problem behaviours, and functional academic skills. This document emphasizes the importance of detailed, well-documented team-based assessment, the articulation of clear goals, followed by delivery of therapeutic interventions that target specific skills/problem behaviours, and ongoing evaluation and documentation of progress.

According to recent reviews of early identification and intervention for children with ASD, features parents should look for include: a theoretical rationale that is based in developmental and behavioural principles, parent involvement, clear articulation of goals and strategies, and adequate intensity and duration of therapy (Bradshaw et al., 2015). Systematic reviews show that where these features exist, children can make significant gains in verbal and nonverbal communication, social engagement, and reductions in autism symptoms (Bradshaw et al., 2015; Reichow, 2012), however, it is widely agreed that more research is needed for the "essential ingredients" to be identified, and no early intervention approach has been acknowledged as universally suitable for all children with ASD. It has also been noted in review studies that as severity of ASD features increases, so too, treatment fidelity (accurate adherence) decreases, which is not surprising given the considerable demands such programmes place on parents' time, and physical and mental energy (and depending on funding processes, on their financial resources also). We agree with the Royal Australasian College of Physicians (RACP) that parents need an opportunity "…to raise and discuss the role of Complementary and Alternative Interventions" (RACP; Paediatrics and Child Health Division, 2008, p. 4); however, we take a stronger line and advocate that clinicians should counsel *against* approaches for which an evidence-base (or at the very least, a scientifically-plausible theoretical rationale) does not exist, in order to prevent squandering precious time and financial and emotional resources, none of which can be replenished. As noted in Chapter 10, there is a conflict of interest for some mainstream health professionals, such as pharmacists, in the promotion and sale of unscientific CAM products. We believe all children deserve better protection in this space.

We encourage all parents to seek out local toy libraries (www.itla-toylibraries.org), whether or not they have a child with a developmental disorder. These not-for-profit services are present in many communities, and promote optimal child development through play. Few families have the money (or space) to provide an endless supply of ever-changing toys for their children, so toy libraries are a wonderful community-based resource. Membership fees are modest, and the toys are selected for their educational value with respect to sensorimotor and language skills across a range of developmental levels, generally up to preschool age. Some toy libraries cater specifically to families with a child who has special needs, and can be valuable sources of both education and social support to parents.

"Talk" Therapies

Cognitive-Behaviour Therapy (CBT)

Several so-called "talk therapies" have undergone significant development and research-led refinement in recent decades. Here, we highlight just two approaches that have merit in assisting children with developmental difficulties, and their families, to deal with mental health problems such as anxiety and depression – sometimes best delivered in modified form to accommodate cognitive and communicative barriers. Such problems have significant implications for family members, who may also derive some benefit from knowledge and/or use of psychological therapies.

CBT is rooted in the teachings of the stoic philosopher, Epictetus, born in what is now modern-day Turkey around 55AD (Hofman, 2011). Surviving an early life of adversity and hardship, Epictetus articulated his fundamental principles for a "good life". The principles intimated that, while we can change very little of the world around us, we do have agency to change the way we *react* to people and events, and until we truly understand this, we cannot achieve inner tranquillity or outward effectiveness. He also taught that circumstances and events do not arise to meet our expectations or desires (otherwise expressed as "the rest of the world does not get up in the morning with a view to making us happy"), so it is pointless for us to make "rules" and expect the rest of the world to comply. To do so, he argued, is to invite disappointment and misery. In the mid-20th century, these principles were adapted by Albert Ellis (b. 1913 d. 2007), a US psychotherapist who was dissatisfied with conventional (Freudian) psychotherapy, observing that despite years of intensive therapy, many anxious, depressed people failed to make material gains, and simply remained depressed and anxious (if financially and emotionally depleted for

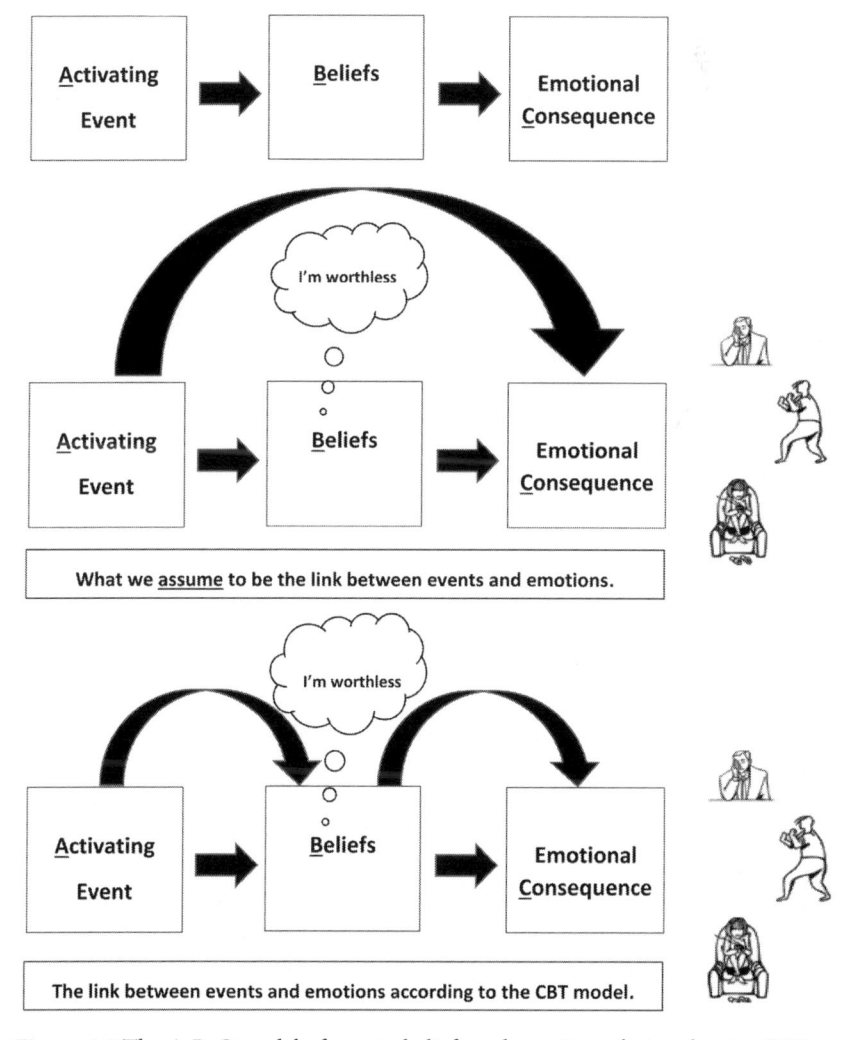

Figure 5.2 The A-B-C model of events, beliefs and emotions that underpins CBT.

all those years of psychotherapy). Ellis developed a psychotherapy that became known as Rational Emotive Therapy, and this, together with the work of father and daughter team Aaron (b. 1921) and Judith (b. 1954) Beck culminated in today's CBT.

A simple way to conceptualize CBT is to use Ellis' A-B-C model of the relationship between events, thoughts, and feelings, as illustrated in Figure 5.2. We might judge that we feel a particular way because something upsetting or confusing happened to us, but the CBT model teaches us to interrogate our beliefs and assumptions (B) about what happened (A), and to then *link that belief* to the emotional outcome (C), rather than linking the activating event directly to the emotional outcome. For example, you text a friend, asking if she would like to see a movie that you discussed recently, together tonight. An hour passes, but she does not reply. If your cognition (thinking) around this says your friend was probably just being polite, and she's probably seeing the movie with another friend *right now*, whose company she prefers, you will feel upset/angry/hurt and/or betrayed. If, however, your cognitive processing yields, "Oh, she must be busy. She'll get back to me eventually. I doubt we'll make it today, though", then you will not experience a strong emotional response in either direction.

CBT focuses on identifying and responding to unhelpful and/or unrealistic automatic thoughts that reflect a person's core beliefs about themselves, their world, and the future, but it is *not* to be construed as "positive thinking" or Pollyanna-ism. As well as focusing on thoughts and beliefs, CBT includes social skills training, assertiveness training, and practice giving and receiving feedback. The approach is active, so homework and graded practice are important. CBT has an impressive evidence-base for its use in treating high-prevalence conditions such as anxiety and depression (Bennett-Levy et al., 2010), happily, without the side-effect profile associated with drug treatments. Unlike drug treatments, CBT's gains persist after treatment ends, though periodic "top-up" therapy may be necessary.

For children and adolescents with developmental disabilities, CBT may need modification (simplification) to be effective, because CBT is a *verbally-mediated* intervention or "talk therapy". There are obvious barriers to implementation for children with expressive and/or receptive language difficulties. There are few situations as verbal as sitting with a (verbally competent) counsellor to talk about thinking about your thinking, and then to do thinking homework. We recommend, therefore, that visual "props" such as pictures are considered, ensuring that key words are written on a whiteboard or tablet computer, perhaps accompanied by a helpful icon or symbol to facilitate comprehension. It may be necessary to slow the pace of therapy, building in specific repetition and additional opportunities for consolidation of new skills; however, children and adolescents with developmental disorders should not automatically be excluded from provision of psychotherapy (Taylor, 2010).

Solution-Focused Brief Therapy (SFBT)

As its name implies, SFBT focuses on outcomes and is short-term. Developed by husband and wife social-worker team, Steve de Shazer (b. 1940 d. 2005) and Insoo Kim Berg (b. 1934 d. 2007), SFBT emphasizes the present and the future, assisting clients to set their own goals as a way of identifying solutions that either remove a problem or make it easier to live with, in the context of their own lives. SFBT eschews key traditional elements of psychotherapy: long discussion of the problem and its history, and positioning the clinician as "the expert". In SFBT there is overt recognition that, as clients know their lives better than anyone, they are the real experts in the room and have resources that make achieving some form of solution possible. The therapist is like a muse, asking questions, complimenting the client on gains already made, and inviting reflection and self-determination through the discerning use of particular types of questions, most notably:

1. **The Miracle Question**: "Suppose that one night, while you are asleep, there is a miracle and the problem that brought you here is solved. However, because you are asleep you don't know that the miracle has already happened. When you wake up in the morning, what will be different that will tell you that the miracle has taken place? What else?"

2. **The Scaling Question**: Here, the clinician asks clients to visualize an imaginary scale from 0–10, and asks them to identify how "bad" the problem is on the scale, or how well they are managing the problem. This information is used in subsequent conversations to identify next steps. For example, if the client rates their current coping as a 4, the clinician might ask what they will be doing differently, or what others will notice about them, when they move up to 5.

3. **The Exception Question**: This approach invites clients to think about times when the problem is not present, or when its impact is lessened in some way, to foster understanding of factors that might be under the client's influence, to leverage even small degrees of change.

SFBT has been applied to a range of highly complex clinical scenarios, e.g., substance abuse, domestic violence, school refusal, and child maltreatment, as well as high-prevalence issues such as depression, anxiety, and relationship difficulties. SFBT has been shown to be effective for use with people with widely varying educational levels and with client groups often considered "unsuitable" for psychotherapy (MacDonald, 2011). Although SFBT has been subjected to less research than CBT, we see it as having potential to assist families to deal with complex emotional and behavioural difficulties, where gains can be slow and more conventional approaches may have failed to deliver meaningful change, either in challenging behaviours or in the response of family members to them.

We note too that there are *many* other forms of evidence-based psychotherapy for commonly-occurring mental health problems, e.g., Interpersonal Therapy, Acceptance and Commitment Therapy, Mindfulness Based Therapy, Family Therapy, Narrative Therapy, and Schema Therapy, to name a few. Some psychological therapies are better suited to certain populations than others, and some are concerned with specific phenomena, such as grief, anger management, or sex offending. Peak bodies such as the British Psychological Society, the Australian Psychological Society, and the American Psychological Association are go-to points for information about indications for, and bona fides of, different approaches.

Music therapy

Music impacts human emotions. Whether it is a song that evokes memories of a loved one, or sounds that transport you back to a great opera hall, a rock concert, or a choir you once sang in, music is up there as an everyday conduit to accessing and influencing what and how people feel. Music can soothe, energize, motivate, and create a sense of mutual connection and belonging. Over the last century, music has found a place as a therapeutic medium for children and adults, especially those with limited verbal communication. The Australian Music Therapy Association (www.austmta.org.au) explains that music therapy (MT) is:

> *"...a research-based practice and profession in which music is used to actively support people as they strive to improve their health, functioning and wellbeing...Music therapy is different from music education and entertainment as it focuses on health, functioning and wellbeing".*

MT is a therapeutic service administered by professionally qualified practitioners, while the more general "therapeutic" qualities of music can be accessed universally, provided that a means of either making or listening to music is available. MT practitioners work in both private and public facilities, in aged care, early childhood, health, and special education. A Cochrane Review (Geretsegger, Elefant, Mössler, & Gold, 2014) on the use of MT with children with ASD identified improvements in a range of preverbal and verbal behaviours such as social interaction and initiation, and social-emotional reciprocity. Improved social adaptation skills and quality of parent-child relationships were also reported.

> *"Where words fail, music speaks."*
> Hans Christian Andersen (b. 1805 d. 1875)

While fairytale titan Hans Christian Andersen captured how many of us feel about music in our 21st-century lives, it is important to note that MT as a profession does not make grandiose claims about what it can offer to children with developmental disorders. Rather, it positions itself as an evidence-based profession whose practitioners conduct assessments, set goals, implement interventions (1:1 and/or group), and evaluate outcomes. Music therapists sometimes employ principles of behaviour modification in their interventions, e.g., by pairing a particular musical signal with a desired behaviour such as eye-contact, and fading the music cue as the desired new behaviour becomes established and more spontaneous on the part of the child. MT has shown a pleasing subscription to scientific principles in applying methodological rigour, and grapples with many challenges that are common in allied health research more generally, e.g., employing adequate sample sizes, using well-controlled study designs with adequate follow-up times (including exploration of generalization of gains to everyday interpersonal communication), and having follow-up assessments done by raters blinded to group allocation. Notwithstanding these challenges, there is sufficient evidence for MT to be regarded as a therapeutic modality that promotes developmental precursors to purposeful communication skills, such as eye-contact and turn-taking duration, use of joint attention, and pointing-and-showing behaviours. We recognize that there will be access limitations to MT in different places; however, when provided by qualified personnel, it shows promise as a therapeutic intervention, and we expect its evidence base to grow.

Your Holy Grail or their Golden Fleece

Emotional, social, and behavioural adjustment is something of a Holy Grail in the developmental disorders field, as it unlocks doors to interpersonal, educational, vocational, and economic opportunities across the lifespan. Children do not need to have a developmental disorder for their parents to find behaviour management a challenging aspect of parenting, but it can be more so where special needs exist. Snake Oil merchants are particularly busy and wily in this space, because they see a Golden Fleece in the form of dollars, euros and pounds (etc.!) in parents' desperation. Practitioners who understand and can systematically and painstakingly "unpack" the complexity of an individual child's emotional and behavioural difficulties have a safer pair of hands than those whose one-size-fits-all services promise literally unbelievable results, and charge accordingly.

6 AAC: Controversies, contradictions and change

Human communication is a paradox. It is all around us in the most pervasive ways – as speech: conversations (those that we are part of and those that we overhear), TV, film, radio, podcasts, videoconferences, and voicemail messages; as writing: books, newspapers, text messages, emails, letters, and social media; and nonverbally, as gestures, signs and body language, from the subtle 0.2 second eyebrow flash to the resonant slamming of doors at the end of a rousing domestic dispute. You would have to work very, *very* hard to escape human communication, so much so that its commonplace role everyday life might foster a belief that communication is simple and straightforward, but it is neither. It is incredibly complex and, in many respects, remains something of a mystery to cognitive scientists, linguists, and SLPs/SLTs. Its central role in our lives as humans means that any breakdown, no matter how slight, will be felt in the interpersonal space. When the breakdown is severe, however, it is catastrophic, and searching for solutions can be all-consuming. In this chapter, we focus on persistent controversial approaches to overcoming severe communication impairment that have entered the marketplace (see Hemsley & Dann, 2014, for discussion), and even courtrooms, in recent decades; chief among these is Facilitated Communication (FC). We broadly map the AAC territory and identify key controversies that have dogged the field for over 30 years. First, though, we look at the buoyant, bourgeoning area of augmentative and alternative communication (AAC or AUGcomm) from manual signing and finger spelling to speech generating devices (SGDs).

Augmentative and alternative communication

Augmentative and alternative communication (AAC), sometimes called alternative and adaptive communication (Beukelman & Mirenda, 2005) covers two types of communication systems for people who need either to augment or to replace speech (and its comprehension) for everyday communication purposes. First, there are *unaided* AAC systems (requiring no special "tools" or equipment, just the user's body, e.g., gestures, body language, finger-spelling and/or sign language); and second, *aided* AAC systems, which require tools or equipment *and* the user's body, ranging from the commonplace (e.g., paper and pencil), to devices which require specialist input for their development, e.g., communication books or boards, text-to-speech voice output devices (monolingual or multilingual SGDs) such as the Lightwriter® and/or written output devices, and picture array systems such as PECS™ (Carr & Felce, 2007) as discussed in Chapter 4. Some AAC approaches are "low-tech" (e.g., communication boards), while others are "high-tech" (e.g., electronic devices that may require tailormade access switches). Many systems and solutions are *multimodal* and communication partners must often play an active role in purposefully supporting the AAC user and promoting success.

Clients themselves and their families are integral members of the AAC team and decision-making processes, with evidence indicating that family involvement improves client outcomes (Bailey, Parette, Stoner, Angell, & Carroll, 2006). However, the decision to explore and/or adopt AAC approaches can be complex and anxiety-provoking for families, and many questions will be raised. *Which approach or device will provide my child with maximal independence? Will the use of AAC approaches hinder the development of verbal communication? Can we afford a high-tech option? How acceptable will other people find my child's AAC approach or device? When should options be reviewed and changed?* We obviously cannot address all of these important questions here, but Cress and Marvin (2003) provide sensible and reassuring answers to common questions that parents and teachers ask about AAC. Ethical issues associated with all AAC approaches must be carefully considered, most notably those associated with autonomy and choice, the probability of inequitable access under different funding jurisdictions, and the need for clinicians to be critical and unbiased consumers of scientific evidence so that communication access for vulnerable clients is maximized in ways that are authentic and flexible. Interested readers are referred to Hemsley (2012), Speech Pathology Australia's (2012) *Augmentative and Alternative Communication Clinical Guideline*, and Travers, Tincani and Lang (2014) for further discussion of ethical aspects of AAC provision.

So, before explaining more about what FC entails and why we do not support it (or its descendant, re-badged approaches, Assisted, or Supported Typing, Saved by Typing, Soma® Rapid Prompting, and the Rapid Prompting Method), we need to unpack what it means to be able to communicate via a non-speech means.

Communicating via non-speech means (aided or unaided): What's involved?

When someone has a severe disability (such as cerebral palsy, intellectual disability (ID), autism spectrum disorder (ASD), acquired brain injury, or some combination of disorders) that prevents "normal" communication, the SLPs/SLTs who carry out assessments are not thinking simply in terms of *mechanical barriers* to communication that must be overcome. This is because effective communication, whether via the conventional spoken word or via some form of AAC, draws on *essential* underlying functions in cognition, in memory, in language (including pragmatics), and in social skills. These are briefly outlined below.

Cognitive functions that underpin communication

The most basic cognitive function required for communication is consciousness. Being conscious means being both *alert* and *aware* (Posner, Saper, Schiff, & Plum, 2007). In turn, being alert means being awake, and not drowsy. You know how difficult it is to process details of a conversation when you are falling asleep or, worse still, are woken unexpectedly. Being *aware* means being cognizant of internal states (e.g., hunger, thirst, pain, anxiety) and external events (e.g., the presence of someone in the room). Once we can assume consciousness (which is not always clear-cut in people in minimally conscious or persistent vegetative states after brain injury), we can begin to think about higher-order cognitive skills such as attention and concentration. To communicate, we have to *pay attention to the task at hand* and screen out irrelevant stimuli – the TV or vacuum cleaner in the background, conversations occurring in the corridor, and so on. As discussed in Chapter 3, babies and young children have limited attention spans and are easily distracted. The skills of paying attention and screening out distractions develop over many years, and are highly vulnerable in the presence of neurodevelopmental disorders. Parents and teachers often work hard to reduce distractions in the environment so as to promote communication success and academic achievement, and for good reason. Other cognitive skills that come into play during communication include reasoning and problem-solving, planning and organization, and the ability to self-regulate and curb impulsivity.

Memory functions that underpin successful communication

There are different memory systems that are fundamental to communication success. Long-term memory is, as the name suggests, our store of memories which are more-or-less consolidated from the past, such as where we grew up and went to school. Such memories are established and evoked through conversations or can be called up via conscious recall, and play a major role in forming our sense of self and our life narratives. Short-term memory, and in particular *working memory* (see pages 32–33), constitutes a mental "notepad" that allows us to retain unfamiliar telephone numbers just long enough to write them down, and to follow conversations in real time, but does not in itself send information to long-term storage unless there is some rehearsal or the experience is highly salient to the individual in some way. Features of working memory are its limited capacity, and the rapid decay of memory traces.

Language functions that underpin successful communication

Where do we begin?! We refer repeatedly to the multilayered nature of language, and Chapter 7 gives an overview of the components of language (e.g., the sound system, vocabulary, syntax, etc.) and its two modalities: expressive and receptive. Whether communicating via speech, writing, an electronic device, a picture-symbol board, a formal sign system, or some combination of these, we use the symbols of language. Of course, nonverbal communication, e.g., posture, eye gaze, facial expressions, is important too but these means in themselves are not enough, as anyone will attest who has tried to convey through gesture a complex message to a person – who is trying *hard* to "get the message" – across a crowded and noisy room. So if you are going to communicate successfully, you *need* language tools at your disposal, and these *must* be at least partially present in both the receptive and expressive channels.

Communication beyond the level of basic needs requires mastery of abstract and nonliteral language (metaphor, sarcasm, idiom, inference, humour), the ability to take the perspective of the listener (e.g., to consider a listener's prior knowledge when telling a story) and the capacity to read social cues about interest, offence, boredom and confusion. These are all difficult enough in the best of circumstances via the verbal modality, but fall away quickly in the context of AAC use for a wide range of reasons, some language and cognition-related, some related to the inefficiencies associated with the physical demands of using the device.

Social skill functions that underpin successful communication

In addition to the "underpinnings" already mentioned, as outlined in Chapter 4, successful communication requires us to "swim between the flags" with respect to the unwritten rules of how human interaction works. We are expected to observe politeness conventions (which vary between cultures and social contexts), know when to talk (verbally or by means of AAC) and when to listen, when and how to change topics, wind up a conversation, interrupt, and/or correct our conversational partner. No wonder parents still provide coaching and feedback on these skills well into their children's late teenage years (or even beyond).

Physical attributes needed to use AAC devices

As if all of the above were not demanding enough, speakers who face neuromuscular barriers to verbal communication (e.g., people with severe dysarthria due to cerebral palsy or brain injury), and who have been assessed by an SLP/SLT as suitable for an AAC device, must clear more hurdles with respect to the physical demands of using the approach or device. Most fundamentally, when using a device, they must be able to *look* at it and *see* it, and then they need to *access it* in some way, e.g., by pointing with a finger, hand or foot, or by using eye gaze. These actions require significant motor (physical) functioning (strength, endurance, flexibility, and coordination), drawing heavily on cognitive skills such as attention, planning, concentration, and memory. Successful AAC use is as much about physical access as it is about cognitive and language skills. The balance differs on a case-by-case basis, but both must always be considered.

There is no clear correspondence between degree of physical impairment, and degree of language, memory, and cognitive impairment. Professor Stephen Hawking, a world-renowned theoretical physicist from the University of Cambridge who has a form of motor neurone disease (MND), is one case in point, as is Martin Pistorius, the South African survivor of a brain infection at age 12 that left him with a form of locked-in syndrome. On the other hand, some people with ASD have no discernable physical basis for being nonverbal, and in spite of having no upper limb weakness, do not have an independent means of AAC. Further, it is a vastly different matter to be an *adult* who once possessed a full range of cognitive and communication skills and then acquires a neurological injury (e.g., due to brain trauma) that impairs some of those skills, versus being a *child* who needs to acquire language, cognitive and memory skills *alongside* learning to use an AAC system.

For an individual with severe communication impairment, then, understanding others' messages and expressing wants, needs, information, and ideas through language is rarely a simple matter of bypassing a unitary mechanical blockage or barrier in a system. In fact, clients who present with such barriers are typically equipped with AAC support by an SLP/SLT after detailed, painstaking assessment, and the origin of their messages is not open to debate. Because of the complexity of disorders such as autism, ID, acquired brain injury, and cerebral palsy, however, difficulties at *multiple levels* must be assessed and addressed, and co-morbidities must be taken into account. This is why it typically takes a long time, and much specialist advice, for people with severe disabilities to be equipped with communication systems that are at least partially successful. There are no quick fixes in the field of severe communication impairment. FC's supporters, however, present it as a remarkable one-size-fits-all intervention that somehow overcomes *all* of the barriers briefly outlined above, and in a range of clinical populations. If you're not hearing alarm bells and thinking about ethical practice at this point, you should be.

A short history of the Facilitated Communication world

In the late 1970s and early 1980s, a teacher named Rosemary Crossley worked with a group of young adults in a care facility in Melbourne, Australia, known as St Nicholas' Hospital. The term "hospital" here was a misnomer by modern standards, as it was in fact a state care institution to which families could relinquish babies and young children with severe disabilities. In the mid-20th century, ignorance and stigma dominated thinking around disability, reinforced, unwittingly perhaps, by the then dominant medical model of disability which focused on underlying neurological pathology, and doing whatever could be done to "fix" impairments and barriers to "normal" functioning. Such thinking was well-intentioned, of course, but through the lens of presentism, focusing on medicine's regrettable ignorance in the past compared with the more enlightened "now", is now generally considered to be paternalistic and inappropriately narrow in its focus.

Foreshadowing more progressive times, 1981 was proclaimed by the United Nations as the International Year of Disabled Persons. This heralded (and to some extent reflected) the beginnings of a global shift in societal thinking about people with disabilities and the social model of disability grew a little more influential in public policy, health, and education – at least in industrialized nations. And so it was that, when Rosemary Crossley asserted that the residents of "St Nick's" (as it was known by Melbournians) not only had a right to a better standard of care, but were in many cases, bright, competent people trapped in extremely physically disabled (and in some cases malnourished) bodies, she captured the zeitgeist in ways that few at the time anticipated.

Among others at St Nick's, Ms Crossley (to become Dr Crossley in 1997 when she completed her PhD at Victoria University, Melbourne) worked with a young woman named Anne McDonald (b. 1961 d. 2010). Anne was born with severe cerebral palsy, and had been placed in the care of the state by her family, who lived in a country town and were unable to support a child whose physical impairments meant that she was completely dependent on around-the-clock, full care. When Dr Crossley began working with Anne in the late 1970s, Anne spent most of her time on a beanbag, weighed only 12kg, and had no immediately obvious means of communication. Sadly, this scenario was not unusual at the time. The Dark Ages extended well into the 20th century where understanding of disability was concerned.

History records (and Google searches reveal) that Dr Crossley went on to claim that Anne was an intellectually bright young woman, essentially trapped inside an uncooperative body. Anne's cerebral palsy resulted in a range of disabilities, including severe dysarthria, so she had no speech. Dr Crossley maintained, however, that when she provided physical support to Anne's arm, she was able to point to letters on a board to spell out meaningful messages, causing immediate and astonished reactions in health and education circles, as Anne had received no formal education. They puzzled, for example, over how she had learned to spell. Interestingly, this form of support was initially given a much more "what it says on the packet" name: *Assisted Communication*, a fact that has almost been lost in the mists of time. The Supreme Court of Victoria ultimately accepted that Anne's communication was her own, and granted her application to leave St Nick's and move into the home Dr Crossley shared with her partner, where she lived in their care until her death (*Sydney Morning Herald*, 2010).

It is not the purpose of this chapter to critique or contest claims that were made about one particular nonverbal client with severe cerebral palsy. We have both been in the health/disability field long enough to know that many decisions were made in earlier decades which we now regard as ill-informed at best and plain wrong and downright harmful at worst. Such is the price we pay for imperfect knowledge and the slow march of progress. We applaud the advocacy work that Rosemary Crossley has done since the early 1980s for people with severe communication impairment, but contest the "science" underpinning what came to be known as Facilitated Communication (FC). Ironically, while many would see the closure of large institutions such as St Nick's as (on the face of it at least) a positive move, the global push that commenced in the 1980s to de-institutionalize people with disabilities and/or long-term psychiatric illnesses is no success story. Expect eye rolling, indignation, and exasperation if you ask any parent or sibling of an adult with severe disabilities or psychiatric illness whether adequate specialized support, stimulation, and sometimes, just basic safety, are provided in community residential settings.

What does FC look like in action?

The easiest way to find out is to go to YouTube™ and enter "Facilitated Communication" as a search term. You will see several examples that are, quite literally, in-credible, and, if you will forgive us for spelling it out, by that we mean un-believable. You will see young people sitting at tables, moving restlessly, eye-gaze all over the room but rarely on their communication devices, arm or hand supported by facilitators, and supposedly producing independent messages. Other examples are of what appear to be quite clear, autonomous communication, with a facilitator sitting nearby, perhaps a hand on the client's shoulder. If any one of these clients is in fact communicating, it is a result of the cognitive, linguistic, memory, and motor skills outlined earlier in this chapter, *not because of a hand on their shoulder*. We are reminded of editorial commentary in an early paper by Prior and Cummins (1992) on FC:

> *"Current promoters of this technique have been unwilling to differentiate those clients for whom a facilitator is useful, from those who can learn spontaneous communication on their own…In addition, the ideologues promoting – 'Facilitated Communication' – use an especially pernicious form of sales technique. They claim that – 'Facilitated Communication' –*

requires faith and a trusting relationship to be effective. They claim that research is inappropriate because it interferes with the trusting relationship" (p. 336).

Controversies, and ethical and legal minefields in FC

From its earliest days at St Nick's and its central role in the Anne McDonald court case, FC has been controversial and divisive, among academics, clinicians, parents, teachers, client advocacy groups, the courts, media, and funding bodies. While we can say with confidence that it is a technique that has been widely and resoundingly discredited, that in itself, dear reader, is not enough to see it exit stage left from the disability marketplace; on the contrary, as noted by Chan and Nankervis (2014), the real work may have only just begun.

An early boost to FC was its endorsement by Dr Douglas Biklen, a special education academic who is now an Emeritus Professor of the School of Education at Syracuse University in New York. Dr Biklen's support for FC was important not only for the reflected respectability associated with an academic endorsement, but because his own particularly ill-informed spin on communication impairment in autism, i.e., that it was a disorder of praxis, or skilled movement (Biklen, 1990), was a convenient retrofit on FC. A teacher invented a technique and an academic invented a rationale as to why it "worked". The rest, as they say, is history. Never mind that the scientific method requires us to develop practice out of theory. That is a minor detail that has also been lost in the mists of time.

As you might expect with a communication technique that is completely reliant on the active assistance/support/facilitation of another person, from its beginnings the origin of the messages conveyed via FC was contested. Bear in mind, too, that there was often an enormous mismatch between what was previously known about a client's language and cognitive skills and the complex content and structure of the messages they were suddenly (you could even say, miraculously) conveying via FC, so the question of how they learned to spell remains unanswered.

> "They were making their wishes known, from the mundane 'I want ice-cream' to the profound 'I want society to accept us for who we are and not to judge us'."
> Schreibman, 2005, p. 205

At odds with the cognitive science on reading acquisition (see Chapter 9), extraordinary claims were made early on that children with autism and ID "…may have learned spelling through occasional print exposure" (Crossley & Remington-Gurney, 1992). It is also notable that FC messages conveyed by children with ASD are said not to display the typical linguistic markers, such as pronoun inversion and echolalia, seen in the spoken language of children with autism (Crossley & Remington-Gurney, 1992); however, no theoretical basis for this surprising anomaly is offered. These logical inconsistencies and telling discrepancies, together with observations that the child's eyes were often not even directed at the communication device, had led psychologists, in the previous 20 years, to devise rigorous experimental conditions that *should* have laid matters to rest. Montee, Miltenberger and Wittrock (1995), for example, conducted an investigation of seven adults with moderate or severe ID across three communication conditions: (a) the facilitator and client had access to the same information; (b) the facilitator did not have access to the picture or activity; and (c) the facilitator was given false information about the picture or activity. They concluded that "…no communication came from the client through facilitated communication", and "the facilitators controlled the typing" (p. 197). Bear in mind that academic researchers typically couch their conclusions in somewhat qualified language ("it appeared that", "the results suggest that"); however, no such qualification was needed here. So that was 1995, but the FC roadshow persisted unabated, and in 2014 an internationally authored systematic review (Schlosser, Balandin, Hemsley, Iacono, Probst, & von Tetzchner, 2014) came to an identical conclusion, citing "…robust evidence that FC is not a valid technique" (p. 366), with even more evidence on which to base their unequivocal assessment. Further evidence of the scientific sidelining of FC lies in its exclusion from a recent Cochrane Review protocol on communication interventions for minimally verbal children with autism (Brignell et al., 2016). Brignell et al. note that, "We will only include interventions that involve the child independently communicating" (p. 5). We take this to mean that it has already been established that FC users cannot be assumed to be communicating independently, and the field needs to move on in its search for approaches that do deliver evidence-based communication capacity.

More recently, Saloviita (2016) applied the science of linguistic analysis to the question of message authorship in FC, concluding that alleged stylistic differences between the language use of facilitators and clients probably reflect a form of code-switching by the facilitator rather than some form of idiosyncratic language use that is specific to FC, strangely not present in other

Table 6.1 The AAC vs. FC balance sheet (after Travers, Tincani, & Lang, 2014, p. 199).

Criteria	Alternative and Augmentative Communication (AAC)	Facilitated Communication (FC) and its derivatives
Theoretical basis	Embedded in current understandings of the neurobiological basis of different forms of communication breakdown, whether congenital or acquired, and the role of different forms of AAC for different disability types.	Based on Biklen's (1990) unsupported theory that communication impairment, in ASD specifically, is a disorder of praxis. Greatly reliant on nebulous variables such as the quality of the relationship between the facilitator and the client. Poor differentiation of disability types. Disproportionate emphasis on "manual dysfunction" and need for emotional support.
Aim of the procedures	Maximal independence in a range of communication contexts.	Stated aim is independent communication but continued reliance on facilitator is usual. Stronger movement of the facilitator than the client is tolerated during training.
Practitioner training/skill set	Qualified SLPs/SLTs with specialist AAC expertise in leadership roles within care teams.	Training is often provided to non-specialists in AAC by non-specialists in AAC.
Assessment process	Based on scientist-practitioner model. Detailed consideration of supporting processes (see pages 151-154) involved in AAC use. Use of standardized assessment and observation tools where appropriate.	May be done using facilitation, so assessment "findings" are inherently questionable. The facilitator's observations are valued over formal assessment procedures.
Training techniques	Tailored to physical, cognitive and communicative needs of the individual. Considers roles for both low and high-tech approaches. Techniques change over time, as user's skills and needs change.	Physical touch or support (e.g., to hand, arm, shoulder) when user is "accessing" a device. Variable expectation of "fading" of facilitation.
Typical outcome measures	Degree of independence in a range of communication settings; acceptability and functionality for communication partners.	Not differentiated for different groups of users.
Evidence	Variable, as a function of degree of research and degree of supporting evidence for different approaches. Some dramatic case accounts popularized in mainstream media (e.g., Stephen Hawking). More rigorous, empirical research is needed.	Highly reliant on anecdotal accounts. Clearly and repeatedly shown to be non-evidenced based. Messages emanate from the facilitator, not the client. Frequently referenced in peer-reviewed literature as "pseudo-science". No further empirical work is warranted given weight of current evidence.
Ethics	Major advances in last two decades; client autonomy and choice are central. Professional bodies explicitly recognize ethical pitfalls in AAC design and use.	Highly problematic. Associated with harm to clients and families. Rather than providing access to communication, the user's voice is "stolen" by the facilitator.

reports of the written language forms and idioms used by people with autism (e.g., Dockrell, Ricketts, Charman, & Lindsay, 2014).

If you are in any doubt about the implausibility of claims made about FC as a means of communication, get hold of a head-pointer, and try to type a message on your tablet (iPad or android). We say tablet device here rather than "desktop" computer, because many of the early claims about FC's success were made on the basis of messages purportedly conveyed via a device known as the Canon Communicator (see Vanderheiden, 2002), operated either by hand or by using a head-pointer. Canon Communicators, in production since 1974, are somewhere between a tablet and a cellphone size-wise, with a keyboard arranged in alphabetical order. A rudimentary understanding of the cognitive-linguistic-memory-motor-visual demands of communication will call into question the claims made about the capacity of people who had apparently never had a verbally-based means of communication before, but could now convey conceptually and linguistically complex messages at the press of a button – provided someone else was supporting or moving their hand or arm, or holding and moving the communication device.

In Table 6.1, we have adapted and expanded a summary table published by Travers et al. (2014, p. 199) to offer a "balance sheet" on the current state of play in AAC and FC practice and research.

FC and allegations of sexual abuse/assault

Allegations of sexual abuse (e.g., "Ben's communication", page 69) or assault made via FC are highly problematic. It is well known that the care and safety of people with disabilities in residential care settings worldwide is sometimes far from optimal, and in fact there have been recent prosecutions in the state of Victoria in Australia, some involving quite senior staff, of major service-providers (Victorian Ombudsman Report, 2015). One of the sources of community and media outrage, shame and distress in such circumstances is our understanding of the compromised communication skills of many people with severe disabilities, together with the low likelihood that (a) they will make allegations, (b) these will be believed and taken seriously, and (c) they will form the basis of legal testimony that results in a successful prosecution of alleged offenders. In fact, even in the absence of disability, children's testimony is highly vulnerable and is often elicited by adults in ways that mean it is easily contested by defence counsel (Snow, Powell, & Sanger, 2012). The deck is well and truly stacked against the person with severe communication impairment in such circumstances and this is a wrong that must be righted. However, FC has definitely not leapt to the rescue in this most complex arena. The following humbling and painful confession (her word) by a brave former SLP and former FC practitioner, Janyce Boynton, lays bare the tragic reality of what can happen when interventions are implemented ahead of science in an area of practice as high stakes as allegations of sexual abuse:

> "Twenty years ago, I was the facilitator in the Wheaton case, a story featured on Frontline's Prisoners of Silence and, later, in a 20/20 episode with Hugh Downs. … I held Betsy Wheaton's hand and typed out accusations against her family members. Graphic depictions of rape and sexual assault that had no bearing in reality. The family was innocent. Betsy was well cared for. No physical evidence of abuse existed. But my words, typed through the guise of FC, put in motion events that caused serious damage to a lot of people. Betsy and her brother were removed from their home to foster care, while her parents were charged. Authorities questioned the brother's role in the alleged abuse. Was he victim? Perpetrator? Both? Lawyers were hired to defend the parents and look out for the children's best interest. Vicious rumors circulated about the family in their small town, lingering even after the charges had been dropped and the children had returned to their home. All this irreparable heartache was caused by my unshakeable belief in FC."
>
> Boynton, pp. 3–4

FC breaks the foremost rule of helping: *first do no harm*. FC's discredited status means that its use as a vehicle for abuse allegations is likely to only further marginalize and silence the voices of people with disabilities who experience physical and/or sexual assault at the hands of so-called carers. A number of compelling but deeply disturbing feature articles in mainstream media have been written recently, profiling in tragic, sometimes bizarre detail, cases involving FC and allegations of sexual abuse or assault of clients. See, for example, David Auerbach's 2015 piece in *Slate* and Daniel Engber's 2015 article in the *New York Times Magazine*. The Anna Stubblefield case (described briefly by Auerbach and in detail by Engber) is particularly troubling, in its own right, as a case of substantiated rape of "D.J.", a young man with severe physical and communication disabilities by Rutgers University pro-FC disability studies professor, Dr Anna Stubblefield. However, as recently noted by Sherry (2016), the case also raises troubling ethical challenges for the disability academics and advocates who supported Stubblefield during (and since) her trial. Sherry observed that:

> *"I never saw anything to support the black disabled man who was the victim of this sexual assault. I even witnessed disability scholars soliciting contributions to (Stubblefield's) legal defense fund, but I never saw a single effort to support the victim. In my view, this response to rape is not only misdirected, it is unethical and shameful. The lack of concern for the victim and his family was chilling, disturbing, and alarming"* (p. 6).

Position statements on Facilitated Communication

A number of high-profile national bodies have released position statements on FC in recent years, and the key theme of these is their lack of support for the approach. Prominent examples include that of the American Speech-Language Hearing Association (1995), which states, in part:

> *"It is the position of the American Speech-Language-Hearing Association (ASHA) that the scientific validity and reliability of facilitated communication have not been demonstrated to date. Information obtained through or based on facilitated communication should not form the sole basis for making any diagnostic or treatment decisions."*
>
> ASHA, 1995

In its 2012 Clinical Guideline on Alternative and Augmentative Communication, Speech Pathology Australia states (p. 9):

> *"...FC remains an approach with little supportive evidence and a preponderance of evidence that contraindicates its use, and its use is not recommended."*
>
> SPA, 2012

Similarly, the International Society for Augmentative and Alternative Communication (ISAAC) does not support the use of FC, and noted in its 2014 position statement that:

> "The main issue that is being disputed is whether the output produced when persons with disabilities are being facilitated is expressing their communicative intentions, or whether the source of the output is that of the facilitators."
>
> ISAAC, 2014

In spite of these position statements and the enormous volume of scientific evidence discrediting it, FC lives on, and in some cases even thrives, in various academic, clinical, education, and client advocacy circles. The reasons for this are as complex as they are troubling, as outlined by Lilienfeld, Marshall, Todd and Shane (2014). These workers point out that academics cannot assume that amassing robust scientific evidence is enough to end an education or clinical practice fad. False hope, cognitive bias, rejection of the scientific method, and the seductive belief that "...an intellectually intact person lurks beneath the normal exterior, merely waiting to be discovered by FC" (p. 88) all conspire to burden the disability community with FC for some time to come. This latter assumption aligns with the pro-FC stance (appealing on the face of it) that we should "presume competence" on the part of people with severe communication impairment (Biklen & Burke, 2006). Presuming competence, however, promotes confirmation bias on the part of clinicians, parents, and teachers, and contrasts with the scientist-practitioner model of not making any *a priori* assumptions, instead simply dealing with painstakingly collected observations and other data points.

A curious inconsistency

The International Communication Project (ICP) (www.international communicationproject.com), initiated in 2014, is an ongoing joint venture of a group of national, member-based organizations that support the common goal of raising the profile of communication disabilities globally, and of the professionals who can help. The six founding organizations, which share the task of running the project's informational and consciousness-raising website, are the mutual recognition agreement (MRA) signatories (see page 307): ASHA, IASLT, NZSTA, RCSLT, SAC-OAC and SPA. As well as the *founding* organizations, there are 48 (as of March 2016) *participating* organizations. They include several that expressly advocate for the rights of AAC users, for example AGOSCI and the Cerebral Palsy Support Network in Australia; Communication Disabilities Access Canada; the Essential Learning Group in

China; CENMAC, the Council for Disabled Children, ICAN, KIDS, PACE, and the Communication Trust in England; ISAAC internationally; Afasic, Commtap, The Children's Society, The Royal Mencap Society, and UK Connect in the United Kingdom; Allied Health Media in the United States; and the Trinh Foundation in Vietnam.

> *"The Opportunity to Communicate is a Basic Human Right. Communication is the most fundamental of human capacities. People need to be able to communicate to fulfill their social, educational, emotional and vocational potential. Everybody has the potential to communicate."*
>
> International Communication Project

There is an invitation on the ICP website to "share your story", noting that, "It may take up to 3–5 business days for your story to be posted". Among the 36 stories, at the time of writing, are *Typing to Communicate – Overcoming Stigma*, extolling the virtues of FC; *Helping Others Speak Through Facilitated Communication* in which the writer "knew in the core of her soul that FC was real"; and *Speaking through a Letterboard* about the Rapid Prompting Method (RPM): don't be led astray, RPM is the same FC mumbo-jumbo under a different moniker.

Now, we do not know *who* took the decision, and up to 3–5 business days to post these three inappropriate stories (after *we* signed the online document in support of the ICP), but were surprised and disappointed to see the ICP providing a platform on which to applaud FC use, thereby lending its implied support to FC's practice. We also wonder how many of the ICP partner organizations, individual SLPs/SLTs and audiologists, and thinking consumers of their services, would re-consider their endorsement if they were aware of this. As bloggers (Snow, 2013) and website owners (Bowen, 1998), we know that it takes just moments, and does not cause a web presence to fall apart, to remove content we regret. However, repeated overtures to the ICP and founding organizations in 2015 and 2016 to take these three stories down have drawn no response to date. The price of (Internet) freedom is eternal vigilance for users.

The ICP site lacks a search tool, but extensive browsing of it failed to yield any mention of "evidence-based practice" or "ethics". Perhaps they are there, but are so well concealed that we could not locate them. Either way, they are not a prominent feature of the project's approach.

Resisting the FC faithful

It is not enough to ride the wave of social and political change that quite rightly discards dated, ableist, paternalistic ways of thinking about disability, in favour of the language of inclusion and respect for diversity. The enormous weight of evidence regarding FC indicates that it is *not* an efficacious means of accessing the wants, needs, thoughts, and ideas of people with severe communication impairment. Sadly, in some cases, such wants, needs, thoughts, and ideas may exist only at very low levels or even be non-existent, by virtue of the severity of the underlying (if as yet poorly understood) neurological impairment. That so many studies have shown that authorship of messages belongs with the facilitator and not the client is a bitter twist on the progressive social inclusion narrative promulgated by FC advocates. Rather than gaining a "voice", many people with severe communication impairment have, by virtue of their vulnerability, become non-consenting players in what is best described as a travesty.

Families have had hopes raised and dashed (interspersed with enormous confusion and often major friction between family members, and palpable hounding, trolling and bullying in social media), and more fruitful opportunities for maximizing functioning and quality of life have been missed. In extreme cases, parents have had their children removed from their care as a result of false allegations of sexual abuse made via FC. Rather than miraculously "unlocking" the voices of people with severe disabilities, FC is now seen not only as an approach that *does not work*, but also as one that is *unethical*. Tostanoski, Lang, Raulston, Carnett and Davis (2013, p. 221) caution that:

> *"FC is commonly seen as the epitome of deceptive and dangerous treatment because of its tragic history of depriving children with autism of the right to self-expression and for destroying families with false accusations of abuse."*

When an intervention has been around for more than 35 years and is still mired in controversy, parents, teachers, advocacy groups such as the International Communication Project, and policymakers should step back. FC shows many features of other forms of pseudoscience, most notably by presenting itself as a one-stop shop for severe communication impairment across the board

(ASD, ID, brain injury, cerebral palsy, etc.). In addition, however, "faith" in the technique is required, and poor outcomes are cruelly attributed to lack of skill, belief, or commitment on the part of the facilitator. This, and the resistance of FC advocates to "play ball" with the scientific method, means we recommend that you stay right away from it.

AAC developments to watch

In the constantly-changing AAC landscape, practice can easily become uncoupled from research, so that AAC users are introduced to methods that seem to have good "face validity" but which have been subjected to little or no ethically and methodologically acceptable research scrutiny. We are critical, in *Making Sense of Interventions for Children's Developmental Disorders*, of those behind approaches who quote bogus evidence or evidence that is so flawed as to be laughable in any other context. We are also aware that, in many cases, the necessary research simply has not been done, and inevitably (though not ideally) clinical practice will march ahead in its absence. In ideal circumstances, skilled clinicians operate as scientist-practitioners, generating and then carefully testing clinical hypotheses about their clients and which approaches will "work".

Research in non-speech communication is hardly a "sexy" funding target[1]. There are no big pharmaceutical companies spending millions of Research and Development funds on it, and academics whose research focus is AAC must compete in funding rounds for grants with their colleagues working in a raft of other health priority areas (think: diabetes, HIV/Aids, mental health problems, asthma, dementia, cancer, etc.). Hence, we are mindful and respectful of the axiom that *absence of evidence does not mean evidence of absence*, i.e., in situations where research has not yet been done, or is only in its infancy, we recommend watchful waiting. We do so advisedly, and only for approaches whose theoretical rationales align with current knowledge about communication sciences and ethical issues in AAC provision. Approaches that fall into this category include Talking Mats® (www.talkingmats.com), the Pragmatic Organization Dynamic Display (PODD) system (Porter &

---

1 While ASD, cancer, and the vaccination debate are "sexy" in the sense of being exciting, appealing, newsworthy research-funding magnets, research areas that are no less deserving of publicity and financial support, like AAC, Developmental Language Disorder (DLD) and Special Education are generally considered to be "unsexy" and "un-vote-grabbing".

Cafiero, 2009) and Language Acquisition through Motor Planning (LAMP; www.aacandautism.com/lamp).

It is pleasing to see peer-reviewed studies on Talking Mats®, and in particular to note that (a) innovative research methodologies are making it easier for young people with AAC needs to be *participants in* rather than *subjects of* research using Talking Mats® (e.g., Germain, 2004), and (b) the approach has been subject to evaluations that conclude that it has *graduated* (rather than one-size-fits-all) suitability for people with AAC needs (e.g., Murphy & Cameron, 2008).

Talking Mats® is noteworthy for offering easy access to publications about the approach via its website. We note, however, that the "portfolio of over one hundred research publications" referred to (www.talkingmats.com/research-consultancy/publications) includes papers in publications at varying points on the research dissemination ladder (e.g., professional bulletins, unpublished research reports, and refereed journal articles). We are particular about this because the same exacting evidence standards must be applied across the board in AAC.

Beyond descriptive papers and case reports (which constitute low levels of evidence), little is known about the effectiveness of PODD and the same must be said for LAMP. Hence we view these as interventions to watch, being attentive (as with all AAC approaches) to the extent to which they are embedded in current theory about the disorders they target (e.g., ASD) and are genuinely client-focused in maximizing, rather than constraining, clients' choices.

Advances in the last decade in mainstream technology, most notably the advent of smart phones and tablet computers, such as the Apple® iPad® and its android counterparts have generated much interest in AAC circles. Bradshaw (2013) notes that such devices have the immediate appeal of being relatively low cost, and by virtue of being in widespread community use are considered "normal gadgets" by AAC users. They do, however, require physical access and visual acuity, both of which may be compromised for AAC users. Further, in spite of their appeal and functionality, the reality for many AAC users may be that lower-tech options offer maximum flexibility, and/or a combination of approaches is needed. As Mirenda (2014, p. 24) has observed:

> "...the vast majority of research on the use of the latest AAC 'trend' – portable touch screen devices (e.g., iPad®) – has (merely) demonstrated that school-aged individuals with IDD [intellectual or developmental disabilities] can use

> them to request desired items and activities from adults...
> Research on the effectiveness of these emerging AAC strategies
> in home, school, community, and work settings, to teach
> communicative functions that go far beyond requesting, is
> crucially important in order to insure that clinical decision-
> making conforms with practices that are evidence-based."

Sitting alongside these technological advances, there has also been progress in recent years in the development of clinical scales designed to bring some order and objectivity to the assessment of children and adults with severe communication impairments. Examples include the *Checklist of Communicative Competencies for Adults with Severe and Multiple Disabilities* (Triple C; Iacono, West, Bloomberg, & Johnson, 2009) and the *Communication Complexity Scale* (Brady et al., 2012). Some of these scales are mainly reliant on parent or caregiver report, while others are based on direct clinical assessment of communication behaviour under relatively controlled circumstances. Their strengths lie in the structure they place around assessment and the fact that they provide data which can be shared and discussed by all team members (which, in our world, always includes family), as well as forming a baseline against which progress can be monitored.

It is also pleasing to see greater focus on systematically understanding and addressing the needs of communication partners of AAC users, including the partners of children. In a meta-analysis, Shire and Jones (2015) highlighted the importance of factors such as partner training and its timing, including device training and enhancing partners' understanding of communication targets. In her commentary on this review, Stephenson (2016) observed that explicit training protocols are needed, and capacity for measuring generalization and maintenance of gains should be developed, alongside efforts to improve AAC users' receptive language skills, and the success of children's AAC use with different partners, such as teachers. Stephenson also pointed out that most of the children in the studies reviewed were preschool age, with research activity dropping off sharply at adolescence and beyond. Hence the training needs of partners of adolescent AAC users must also be studied, so that spontaneous use of a full range of pragmatic functions can be promoted for such users.

AAC frontiers and challenges ahead

We are guardedly encouraged by two frontier developments in AAC: the technological advances that are providing incremental improvements in communication access to people with severe disabilities, and the growing sophistication evident among those involved in consideration of ethical issues in AAC. Technological advances may occur more rapidly for those whose communication impairments are acquired due to illness or injury (such as Stephen Hawking and Martin Pistorius, whom we mentioned briefly earlier), than for children with ASD and/or ID. Adults and children with acquired neurological disabilities are likely to be better positioned than those with congenital disorders to take advantage of developments such as eye-tracking, because of the nature of their underlying neurological impairments as well as the presence of preserved skills that can be drawn on to promote AAC success. As long as the neuropsychological basis of disorders such as ASD continues to elude our understanding, AAC advances for those clients will be less dramatic. Nonetheless, through close involvement of families and significant others, and careful responsiveness to their everyday observations, incremental gains in skills that support successful communication can be made.

Communication sciences and disorders and societal attitudes have come a long way in the last thirty years in refining our understanding of the ethical responsibilities attached to providing AAC to people with complex communication needs , in the context of where such users live, go to school, and spend their time during the day as adults (Mirenda, 2014b). SLPs/SLTs and their professional bodies have a more nuanced and explicit grasp of the need for painstaking and persistent data-led approaches to AAC provision. We are also considerably more conscious now than thirty years ago of the dreadful pitfalls that await those who do not adhere closely to scientific principles in their work with clients who cannot communicate independently without some form of AAC. Ironically, we have FC's legacy to thank for some of these ethical advances and shifts in thinking.

Much remains to be achieved, however, not only in advancing technology, but also in advancing the equitable access of AAC users to that technology, and to specialist early intervention clinical and technical services to enable its effective use (Romski, Sevcik, Barton-Hulsey, & Whitmore, 2015). In Australia, some funding programmes are state-based and some are federal, meaning that families must contend with multiple bureaucracies. Still others depend on eligibility (often narrowly defined) for particular funding programmes, and in the UK it has been observed that both parents and professionals expend significant resources on lobbying for AAC devices for the estimated 0.5% of the population who require them (Communication Matters, 2013). If we are to walk-the-walk of communication being a human right, then these bureaucratic barriers and hurdles must go.

7 Voice, language, speech and fluency

When a child is referred to an SLP/SLT for assessment of a communication or swallowing disorder, two important things happen. First, it is routine in most settings for the child to have an audiogram – a hearing test with headphones, administered by an audiologist or an appropriately qualified SLP/SLT who may also perform a tympanogram, investigating middle ear health and function, checking for "glue ear". Second, even though individual SLPs/SLTs do not typically see a caseload that encompasses *all* potential client groups (see page 307), they are obliged to *screen* across all areas of communication and swallowing.

For example, a child might be referred with a request for "help with articulation", but the SLP/SLT would not take this entirely at face value. Rather, they would first make *educated* screening observations of the child's *voice, language* (including the *pragmatic language skills* displayed in Figure 4.1 on page 60, and, depending on the child's age), *literacy, speech* (including articulation), *fluency, eating* and *drinking*. If screening revealed more was amiss than the "help with articulation" request suggested, those problem areas would then be assessed in detail. Equally, a parent cannot call an SLP/SLT and say, "My child needs XYZ therapy" and expect to receive it without the clinician performing an evaluation to identify any difficulties, to see if the requested intervention is suitable, and to suggest alternatives if not.

This meticulous process of screening, detailed assessment, and choosing an intervention that matches the child's needs is lacking in many fad interventions, where all a parent need do is "self-diagnose" a difficulty (e.g., stuttering), locate a product or service, pay the money, and live with the consequences. In this chapter we explain what *voice, language, speech* and *fluency* mean in SLP/SLT terms, outline the communication disorders associated with them, and explore ways of assessing, treating and managing them.

Voice

Voice is the sound produced by the delicate vocal folds (vocal cords[1]), inside the

---

1 The vocal folds, or vocal cords, are folds of membranous tissue that project inwards from the sides of the larynx to form a slit across the glottis in the throat. The cords, often (amusingly) misspelled "chords", vibrate in the airstream from the lungs to produce voice.

larynx, and voice disorders are medical conditions affecting voice production. SLPs/SLTs do not assess or treat adults or children with voice disorders until an Ear Nose and Throat (ENT) specialist has inspected the patient's larynx, diagnosed the source of the problem, and ruled out (or in) potentially life-threatening conditions, including cancer. Sometimes, the ENT and the SLP/SLT request referral to another specialist, such as an allergist, endocrinologist, geneticist, paediatrician, physiotherapist, psychologist, or respiratory physician, or to a sleep disorders unit.

Voice disorders in children

Estimates vary, but probably 7–9% of children have voice problems at some point. The most common childhood voice disorder is chronic or intermittent hoarseness, which may or may not be associated with vocal cord thickening or vocal nodules: benign, noncancerous swellings on either or both cords. The preferred treatment for vocal nodules ("nodules") is voice therapy to train the child to use the voice optimally for speaking and singing without forcing or over-use. With cooperation from child and family, this reduces vocal load, causing the nodules to soften, reduce in size and eventually go. Recovery from nodules is analogous to what happens when a shoe has rubbed, causing a blister. You stop wearing the shoe, or do something to eliminate the irritation, and the blister gradually changes and then goes away.

Many children who develop nodules are extreme voice users: not just to talk, and make "silly noises" and sound effects, but also to express emotion: shouting, screaming and crying loudly, and at length. Their voice therapy is strictly the job of an SLP/SLT with an appropriate clinical background and not, for example, a speech, drama, English or singing teacher, a choir director, or a voice coach working without SLP/SLT and ENT input. That said, all these can be invaluable allies in intervention.

Voice therapy is based on painstaking *in-person* SLP/SLT assessment – incorporating the ENT's recommendations – specifically geared to the child's needs, with the goal of behavioural change. There is no "off-the-shelf", one-size-fits-all intervention, or treatment administered on the basis of an online questionnaire. Surgery to remove nodules in children is a rare last resort, because they will likely recur if the excessive vocal load continues or resumes. The SLP/SLT may work collaboratively with a family therapist, who is often a qualified psychologist or social worker. Family therapy (Bitter, 2013, 2015) and professional family counselling are particularly relevant when a child's voice overuse derives from a family pattern of loud, dysfunctional acting-out, distress, and *excessive* conflict (*all* families tussle at times). The family, not the child, is "the client", and no individual is scapegoated or blamed for all the uproar, or the nodules.

Will you have Monastery Herbs with that?

Treatment of voice disorders in children does not incorporate "remedies" like:

- *Dietary adjustments*: eliminating gluten, citrus or dairy, or introducing wonder foods (certified dieticians advise, and common sense decrees, a healthy diet and reasonable portion control, and avoiding known allergens specific to the child in question);
- *Patent medicines*: cold cures, cough drops, decongestant nasal drops and sprays, Friar's Balsam[2] inhalations, mentholated sweets, (lollies/candy) and volatile chest rubs;
- *"Natural remedies"*: echinacea, fish oil, garlic, lemon thyme, Oregon holly grape, slippery elm, and witch hazel, and amalgams of beeswax, black cohosh, black pepper, burdock, camphor, fennel, holy basil, honeysuckle, marshmallow root, mistletoe, Monastery Herbs, myrrh, nettles, okra, oranges, oregano, paico leaf, peppermint, quercus alba, rosemary, sage, seaweed, sumac, thyme, vinca, vinegar, water lily or yarrow;
- *Acupuncture, acupressure, aromatherapy, astrological psychology, Anthroposophic Therapeutic Speech, Bach flowers, chirophonetics* (www.chirophoneticspacific.com) or any *chiropractic* intervention, *exorcism, healing gemstones and crystals, homeopathy, naturopathy,* or *Vocal Science*™ from the Royans Institute for Non-Surgical Voice Repair (www.vocalscience.com/www.repairyourvoice.com).

Homeopathy

> *"I do not expect that homeopathy will ever be established as a legitimate form of treatment, but I do expect that it will continue to be popular."*
>
> James Randi, 2014

Homeopathy is a pseudoscientific intervention based on using animal, vegetable

---

2 Over 600 years, Friar's Balsam has been known as Balsamum Traumaticum, Balsamic Tincture, Jerusalem Drops, Jesuits' Drops, and Commander's-, Persian-, St. Victor's-. Swedish-, Turlington's-, Wade's-, and Wound- Balsam.

and mineral constituents, mixed with alcohol and vastly diluted in water, that "homeopathic doctors" claim can stimulate the body to self-heal. It is based on two cornerstone principles, *like cures like*, and *succession*, a process of *dilution* in water and *shaking* the resultant suspension. In the late 18th century, German alternative medicine pioneer, Christian Friedrich Samuel Hahnemann (b. 1755 d. 1843), a disenchanted village physician, abandoned medical practice to develop it. Like Dr Hahnemann, today's homeopaths believe that an ingredient that causes certain symptoms can also help eliminate them, and that the more a *mother tincture* (*teinture-mère*) is subjected to succussion (causing *dynamization or potentization*), the greater its healing power. A mother tincture is an extract of plant material macerated in alcohol, after which water is added, and added. Homeopathic dilutions have had water added so many times that no, or almost no, trace of the original mother tincture remains. Dilutions – purported to have a "memory" of the original substances – are usually administered as sugar pills, pilules or globules, or liquids (drop doses) taken orally, but they also come as skin creams, granules, injections, lotions, mouth sprays, ointments, olfaction doses (nasal drops or sprays), powders, suppositories, and tablets.

> "I keep washing a bottle of #homeopathic medicine I have, but contents keep getting stronger. Help!"
> Simon Chapman @SimonChapman6, in
> Twitter 26 Dec 2015

Disturbingly, over 40 homeopathic dilutions are commonly used by homeopaths to treat vocal nodules in adults and children. Their mother tinctures include arnica, arsenic, arum, belladonna, borax, capsicum, iodine, iron, nitric acid, phosphorus, spider venom, squid ink, sulphur, and zinc. In an industry that is erratically regulated around the world, these dilutions can be bought for home remediation from chemists, drugstores and retail pharmacies, where white-coated pharmacists, and uniformed, nurse-like sales assistants lend them an air of propriety, and a fresh feeling that you have walked onto the set of a mouthwash commercial (see pages 258–259). They are also available online, worldwide, from thousands of retailers and stockists.

There is no credible evidence that homeopathy is effective in treating vocal nodules, or *any* health condition in children (Altunc, Pittler, & Ernst, 2007) or adults (National Health and Medical Research Council, 2015). Because they are comprised of water, an excipient, medium or vehicle, and a miniscule mother tincture (if any is left), homeopathic dilutions are generally considered safe

– and something of a joke by various detractors – with a low risk of adverse side effects. But the inherent dangers (Posadzki, Alotaibi, & Ernst, 2012) are no laughing matter. Mother tinctures require safe storage away from children and pets as they may be highly toxic (e.g., if they contain arsenic, scorpion or snake venom, or strychnine), and some homeopathic remedies may contain unsafe substances that interfere with the effectiveness of other medicines.

Homeopaths are untrained in *diagnosing* voice problems, or indeed communication and swallowing disorders of any type; *eliminating* head and neck cancers, gastroesophageal reflux disease, HIV infections, and thyroid disease; *advising* properly on treatment; *referring* appropriately to mainstream professionals (though they may be pretty good at sending you to other CAM practitioners); or *providing* treatment. Once someone is convinced of the benefits or superiority of homeopathic fabrications over scientifically-based treatments, there are further risks in terms of disease control and prevention, and public health. For example, parents who have grown up with homeopathy or who are converts to it, may be swayed to give their children homeopathic "vaccinations" that offer false reassurance and no safeguards whatsoever from communicable, *preventable* killer diseases: diphtheria, measles, poliomyelitis, rubella, tetanus, tuberculosis and pertussis (whooping cough).

Language

Language has been called the symbolization of thought, and our most human characteristic. It is a learned code that lets us think about our world; generate, remember, share and understand information; appreciate knowledge, ideas, literature, science and the arts; enjoy leisure pastimes; express political and religious convictions, humour and emotion; reveal our personalities and needs; and survive in today's society. It is partly innate and partly learned. Infants have the inborn capacity to develop language and this potential is fostered as they grow and interact with the people who care for and communicate with them.

Language has two main "channels": receptive language: understanding speech, writing or gesture; and expressive language: speaking, writing or gesturing. Gestures range from simple actions, like nodding or shaking your head, or rolling your eyes to agree, disagree or emphasize a point, or miming drinking from a vessel, through to finger spelling, Amerind, MAKATON, and sophisticated sign language.

Language disorders[3] negatively influence any or all facets of receptive language, expressive language, or both, in all their forms. Toddlers and preschoolers may be "late talkers" with "delayed language development" (or not: McKean et al., 2015); older children from the age of about 4 or 5 may be diagnosed with Developmental Language Disorder (DLD) (for discussion see Bishop, 2014; Bishop, Snowling, Thompson, & Greenhalgh, 2016), also called Specific Language Impairment (SLI) (Rice, 2014); and school students may have significant language-related difficulties with literacy, impacting some combination of their phonemic awareness, phonics knowledge, reading fluency, reading comprehension, spelling accuracy, and written expression.

How reassuring it is to know from the Early Language in Victoria Study (ELVS) investigators (McKean et al., 2015) that 2-year-old "late talkers" can catch up, so that their language skills at age 5 are in parallel with those of children who produced more words at the age of 2. It is also helpful, though troubling, to know that McKean and colleagues found that late talkers who continued to have difficulties with language at 5 were likely to have memory skills that were less advanced.

Developmental Language Disorder (DLD)

Two jobs of the paediatric SLP/SLT are to assess, diagnose and treat *developmental language disorder (DLD)* and *reading difficulties* (see Chapter 9). Language intervention begins with a structured assessment protocol that combines a case history interview, information gathering, expert observations and standardized tests (if the child has the capacity to do them) and informal tests, administered in one, or over several sessions.

Assessment of younger children's language development may be quite quick, mainly comprising skilled observations, and objective comparisons with typical language development ("the norms" or "normative data"), with parents present throughout. The conclusion may be that the child is progressing typically, or confirmation that language development is delayed, or that the SLP/SLT diagnosis must wait until a "trial of therapy" or "watchful waiting" has

---

3 We use "language disorder" to refer to a profile of difficulties that interfere with everyday life activities, and which is associated with poor prognosis. "Developmental Language Disorder" (DLD) is used where language disorder is not associated with a known biomedical cause (aetiology). The presence of risk factors (biological or environmental factors with a weak statistical association with language disorder), however, does not rule out a diagnosis of DLD. DLD can co-occur with other neurodevelopmental disorders, and a DLD diagnosis does not require a discrepancy between verbal and nonverbal IQ.

occurred, or that there is more going on than language difficulties alone and that the child requires additional assessment (e.g., if ASD or ID are suspected).

Initial language assessment of school students can take one to four hours or more, and parents may or may not be present as participant-observers, while standardized and informal language tests are administered. Again, the results of testing may not lead to immediate, diagnosis. The SLP/SLT prepares a *comprehensible* written report (Leitão, Scarinci, & Koenig, 2015) with recommendations for treatment and possibly for further assessment. The report is discussed with parents, and the child where appropriate, and distributed at their discretion to other professionals (e.g., the child's teacher and GP). Assessment is ongoing as intervention proceeds, with the SLP/SLT probing at intervals in order to measure headway.

Intervention comprises evidence-based procedures to assist with the aspects of language that are difficult for the child. This may encompass work on comprehending spoken and written language, conversation skills (discourse and narrative), forming sentences (syntax), learning grammatical rules (morphology), inferring information, understanding figurative language and other literary devices, using pragmatic language skills, developing vocabulary (semantics), word retrieval skills, and written expression – in treatment sessions and also in everyday situations.

Some children with DLD benefit from special educational placements, such as the Moor House School and College in the UK for children and young people with speech and language difficulties. In that particular supportive environment, teachers and SLTs work collaboratively with care staff, teaching and SLT assistants, psychologists, literacy specialists, OTs, OT assistants, physiotherapists, and psychotherapists, to meet the needs of day pupils and boarders. Such specialist settings are rare and, unfortunately, most children with DLD must make do with resources mobilized in their school settings. These are highly variable and often short-term.

Language disorders and pseudoscience

Among the non-evidence-based, pseudoscientific "therapies" that parents of children with language disorders, including DLD, may encounter are bodywork, craniosacral therapy, holistic coaching, kinesiology, polarity therapy, reflexology, and Reiki. Two that stand out – not because they work but because SLPs/SLTs are often attracted to including them in their intervention repertoires – are Auditory Integration Therapies (e.g., Berard AIT, Johansen

Individualized Auditory Stimulation (JIAS): "sound therapy", The Listening Program®, Therapeutic Listening™, Tomatis®) and interventions targeting *executive function*, discussed in Chapters 8 and 3 respectively.

Specialist teachers and adequately qualified clinical and educational psychologists also have fundamental professional roles to play with children with *reading difficulties*, but it is not a job for passionate amateurs, and those dispensing gimmicky "methods" (e.g., the Arrowsmith Program™, BrainWoRx, Cellfield™, Interactive Metronome®, iLs Integrated Listening Systems, MNRI®, Primary Movement®, NOW!® Programs, or ReadingWise). Neither is it the job of tutor schools like Kip and Storm McGrath's KipOnline; self-appointed "reading experts" including behavioural optometrists, intrinsic touch therapists, neurofeedback therapists, and sound therapists; retired or moonlighting English or primary school teachers with rich experience but no specialist qualifications; or university students tutoring in subjects they were "good at" at school. Nor is it a suitable job for anyone in Whole Language or Reading Recovery™ blinkers (see pages 226–229 and 232–234), or advocating Xlens ("the original dyslexia colour filters"; www.xlens.com) or Irlen® lenses. Unlike "psychologist" which, by law, can only be used by appropriately qualified practitioners, there is nothing to stop any well-intentioned (or not) wannabe from hanging out a shingle as a so-called literacy expert.

Speech

As the spoken medium of language, speech is comprised of audible consonants and vowels (speech sounds or phones); their underlying representations in the mind (phonemes); syllables, words, phrases, sentences, narrative and discourse: all uttered with appropriate articulation, tones (in tonal languages like Cantonese, Hmong, Mandarin, Thai and Vietnamese), clicks (as in Gciriku, isiZulu and Xhosa) and prosody[4]. Typical speech acquisition is gradual, with predictable milestones. It encompasses five "levels" of function: anatomic or sensory, motoric, perceptual, phonetic and phonemic. Figure 7.1 is a simple depiction of how the levels relate to the four types of speech sound disorder (SSD): childhood apraxia of speech, the dysarthrias, articulation disorder, and phonological disorder.

Any, or all, of the five levels of breakdown can co-occur (e.g., a child can

---

4 Prosody: Variations in the duration of words and longer utterances, and the duration of pauses, increases and decreases in loudness, and the rise and fall of the pitch of the voice that are used to convey meaning and emotion.

have phonetic *and* phonemic *and* perceptual problems), and any, or all, of the four types of SSD can co-occur (e.g., a child can have CAS *and* phonological disorder) in varying degrees. SSD can co-occur with other communication disorders (e.g., articulation disorder *and* stuttering), and with other conditions (e.g., phonological disorder *and* ID).

1 Anatomic and sensory levels

The child's *anatomy* (body structure) and sensory systems must be adequate in order for speech and language to develop. Structural difficulties that can impact speech are ankyloglossia (a short lingual frenulum, often referred to as "tongue-tie"), cleft lip and palate, hearing impairment, dental malocclusion (misaligned teeth), and the head and neck characteristics that may be present in some syndromes. Ankyloglossia *can* cause articulation difficulties, but rarely. Cleft palate and more extensive facial differences, even after repair, may be associated with articulation and phonological disorders and, to complicate matters, children with craniofacial anomalies often have impaired hearing. *Sensory* difficulties include hearing impairment, and children with hearing impairment are prone to articulation and phonological disorders.

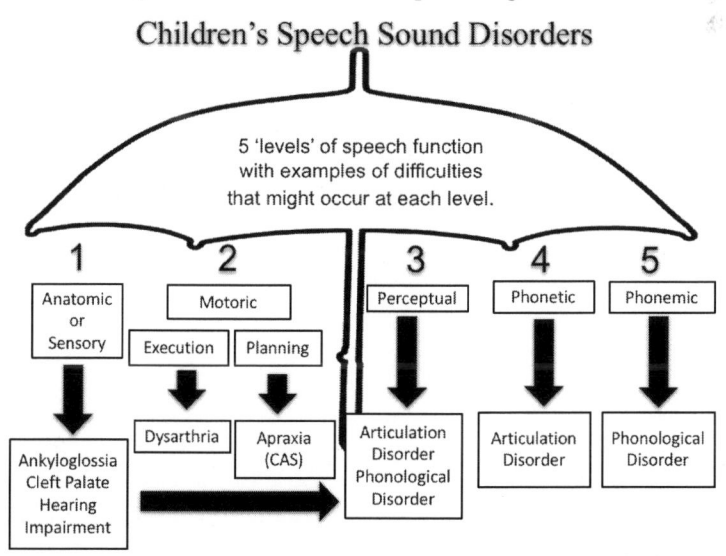

Figure 7.1 Five potential levels of breakdown underlying children's speech sound disorders (SSD).

2 Motoric levels

The *motoric* level entails motor *planning*: organizing, sequencing, integrating and producing speech movements; and motor *execution*: performing the required movements.

Motor planning

Childhood Apraxia of Speech (CAS) is a relatively rare, severe, lifelong SSD whose incidence is estimated to be less than 1% of a typical SLP/SLT child caseload. Children with CAS have difficulty planning and sequencing the movements required for speech, and difficulty with prosody. Most children with CAS have language difficulties in addition to their SSD, with a receptive-expressive gap. This means they comprehend language better than they can use it to express themselves. Despite the similar sounding name, CAS is a different disorder from Apraxia of Speech in adults (typically after a stroke), with different characteristics.

ASHA's preferred term is CAS, and their definition of it (ASHA, 2007a, b) subsumes apraxia of speech in children irrespective of the cause. By contrast, in 2011 the Royal College of Speech & Language Therapists officially adopted the term Developmental Verbal Dyspraxia: DVD (RCSLT, 2011). DVD refers *only* to children whose motor speech disorder is *idiopathic* or *functional*, having no currently known cause, and a distinction is made between these children and children who have apraxia of speech due to a *known* cause. "CAS" is now used in most professional literature to refer to apraxia of speech in children in all its manifestations, whether genetic, idiopathic, metabolic or traumatic in origin. So, when turning to journals for information about apraxia in children, it is important to know that, regrettably, the term "CAS" and "DVD" are not synonymous and cannot be used interchangeably.

Because children with CAS develop speech slowly, and because *speech* observations are an obligatory aspect of assessment, the challenging task of differentially diagnosing CAS is lengthy for the SLP/SLT, and frustrating for parents who, understandably, want answers. *Fortunately*, there are theoretically sound, child-friendly procedures that the therapist and family can employ if CAS is suspected but not confirmed. *Unfortunately*, the protracted diagnostic process, diagnostic uncertainty and use of the term "suspected CAS" (sCAS) can create an environment in which parents are prompted to search for definitive answers on the Internet – where it is easy to find operators who will "diagnose" and treat CAS on the basis of parents' replies to a handful of leading questions (in lieu of professional assessment), and their preparedness to pay. Furthermore, there are practitioners, including SLPs/SLTs, who will "diagnose" CAS in nonverbal children, particularly children on the autism spectrum, reasoning that the *absence of speech* is due to CAS – this, of course, is absurd.

Motor execution

"Dysarthria", or more accurately "the dysarthrias", denotes lifelong speech impairment due to neurological damage (e.g., in cerebral palsy and foetal alcohol spectrum disorder), or injuries (e.g., brain trauma due to traffic accidents), or conditions (e.g., Fragile-X syndrome, Friedreich's ataxia, neurofibromatosis, subacute sclerosing panencephalitis, and Wilson's disease: hepatolenticular degeneration), that affect the nerves and muscles involved in speaking. Mild, moderate or severe dysarthrias may be present in conditions like cerebral palsy, muscular dystrophy, or following acquired brain injury due to neonatal stroke, trauma, or brain infections. There is a prevalent misconception that individuals with Down syndrome (see pages 195–197) commonly have a dysarthria; they *may*, but only at the same rate as the general population (Rupela, Velleman, & Andrianopoulos, 2016). Five dysarthrias that can occur in children are the spastic, flaccid, ataxic, hyperkinetic, and mixed dysarthrias. Hypokinetic dysarthria predominates in Parkinson's disease in adults.

Generally-observed characteristics of childhood dysarthrias are: difficulties regulating the pitch of the voice; difficulties using appropriate intonation patterns to convey meaning; effortful speech due to breathing coordination difficulties; shallow breathing; excessively quiet or loud voice, or erratic variation between the two; imprecise articulation; slowed speech; slurred "unsteady" speech; and some combination of hoarse voice quality, hypernasal voice quality (excess nasal resonance), or breathy voice quality. Some children with dysarthria have dysphagia (eating difficulties; see pages 260–262), also requiring SLP/SLT assessment and management.

Intervention for the dysarthrias

Following detailed assessment (Skinder-Meredith, 2015), and screening for other difficulties, the SLP/SLT treatment for dysarthria (Hodge, 2010) may encompass compensatory activities to improve intelligibility, voice (pitch, quality and loudness) and prosody, while helping the child, if necessary, to: look at the person they are talking with, take a breath before speaking, slow down, speak in short utterances, and pause deliberately between utterances. The SLP/SLT collaborates within a team of medical and allied health professionals, and also works closely with family, school personnel, carers if applicable, and others, to help the child communicate more easily and effectively. Usual strategies are: giving the child feedback when parts of utterances are unclear and providing feedback for communicative success; asking the child to *show* their listener what they want (if words are unclear); and training communicative partners to stop and make time to listen actively and attentively.

In performing a Cochrane Review, Pennington, Parker, Kelly, and Miller (2016) were unable to locate randomized controlled trials (RCTs) or group studies of the effectiveness of speech and language therapy interventions to improve the speech of children with "early acquired" (before the 3rd birthday) dysarthria. Calling for rigorous, fully powered RCTs into any positive and generalizable changes wrought by SLP/SLT services, they concluded that, "Research should examine change in children's speech production and intelligibility. It must also investigate children's participation in social and educational activities, and their quality of life, as well as the cost and acceptability of interventions" (p. 8).

If a child is essentially nonverbal due to the severity of their dysarthria (with or without complicating factors like ID, hearing impairment, or ASD), or their intelligibility is severely impaired, the SLP/SLT may be able to provide support by initiating an individualized alternative and augmentative communication (AAC) system. Such systems, described in Chapter 6, can be high- or low-tech, taking in various combinations of gestures, signs and picture boards, through to electronic voice output devices. Among the independent AAC users who are famously successful communicators, and who have written about the lived experience of relying on communication devices, are UK theoretical physicist and cosmologist Stephen Hawking (Hawking, 2013), and South African web designer and developer Martin Pistorius (Pistorius, 2013).

3 Perceptual level

Difficulties at the perceptual level may account partly or entirely for articulation and phonological disorders in some children, whether or not they have normal hearing acuity. Numerous studies, implemented by Susan Rvachew and colleagues (reviewed by Rvachew & Brosseau-Lapré, 2012) demonstrate that many children with SSD cannot distinguish the phone (consonant or vowel) they need to say (e.g., /s/ in *symbol* or /ɹ/ in *rock*[5]) from their customary pronunciation (e.g., *thimble* and *wok*, in this example).

4 Phonetic level

The phonetic or articulation level is concerned with the motor act of producing phones, to ensure a repertoire of all the consonants and vowels needed in order to speak our language(s). An articulation disorder is an SSD affecting the phonetic level, in which the child has difficulty saying some consonants and/or vowels. The reason for this may be unknown (e.g., in children with articulation disorders with *no* serious problems with nerve-muscle function), or known (e.g., in children with a dysarthria who *have* serious problems with nerve-muscle function). Usually, children diagnosed with articulation disorder of unknown origin have difficulty with a small selection of sounds, and their speech is easy to understand. In English, commonly affected phones are [s] as in *see*, [z] as in *zoo*, [ɹ] as in *rye*, [l] as in *low*, [θ] as in *thaw* and [ð] as in *the*. Untreated, or unsuccessfully treated, articulation disorders can persist into adulthood, sometimes interfering with the acquisition of reading and of spelling rules.

5 Phonemic level

The phonemic or phonological level, in the mind, is responsible for the brainwork that goes into organizing speech sounds into patterns of sound contrasts. A child with a phonological disorder may be able to produce all sounds (i.e., the phonetic level is fine), but has difficulty organizing the system of contrasts. The sounds need to contrast with each other, or be distinct from one another, so that we can make sense when we talk. For example, if a child pronounced *sip, zip, ship, chip, tip, trip,* and *drip* homophonously as "dip", replacing every /s/, /z/, /ʃ/, /tʃ/, /t/, /tɹ/, and /dɹ/ with [d], their speech would make little sense. The phonemic or phonological level is sometimes called "the linguistic level", "a language level" or "a cognitive level", with some scholars thinking of phonological disorder, as we do, as a *language* disorder affecting speech. As in CAS, from a listener's perspective, the obvious feature

---

5 In phonetics, the upside-down-r, /ɹ/ denotes a voiced alveolar approximant, as in "rock", "rye", and "Kerry" while the right-way-up-r, /r/ signifies a voiced alveolar trill, or "rolled-r". The /r/ is found in Spanish, Russian and Italian, and in the English of some Scottish and Welsh speakers.

of phonological disorder is the child's poor intelligibility due to error patterns involving sound substitutions and/or syllable structure.

Substitution errors, also called systemic errors, might involve a pattern of exchanging the fricatives, displayed in the Place-Voice-Manner (PVM) Chart in Figure 7.2, with stops, so that the child produces *fun* as *pun*, *so* as *doe*, *shoe* as *do*, and *zip* as *dip*. This is a phonological pattern, or phonological process called stopping. Other substitution error patterns are fronting (e.g., *key* pronounced as *tea*, and *get* pronounced as *debt*), backing (e.g., *tea* pronounced as *key*, *debt* pronounced as *get*, gliding (*one* for *run*; *yet* for *let*), and pre-vocalic voicing (*bee* for *pea*, *do* for *two*, *ghee* for *key*). Syllable structure errors, or structural errors involve changes to syllables, as in final consonant deletion (*tie* for *time*), initial consonant deletion (*up* for *cup*), weak syllable deletion (*effant* for *elephant*) and cluster reduction (*boo* for *blue*). "Errors" like these are normal in young children, but are abnormal past certain (approximate) cut-off ages, shown in a series of four tables at www.speech-language-therapy.com.

Selecting an intervention approach

Ethical SLPs/SLTs do not knowingly implement a treatment unless they believe

PVM Chart: English			PLACE							
			LABIAL		CORONAL				DORSAL	
	MANNER	VOICING	Bilabial	Labiodental	Dental	Alveolar	Postalveolar	Palatal	Velar	Glottal
OBSTRUENTS	Stop	Voiceless	p			t			k	ʔ
		Voiced	b			d			g	
	Fricative	Voiceless		f	θ	s	ʃ			h
		Voiced		v	ð	z	ʒ			
	Affricate	Voiceless					tʃ			
		Voiced					dʒ			
SONORANTS	Nasal	Voiced	m			n			ŋ	
	LIQUID Lateral	Voiced				l				
	LIQUID Rhotic	Voiced						ɹ		
	Glide	Voiced	w					j	w	

Figure 7.2 English Place-Voice-Manner chart.

that it is going to work in the client's best interests. With this in mind, Clark (2003) discussed a two-question method that SLPs/SLTs might adopt when selecting an intervention. Question 1 is, "*Does* this therapy work; is it evidence-based?" To answer it, the clinician searches the scientific literature for answers – "proof", if you like. If evidence is not forthcoming, all is not lost. Not every important clinical question has been subjected to research interrogation, and the clinician can ask question 2, "*Should* this therapy work; is it theoretically sound?" and seek an understanding of how the intervention is *supposed* to work. For question 2 to succeed, the clinician must have a clear understanding of the therapeutic mechanism or "active ingredient" of the intervention, and consider its plausibility. Is the theoretical proposition credible, is it biologically plausible, and does it fit logically with the scientific knowledge-base; or is it mystical, pseudoscientific hot air, or just plain mad?

Interventions for speech sound disorders

There is a huge range of evidence-based and/or theoretically sound interventions that SLPs/SLTs can employ to work with children with SSD. Good outcomes can be expected in treatments for articulation and phonological disorders, administered as intended by those who devised and tested them, frequently enough and for long enough. Motor speech disorders persist for a lifetime. The dysarthrias can be treated by teaching compensatory strategies that enable more intelligible speech or, if that is not possible, by introducing AAC, or a combination of AAC and speech. Some children with CAS progress to the point that their speech is so "normal" that society (excluding SLPs/SLTs who are alert to subtle giveaway signs) would not suspect their early struggle to speak (Hennessy & Hennessy, 2013).

Effective interventions include:

- for ***articulation disorder***: some combination of Perceptually Based Intervention, Phonetic Intervention, and Auditory Input (Naturalistic) Intervention;

- for ***CAS***: Dynamic Temporal and Tactile Cueing, Integral Stimulation, Rapid Syllable Transition Training (ReST), and the Nuffield Centre Dyspraxia Programme; and

- for ***phonological disorder***: Core Vocabulary Therapy, the Cycles Phonological Patterns Approach, Imagery Therapy, Metaphon, Parents and Children Together (PACT), Phoneme Awareness

Intervention, Phonemic Intervention (Conventional Minimal Pairs, Multiple Oppositions, Maximal Oppositions and Empty Set, and Vowel Remediation), Psycholinguistic Intervention, and Stimulability Therapy.

All of these approaches are described in Bowen (2015) and Williams, McLeod, and McCauley (2010), and most of them in Rvachew and Brosseau-Lapré (2012; noting here that a second edition of this comprehensive work is expected in 2018). Among the popularly administered CAS treatments, Nancy Kaufman's approach is undergoing independent evaluation by researchers at the University of Sydney at the time of writing (July 2016), Deborah Hayden's PROMPT© approach is popular but supported by slim evidence, David Hammer's Multisensory Approach is theoretically sound but not currently evidence based, Margaret Fish's PRISM awaits evaluation, and the various oral motor therapies (NS-OME, NS-OMT, OPT from TalkTools®, etc.) have testimonial support only.

Articulation therapy/phonetic intervention, and perceptual intervention

Treatment for articulation disorder involves the phonetic (production) *and* perceptual (auditory discrimination) levels. Expertly guided by the clinician, a child with an articulation disorder learns to discriminate error from "target" – the correct sound – using perceptual techniques, and is shown how to produce the target correctly in terms of place, manner and voice, gradually replacing their error with the newly-introduced target, and stabilizing it in increasingly difficult contexts (sound-syllable-word-phrase-sentence-etc.) until they can use it all the time in everyday speech, without needing to concentrate unduly.

Phonological intervention/phonological therapy, and perceptual intervention

In treating phonological disorder, the SLP/SLT addresses phonemic *and* perceptual levels (*and* sometimes the phonetic level) basing activities on the expected system(s) of sound contrasts in the child's language(s). The activities are *conceptual* rather than motoric, and intervention has *generalization* as its ultimate goal, promoting intelligibility. Using word-pairs like the *minimal pairs*: rock-wok, car-tar, ship-sip and gown-down, and *near minimal pairs* like own-bone, bay-bait, blue-boo, and Bess-best, phonological approaches focus on teaching children the function of sounds; that *changing sounds changes meaning*; and making meaning (making sense) is needed for communication. For example, if you said, "The tar is on the road" when you meant, "The car is on the road", or "The twins are Kerry and Donnie" when their names are Kelly and Johnny, you may confuse your listener. In other words, /k/ in car and /t/ in tar; /l/ in Kelly and /ɹ/ Kerry; and /dʒ/ in Johnny and /d/ in Donnie must contrast, or be distinct from each other.

Intervention for childhood apraxia of speech

Intervention for CAS happens at the *motoric level*. The therapist devises activities based on the *principles of motor learning* (Schmidt & Lee, 2011), and maximizes *intensive* client-specific *motor drill* in therapy sessions and for homework, with practice distributed across activities, settings and situations. All children with CAS will require "speech work" at the phonetic level too, and a large proportion need work at the perceptual and phonological levels, *and* intervention to address prosodic difficulties and the receptive-expressive language gap. Many also need help with literacy. The speech aspect of the therapy has *habituation*, and then *automaticity* as its ultimate goal, promoting intelligibility.

Speech sound disorders and pseudoscience

Unscientific treatments for SSD occupy two categories: those that few SLPs/SLTs would consider touching with a barge pole, such as the Apraxia VML Method, and Kill Your Lisp; and those that many SLPs/SLTs embrace enthusiastically and defend, like oral motor therapies and Speech Buddies™, in spite of what the evidence says, and does not say, about them.

Apraxia Verbal Motor Learning Method (VML)

Elad Vashdi has held a Bachelor degree in physiotherapy since 2000 and a Masters in physical education since 2004 from Israeli institutions, and in 2009 was awarded the degree of Doctor of Physical Therapy Entry Level from Nova Southeastern University in Florida, genuinely affording him the title "Dr". But, Nova Southeastern University's 'Entry Level DPT Programs Essential Functions Policy for Admission, Retention, and Graduation' document (www.healthsciences.nova.edu/pt/forms/nsu-dpt-essential-functions.pdf), and the web page: www.apta.org/PostprofessionalDegree/TransitionDPTFAQs from the American Physical Therapy Association reveal that Dr Vashdi is as qualified to practise SLP/SLT as we are to practise physiotherapy. That is, he is *not* qualified to assess, diagnose or treat communication disorders. Calling VML "speech therapy", and a "complete tool to treat CAS" is misleading, but it would be mischievous of us to suggest that you need to *be* a "complete tool to treat CAS" with VML.

Since 1996 (when he embarked on his first degree) Dr Vashdi has provided "private treatments for children with developmental disorders, especially with autism and apraxia of speech". Since 2004, when he was doing his physical education degree, he has lectured on "speech and motor treatment"; and since 2005 has presented papers on "motor speech therapy" at conferences. He says, "The method was built out of field work with autistic children on speech via motor learning principles and touching techniques" and that "hundreds of children" have been treated using the method.

Three YouTube™ (www.youtube) videos of Dr Vashdi working with children are available. The children in the first and third video are engaged and cooperative, and Dr Vashdi has an agreeable, affectionate way of interacting with them, praising and encouraging them in a manner they plainly enjoy. The child in the second video is unresponsive. If the videos represent a fair summation of VML – and why else would Elad Vashdi have posted them to YouTube™ – then it is clear that it meets none of the basic requirements for a CAS treatment (ASHA, 2007a).

The first video, *The VML Method – treating apraxia of speech* shows "sensory techniques" where Dr Vashdi rhythmically presses and stretches the child's lower face and neck while singing *Twinkle, Twinkle Little Star* to her; "breath control" where adult and child share a whistle, a horn, and presumably spit, taking turns to blow; and the child attempts to extinguish a candle with a voiceless bilabial trill ("horse blow"). She is urged to produce approximations of "mummy", "oo", "boat", "bowl" and "bow", and attempts to pop soap bubbles blown by Dr Vashdi with a little stick, and "catches" a small balloon thrown by him, in activities aimed at producing /b/. Then, /g/ is targeted in the word "go": Dr Vashdi squeezes the child's neck and cheeks, and depresses her tongue with toothbrush bristles. Finally, her face is manipulated to produce an unintelligible approximation of "open".

In the second video: *Blowing techniques and speech the VML method*, Dr Vashdi is seen utilizing whistle-, balloon- and candle-blowing, ostensibly to facilitate production of voiceless consonants. The rationale for the activities is explained in a narration that is superficially plausible, but wrongheaded. It ends with text reading, "AFTER SIX MONTHS OF PRACTISING DAILY IT WORKED!!!!!" showing the indifferent child blowing (at nothing) with tactile prompts, while having his nostrils occluded manually by Dr Vashdi, "AND THEN THE NON VOICED CONSONANTS STARTED TO APPEAR", and no further footage.

In the third video, *Vowels techniques – the VML method for childhood apraxia of speech*, Dr Vashdi engages with a cooperative, typically developing "child actor" aged about 9, to imitate, with tactile and verbal prompts, "ah" (amidst boyish giggles and splutters), "or", "buh", "oo", "ee", "ee" in quick sequences while Dr Vashdi presses the boy's tummy with a gentle but sharp pumping action (more chuckles from the child actor), and finally "eh".

Neither communicatively impaired child receiving VML has *any* spontaneous speech, so for them a CAS diagnosis is impossible. The limited observations the videos allow suggest that the nonverbal girl of about 9 has a dysarthria, and the nonverbal boy of about 8 is on the autism spectrum, with little or no communicative intent. In terms of the principles of motor learning, the manoeuvres in the videos are pointless and unrelated to functional communication goals, and the written material on VML is a jumble of buzz words that make no scientific sense. So, why include VML here? Surely people would check credentials, read the technical data, get the picture, and dismiss VML as so much (probably well-meant) hocus-pocus. After all, the Childhood Apraxia of Speech Association of North America (CASANA) sensibly rejected Dr Vashdi's submission to their July 2015 national conference in San Antonio.

Inexplicably, many SLPs/SLTs appear to lend Dr Vashdi, VML, and his MDT method (Multi-Disciplinary Collaboration in Treatment of Children with Severe Developmental Delay) unmerited credibility. Take the California Speech-Language-Hearing Association. At its March 2015 Annual Convention in Long Beach, Elad Vashdi gave a 90-minute presentation and a poster session on "The Correlation between NSOME and Speech Production in CAS Population, a Wide Clinical Retrospective Research" and a 90-minute presentation on MDT. The previous November he presented on CAS at the 2014 ASHA Convention in Orlando. At the 2015 ASHA Convention in Denver he presented a poster: "The MDT Method: A New Integrative Framework for Multidisciplinary Collaboration in Treatment of Children with Autism". Augmenting his perceived credibility, he is associated with two speech pathology practices in Melbourne, Australia, and a certified member of Speech Pathology Australia has contributed a lavish online testimonial endorsing VML and

MDT. With followings in Australia, Israel, Poland and the US, and implicit support from the world's largest SLP/SLT professional association, Dr Vashdi is one to keep an eye on.

Kill Your Lisp

Ari Kreitberg (real name Arjun Lal) is the brains behind the Kill Your Lisp enterprise. His site (www.killyourspeechlisp.com: "eliminate your lisp in just minutes") has a list headed, "Here's what you DON'T need". An identical list appears on Mr Lal's Kill Your Stutter site (www.killyourstutter.com: "eliminate your stuttering in under ten minutes"). The websites are awful enough to be funny for an SLP/SLT in the right mood, but not funny for parents who shell out $US97.00 downloading either product. This is the list: "…

- You do NOT need to spend upwards of $50 per hour – The rate of the average speech therapist!
- You do NOT need to spend time researching or doing things you don't like – I'd rather be spending my precious time with my family or pets!
- You do NOT need to wait for the results to come…it starts working instantly as you go through the technique!
- You do NOT need to be out in the open practicing talking to people to make this work, it can be done from the privacy of your home
- You do NOT need to spend energy using 'will power' to control your speech consciously, there is a scientific reason why people Lisp, and you'll learn how to stop it for good"

Long story short: *here's* what you possibly don't need: "Kill Your Lisp" (and "Kill Your Stutter").

Mouth exercises

Non-speech oral motor treatments (NS-OMT) go by various names and acronyms: Non-Speech Oral Motor Therapy (NS-OMT), Non-speech Oral Motor Exercises (NS-OME), Non-speech Oral Motor Movement (NSOM), Oral Placement Therapy (OPT), Oro-Motor Work, Oral-motor Therapy, and more. As a profession, SLP/SLT prides itself on good communication, and this is generally associated with collegial relationships. So, the debate and polarized standpoints among clinical SLPs/SLTs (e.g., some members of the American Academy of Private Practice in Speech Pathology and Audiology (AAPPSPA), and some academics) and parent-groups, regarding NS-OMT in the treatment of SSD, are noteworthy. In the mix is a considered systematic review (Lee & Gibbon, 2015) and a position paper (McCauley et al., 2009) cautioning that the evidence "for" and "against" is equivocal; and ringing endorsements of Oral-motor Therapy, OPT, Oral-motor Therapy plus OPT, and Myofunctional therapy in an undated position statement authorized by AAPPSPA (www.aappspa.org/documents/AAPPSPA-Oral-Motor-Position-Statement.pdf) and posted to its website in 2015.

Like Lee and Gibbon, and McCauley and colleagues, respected speech researcher at the University of Wisconsin–Madison, Dr Ray D. Kent, is remarkably calm amid the furore. Looking beyond SSD, he is at pains to thwart a premature burial of nonspeech motor tasks for the assessment or treatment of various disorders, believing that outright rejection of these techniques might constrain innovations in clinical practice. Nevertheless, in his welcome narrative review (Kent, 2015, p. 773), he writes, "The preponderance of the evidence does not support the use of NSOM tasks in treating developmental speech sound disorders".

NSOM tasks are embedded in the TalkTools® company's OPT for children with "oral placement disorder", which has not yet been verified as a diagnostic entity. NS-OME and NSOM tasks (not necessarily under the TalkTools® aegis) are used routinely and with good intent by SLPs/SLTs, with children with anatomic sensory, motoric, perceptual, phonetic and phonemic bases for their SSDs. Within that, they are used a *lot* in the management of children with clefts, ID (particularly with children with Down syndrome), and ASD.

The tentacles of NS-OME commerce are prominent on the Internet, in print catalogues, conference trade displays, and CPD events. A seemingly endless range of NS-OME "tools and toys" to suck, blow, chew or wear includes Blow Pens, Bubble Trumpets, Bumpy-Q's, "Dentist-Designed Chewy Fidgets", Frog Whistles, "fashionable chew pendants" (military-style dog-tags for "older students"), straws and horns, Tough Bar Chew Stixx, Z-Vibes and Zipper-Pull Chew Tubes. They are marketed to behaviour analysts, OTs, parents, special educators, and SLPs/SLTs. They festoon clinics, classrooms and university departments worldwide; and quite shockingly, in our *direct* experience, can be found in SLP/SLT workplaces in Australia, Brunei, Canada, Denmark, England, Hong Kong, Indonesia, Ireland, Malaysia, New Zealand, Northern Ireland, Norway, the Philippines, Portugal, Singapore, South Africa, Turkey and the US.

Six rationales for NS-OME and NSOM are generally put forward, namely that they will:

1. *Increase the range, accuracy, strength and speed of oral movements.* Problems: because the exercises are performed outside the context of speech, they cannot impact range, accuracy, and speed; and we do not need strength for speech. Even if we did, the exercises would not "strengthen" because they are not done often enough or against resistance.

2. *Develop voluntary control of oral movements.* Problem: practising non-speech movements cannot transfer to speech movements, as there are differences in nervous system organization for non-speech versus speech movements.

3. *Develop awareness of oral structures.* Problem: no evidence suggests they affect oral awareness.

4. *Develop motor programs underlying specific features of speech sounds.* Problem: the "broken down" bits that oral motor exercises represent will not automatically integrate into speech behaviours. Highly integrated motor tasks must be taught as a whole, not in segregated parts.

5. *Stimulate speech development.* Problem: the evidence shows that non-speech behaviours are not a precursor to later speech learning, so they are not a "foundation" for speech.

6. *Provide a non-threatening way in to therapy for children wary of direct speech work.* Problem: no evidence supports their use in terms of speech outcomes, even for "oral awareness" training (see 3 above). "Warm up drills" *may* be constructive in creating a "fun start" to a therapy session, keeping a child engaged and attentive, but that is as far as it goes.

As Gregory Lof is fond of saying (e.g., Lof, 2011): to improve speech, work on speech.

Speech Buddies™

For $US299.00 you can own the Speech Buddies™ Set, promoted to parents and SLPs/SLTs as "five tools that fix the R, S, SH, CH and L sounds" (sic), packaged in a metal box. Described as an "Exerciser, Non-Measuring" a Speech Buddy is a removable speech appliance used to position the tongue to produce a sound in need of remediation. Instruction manuals and video demonstrations for the five phones are available to download, free, on the Speech Buddies™ website (www.speechbuddy.com), where it reads, "Our clinically-proven practice tools work nearly twice as fast and our speech therapists are the best in the nation" alongside claims as to their efficacy, effects, efficiency and effectiveness (the Buddies', not the speech therapists'). In the explanation for how Speech Buddies™ work, we find "they train the tongue to make the correct shape by providing targets that you can feel". While it is possible that removable appliances might help with phonetic placement, *one aspect* of articulation therapy, with some experimental support for this view, there are three major difficulties with the products other than the odious "hard sell" and reliance on exaggerated testimonials.

First, none of the "evidence" is peer reviewed, even though it says on the site: "Speech Buddies™ have helped patients age four and older with: speech and articulation disorders of all severities and several types, including hearing impairment (with or without cochlear implants), autism spectrum disorder, or no known cause; childhood apraxia of speech; acquired apraxia of speech from stroke or traumatic brain injury (TBI); accent modification where English sounds are misarticulated due to a foreign accent. Speech Buddies™ are still being evaluated for: speech and articulation disorders associated with neuromuscular weakness, cerebral palsy, paralysis, Down syndrome and post-surgical cleft palate." Second, the treatment programme includes no speech perception element, and we know from Rvachew and Brosseau-Lapré's (2012) review that, for many children, for articulation therapy to be effective there must be a perceptual (listening) component. Third, the tools are marketed to parents who, unless they are SLPs/SLTs themselves, are not competent to diagnose the nature of their child's communication disorder.

Fluency

Fluency refers to the smoothness or flow of speech, and the ease with which a child "gets words out". Stuttering, called "stammering" in the UK, is a fluency disorder. Since stuttering disrupts fluency of speech, "stutters" are referred to as "dysfluencies" or "nonfluencies". Stuttered speech is characterized by prolongations and repetitions of sounds, syllables, words or phrases, and "stuttering blocks" when sound ceases as children who stutter try to initiate speech or continue speaking. Additional verbal and nonverbal features (secondary behaviours) may be present: little noises like creaks and squeaks, grunts, filler-words (ah, and, err, I-I-I, uh, um), and unplanned pauses, facial grimaces, blinking and screwing up the eyes, head bobbing and jerking, other body movements, and obvious struggle to speak. These interruptions may be present, consistently or variably, and all children who stutter require *in-person* assessment by an SLP/SLT. Mercifully, a related *fluency and rate* disorder, cluttering, appears not to have caught the eye of fad and CAM practitioners. In cluttering, speech is uttered in abnormally rapid and/or irregular bursts, with some combination of atypical syntax, word use, and excessive co-articulation of sounds, particularly in words of two syllables or more. Words tumble out on top of each other, and the speaker usually appears unaware that this is happening.

Treating stuttering

Treatment for stuttering (Logan, 2014) takes at least three forms. First, there are therapist-guided-parent-administered, or therapist-administered, direct treatments such as the Lidcombe Program for children (O'Brian et al., 2013) and the Camperdown Program for adolescents (Carey, O'Brian, Lowe, & Onslow, 2014). Second, indirect treatments – yielding limited effects – in which an SLP/SLT ensures that "the environment" (parents and teachers) is "managed" to create conditions believed to promote fluency, with the child excluded from the therapeutic contact. And third, there are interventions that combine indirect and direct methodologies, such as the RESTART Demands and Capacities method (RESTART-DCM) (de Sonneville-Koedoot, Stolk, Rietveld, & Franken, 2015), and Palin Parent-Child Interaction Therapy (PCI) (Millard, Nicholas, & Cook, 2008).

Not so long ago, parents of children who stuttered were told that they were part of "the cause" of stuttering, and/or to "ignore it and it will go away", amidst warnings that drawing attention to stuttering would make it worse or make it "stick". We now know that was terrible advice. The Lidcombe, Camperdown, RESTART-DCM, and PCI approaches, all of which have been found through rigorous research to be effective, developed in environments which recognized that: genetic factors underlie stuttering; stuttering is fundamentally different from the normal period of dysfluency experienced by many preschoolers; children who stutter have less capacity for fluent speech than children who do not stutter; and that there is evidence that stuttering can be reduced by (appropriately) calling attention to it.

Fluency disorders in children, and pseudoscience

Most disreputable fluency interventions are spruiked to adults who stutter, and not to parents. But there are several to avoid. We have already introduced

Arjun Lal ("Ari Kreitberg") of Kill Your Lisp and Kill Your Stutter notoriety, so we will not waste words. The whole situation can be summed up with "buyer beware" – or, referring to Mr Lal's style guide: **BUYER BEWARE** (CAPS, **boldface**, underline, *italics*) – and "where is the evidence?" The same applies to Dr Baker (www.askdrbob.org); Dr Vasilka Yurukova, MD (www.homeopathytoday.net) and her homeopathic dilutions of belladonna, causticum, cuprum metallicum, mercurius solubilis, and stramonium; and the Anna Deeter program, *Etalon* (www.livestutterfree.com). Ms Deeter styles herself as the ETALON WISDOM KEEPER (her caps) and she and her chums ask for $US6000–$8000 to sign up for "Skype Treatment". In short, if you see the words Etalon, Anna Deeter or Dr Roman Snezhko, look away. Finally, neither the McGuire Program (www.mcguireprogramme.com) nor McGuire Speech Helper Software are evidence-based.

Down syndrome

The communication abilities of children and adults with Down syndrome (Ds) represent a confluence of most communication disorders addressed by SLPs/SLTs, because a single individual with Ds can have some, or even *all*, of the following characteristics.

> *Babbling*: While infants with Ds often babble on par with typically developing (TD) babies, the onset of their speech is often, but not inevitably, delayed.
>
> *Language*: As a child with Ds grows older, the gap in language acquisition progressively widens between theirs and that of TD peers. Word retrieval difficulties are common.
>
> *Speech*: Intelligibility difficulties are more marked in Ds than in other groups of individuals with ID. Speech comprehensibility may be impacted by limitations in expressive syntax, pragmatics, and "listener experience": i.e., unfamiliar listeners have more trouble decoding the speech of a person with Ds than do familiar listeners; you might easily understand your brother with Ds, but not your friend's sister with Ds. Motor Speech Disorder Not Otherwise Specified (MSD-NOS) (Shriberg, Potter, & Strand, 2011), often mistaken for a dysarthria (Rupela et al., 2016), may be present, giving speech an imprecise quality.

Consistency: Individuals with Ds tend to make variable speech errors. The same word may be pronounced several ways, even within the same conversation (e.g., "stop" pronounced as *stop, sop, top, dop, doh* and *op*) in what is called token-to-token inconsistency.

Speech rate: It is common for individuals with Ds to have a rapid rate of speech, possibly due to poor breath control and a decreased ability to sustain phonation (due to running out of breath).

Auditory processing: People with Ds may have difficulties processing information presented auditorily. It is thought they may *also* have a specific sequential processing problem, leading to difficulty remembering and reproducing information they see and hear in the correct order.

Hearing: About 80% of individuals with Ds experience otitis media (middle ear infections) with effusion (glue ear), and there is a high incidence of sensorineural hearing loss ("nerve deafness").

Anatomy: Many have small, narrow external ear canals, narrow, more horizontal eustachian tubes (the small drain and pressure-equalizing tubes running from the middle ear to the oro-pharynx), a small nasopharynx, and large tonsils and adenoids. They may have a small oral cavity, narrow palate, and less and/or different oral musculature, resulting, for example, in difficulty with lip rounding.

Anxiety: It is common for individuals with Ds to be anxious about speaking.

Fluency: 45–53% stutter, and many clutter.

Prosody: Difficulties with stress and phrasing may be present.

Resonance: Voices may be hypernasal with excess air escaping through the nose during speech.

Voice quality: The person's voice may be chronically hoarse or breathy.

Speech intervention and children with Down syndrome

Because children with Ds have speech errors characteristic of the speech of younger TD children, SLPs/SLTs employ assessment procedures that they would use for any child-speech intelligibility issues. They consider all the contributing factors affecting speech, including hearing, motor speech and anatomic differences, and auditory perceptual, cognitive and language abilities. The clinician establishes the child's word production consistency, analyzes error patterns and vowel production, and evaluates consonant stimulability to 2 syllable positions, and vowel stimulability (stimulability is the child's ability to produce phones if they are given support). Prosodic characteristics are observed and recorded, and MSD-NOS and dysarthria ruled in or out.

Integrated therapy (combining speech, literacy/phonological awareness, and language) is highly desirable. Intervention includes Phonemic Intervention to eliminate error patterns, Core Vocabulary Therapy to target consistency of word production, and Naturalistic Intervention that includes recasting for speech *and* grammar. Visual supports are emphasized: e.g., signs; gestural, tactile, written and pictorial cues. There is a focus on *meaningful, functional* practice across a range of settings to promote generalization; a slowed down rate of speech is encouraged, e.g., using quiet finger pacing; and a core vocabulary is developed of "important" and "powerful" words that they can use effectively to "make things happen" in real life.

Adopting a lifelong learning approach, the SLP/SLT may train conversational partners and support parents to use strategies taught in therapy sessions. Although children and young people with Ds may have complex speech production issues, with focused intervention and meaningful encouragement they can make improvements which will benefit their intelligibility, language and, in many cases, literacy, and improve their social functioning and quality of life.

Children with Down syndrome, and pseudoscience

The parents and grandparents of babies and children with Ds have become magnets for unscrupulous, or perhaps in some cases, poorly-informed, gullible but well-intentioned providers of fad interventions. This much-plagiarized excerpt comes, unedited, from the Ds "what we do" section of a randomly-selected SLP/SLT website: "**Oral-motor/feeding and swallowing therapy**: The SLP will use a variety of oral exercises – including facial massage and various tongue, lip, and jaw exercises – to strengthen the muscles of the mouth. The SLP also may work with different food textures and temperatures to increase a child's oral awareness during eating and swallowing." If you read the section on mouth exercises (pages 191–192) you will understand why that captured our attention. It sounds so scientific, but it is not.

Web searches for strings such as down+syndrome+alternative+medicine, down+syndrome+chiropractic, down+syndrome+holistic, down+syndrome+homeopathy, down+syndrome+oral+motor, down+syndrome+shichida, exhume plenty of interventions with shady credentials. Then again, searches with other strings will unearth gems for parents like *Talk Down Syndrome*: www.talk-ds.org from Jennifer J. Bekins It makes you smile.

8 Auditory processing and learning

Language is a *two-channel* process. Whether we are using signed, spoken or written words, we must consider both *input* as well as *output* channels, as effective communication relies on both. When a child has difficulties in the expressive language domain, it is often obvious to parents, teachers, and peers because they are comparatively reticent and give shorter, less elaborate responses. They may also take pains to avoid speaking under more demanding circumstances at school, such as Show'n'Tell in the early years, or in debating teams in the later years. Receptive language difficulties are not always as obvious, and are easily missed or misinterpreted by parents, teachers, and other professionals. Children with receptive language difficulties may appear inattentive, but closer examination often reveals that they are processing ("taking in") just parts of the speaker's message. So for example, when a teacher says to the class, "After you get your reader out of your bag, put your pencils away and then sit on the floor", Kim, aged 8, who has a Developmental Language Disorder (DLD), hears the nouns *reader, bag, pencils* and *floor*, but is unable to process prepositions or subordinating conjunctions (*after* and *then*) to determine that there is a sequence to follow, and what that sequence involves. The Kims of the world do their utmost in these situations, probably getting their readers out and sitting on the floor, hoping for the best, but missing the pencils step altogether. A concerned teacher tells Kim's parents that significant work needs to be done to improve her concentration. Phrases like "off in her own little world" and "needs to improve her listening", with feedback that Kim's reading progress is slow, leave her parents anxious and concerned that her learning is compromised, and wondering if they need to supplement the school's efforts.

Exploring acronymsЯus territory on the Web, they start to wonder whether Kim has an auditory processing disorder (APD) or a so-called central auditory processing disorder (CAPD, or (C)APD) in addition to the receptive language disorder diagnosed by her SLP/SLT. Or perhaps she does not have a receptive language disorder at all; perhaps the *real* problem is just the APD. Fix that, and her language skills will improve. But wait! Her teacher repeatedly mentions Kim's inattention; so might she actually have ADHD? Could this be in addition to one of the other two problems, or is it a stand-alone diagnosis that accounts for both her inattentiveness and her learning difficulties? Clicking through to more web pages, they ponder whether Kim's problem is weak working memory capacity. Overwhelmed? So are Kim's parents. The chaotic diagnostic landscape and the range of interventions they find generate more questions than answers. A plethora of neurosciencey-sounding programmes they discover all make big promises, supported by glowing testimonials, and some are described as "research-backed". It all sounds too good to be true, and Kim's discerning parents are thinking, "Snake oil?"

In this chapter, we consider some well-oiled examples, and try to unpack the evidence behind their claims. Before doing so, however, we thread ourselves through the eye of a needle and consider some contested and confusing territory regarding the basis of children's auditory processing and comprehension difficulties.

Although as professionals we have long known that debated diagnostic frameworks exist in relation to developmental disorders, this has been accentuated for us while writing this book, with parents' perspectives front of mind. It is one thing for professionals to know the historical basis of different diagnoses and classification systems. We are accustomed to academic debate and can immerse ourselves in interesting theoretical nuances and tussles, understanding that these are generally conducted in the interests of advancing knowledge and (ultimately) clinical practice. For parents, there is no luxuriating in theoretical navel-gazing. Parents want to know what the various disorders are, what they mean, how they are diagnosed and, most importantly, what can be done about them, and the long-term consequences, if any. Sadly, (central) auditory processing disorder (CAPD, (C)APD, or APD) will be among the least navigable terrains for parents, because different professional stakeholders still make a meal of it between themselves. We try to provide a map and satnav system to help you find your way (you may need a packed lunch, too). First though, we need to consider what auditory processing is and how it works.

Auditory processing: What is it and how does it work?

In Chapter 3, we emphasize that focusing and maintaining attention requires a complex set of skills that develop over many years. *Attentional* skills allow us to determine what information coming in via the senses is important ("salient") and what is background, less important, and in need of filtering. *Working memory* enables the temporary storage and manipulation of incoming information from the senses, to support – dynamically – ongoing cognitive activity. Everyday information that a child needs to process, both for social

Auditory processing and learning 201

Auditory Cortex

Cochlea

Brainstem

Sounds are recognized and processed in the auditory cortex

↳ Sound signals are decoded as they travel through the brain

↳ Sound is passed from the cochlea to the brainstem via the auditory nerve

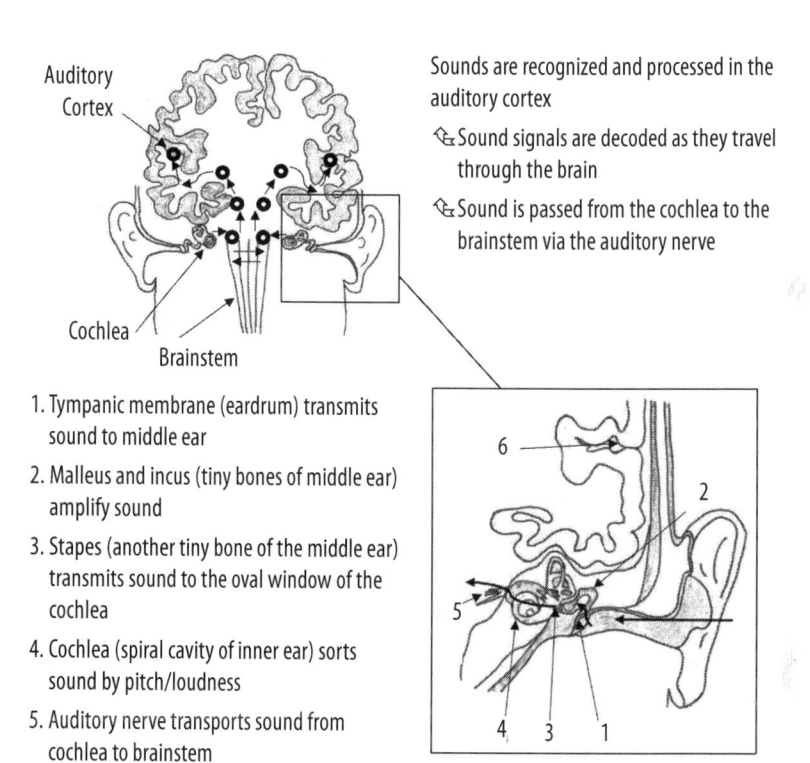

1. Tympanic membrane (eardrum) transmits sound to middle ear
2. Malleus and incus (tiny bones of middle ear) amplify sound
3. Stapes (another tiny bone of the middle ear) transmits sound to the oval window of the cochlea
4. Cochlea (spiral cavity of inner ear) sorts sound by pitch/loudness
5. Auditory nerve transports sound from cochlea to brainstem
6. Auditory cortex

Figure 8.1 The auditory mechanism. Emina McLean

and emotional purposes and for academic success, reaches his or her brain via the auditory-verbal channel; by listening to speech. We need to consider, then, how this information reaches, and is used by, the brain.

Figure 8.1 (above) is a view of the left ear and part of a human head in a coronal section – i.e., as if sliced through the centre, from left-to-right, looking from the front. Broadly, the auditory mechanism has three components: the external, middle, and inner ears, and these roughly correspond to three different systems for transmitting sound: air conduction, mechanical energy, and electrical energy. As Figure 8.1 shows, sound enters the external auditory canal, and travels to the tympanic membrane (eardrum), a taut disc of tissue that reverberates in response to sound, in order to transmit sound-waves into the middle ear. The tympanic membrane is linked to the shell-like cochlear mechanism (in the inner ear) via the three smallest bones in the human body (so tiny, that they would all fit on an adult thumbnail), the ossicles. The ossicles receive sound waves from the reverberating tympanic membrane and direct them to the cochlea.

The cochlea's hair cells transmit what is now an electrical signal to the eighth cranial nerve or "auditory nerve", via which messages are relayed to the auditory regions of the cerebral cortex (in the temporal lobes of both cerebral hemispheres), via important nuclei in the midbrain (the upper part of the brainstem) and the thalamus. The thalamus is a central relay station through which all sensory information from the outside world passes before being directed to specialized regions of the cortex for further analysis, synthesis and integration. These cortical processes support phonological awareness, working memory, and lexical (word) storage and meanings, among many other brain functions. An important distinction the human brain must make in this process is between speech and non-speech sounds, as these are processed by different regions of the brain.

Under typical circumstances, this all happens in milliseconds, without conscious effort or control. Auditory pathways become more refined and better at transmitting signals in the same way that all neural pathways become refined – with repeated firing as a result of environmental exposure and practice. Ideally, such exposure is graduated in terms of amount and complexity, both of which increase incrementally from infancy, through toddlerhood, early childhood, and beyond. We only become aware of the workings of the auditory system when its function is impaired, e.g., due to a middle ear infection (otitis media), when hearing deteriorates with age, or when we battle to communicate against background noise. We are also given pause for thought on the workings of the auditory system when we meet children who, despite normal hearing tests (audiometry and measures of middle ear function such as tympanometry), struggle to make full sense and use of incoming auditory-verbal information (speech) and/or are unusually bothered by noise, whether speech or other environmental sounds.

Receptive language difficulties

In Chapter 7, we discuss receptive language difficulties – problems with verbal comprehension that are not explained on the grounds of hearing impairment. They are typically diagnosed by an SLP/SLT, following assessment by a clinical audiologist, on the basis of careful history taking and administration, scoring, and interpretation of standardized language measures. Receptive language difficulties typically occur in conjunction with expressive language difficulties; however, their presence can go undetected or be misdiagnosed/misattributed (e.g., to distractibility, lack of interest, and poor motivation). Because of the intrinsic links between oral language skills and the transition to literacy, children with receptive language difficulties will invariably experience reading difficulties too, chiefly in the comprehension domain, though it should not be assumed that decoding skills will be spared (see Chapter 9).

Auditory processing difficulties

Predictably, there is considerable overlap between the types of interventions offered for children with reading difficulties and those that are offered for children with receptive language difficulties, some of whom will be said to have auditory processing difficulties. The idea that language comprehension difficulties may have their roots in underlying auditory perceptual difficulties (reflecting dysfunction somewhere between the cochlea and the brain: see Figure 8.1) was first mooted in 1954 by psychologist Dr Helmer Myklebust (b. 1910 d. 2008). He proposed a distinction between children whose comprehension difficulties were *language based* (reflecting problems with the phonological, semantic, syntactic, morphological systems) and those whose difficulties were *perceptually* based (reflecting a breakdown in the physiological processes supporting transmission of speech sounds to the cerebral cortex). This idea was superficially attractive (like so many things in the developmental disability field) because, if right, it suggested that different subgroups of children would benefit from different intervention approaches. Some would require *language-*based interventions to support, for example, phonemic awareness, vocabulary, syntax, and narrative skill development, while others would need assistance with the *perceptual* aspects of interpreting incoming speech signals, e.g., dealing with changes in the rate of incoming signals, the time that elapses between them, their pitch (frequency) and volume, and the presence of competing background noise.

In the 1970s and 1980s, the term Central Auditory Processing Disorder (CAPD) became prominent in the academic literature, fast gaining traction in the international audiological community in particular, although it was also eagerly adopted by some in the SLP/SLT and educational psychology communities. The term "central" was used to emphasize the presence of breakdown in the relaying and interpretation of acoustic features of incoming speech signals once they left the cochlea. Over time, however, the descriptor "central" was gradually dropped, so now the literature predominantly refers to APD.

So, thinking some more about 8-year-old Kim, it is easy to see why a child who has trouble following run-of-the-mill instructions, appears to be easily overwhelmed by routine information-processing requirements, and struggles to learn to read, will create diagnostic dilemmas. Does Kim have an APD? A developmental language disorder? ADHD? Is APD a "bottom-up" way of thinking about comprehension problems, where language disorder is a "top-down" approach? Does Kim have two or more disorders, concurrently? What would be the purpose of assessing Kim? And, perhaps weighing in with far too much importance, who will conduct the assessment?

In proposing the creation of a new diagnostic entity, a primary task of researchers is to show that it has reasonably robust boundaries. We say "reasonably", recognizing that there are many instances in medicine and developmental psychology where the presenting task is one of *differential diagnosis*. Someone exhibiting acute-onset severe abdominal pain may have appendicitis, or a bowel obstruction, or diverticulitis – or one of many other potential reasons for their clinical presentation. The fact that clinical disorders can present in similar ways is not in itself, however, a reason to simply lump them all together and treat them the same. Appendicitis, bowel obstruction, and diverticulitis each need different treatments and the consequences could be disastrous if this were not recognized. Unfortunately, in the context of children's (or adults') neurodevelopmental difficulties, a careful diagnostic process does not automatically lead to an unequivocal diagnosis which will be agreed upon by a range of practitioners, whether they are from the same discipline or from several. This is nowhere more evident than in the realm of auditory processing difficulties. This diagnostic debate is often undisclosed to parents, especially by commercial providers of programmes who typically either over-simplify diagnostic categories or (more commonly) offer their intervention as a one-stop shop for a ridiculously wide range of disorders.

APD is a contested and debated diagnosis. It does not have a place alongside established clinical entities such as ADHD and childhood language disorders in major diagnostic frameworks such as the DSM-5 (American Psychiatric Association, 2013). Its clinical features, the most appropriate diagnostic tests for its identification and measurement, and even its very existence as a useful, stand-alone clinical entity remain controversial and troubling.

While authors of "parent information" on some websites attempt to differentiate related disorders (see, for example, www.auditorycenter.com, www.additudemag.com, or https://www.hearing.com.au/central-auditory-processing-disorder), we think site visitors will feel *more* rather than less confused after consulting them. In practice, it is just not possible to group children into separate camps for "pure" APD, "pure" receptive language difficulties, and "pure" ADHD. It must be noted, too, that auditory processing difficulties of various forms, particularly hypersensitivity to sound, are common features in Autism Spectrum Disorders (ASD). At best, all we can say currently is that children diagnosed with receptive language disorder, and those diagnosed with ASD and/or ADHD, may, on testing, display test profiles that some practitioners would say are also consistent with a diagnosis of APD. This does not mean, though, that APD is a clear, stand-alone diagnostic entity; nor does it mean that its diagnosis will lead to more targeted and effective interventions that result in improved functioning in domains that are important for social and academic success.

Because of the debate and disagreement around terminology for auditory processing difficulties that existed from their earliest descriptions, at the beginning of the 21st century, an attempt was made by a large group of researchers to achieve common understandings. In their 2000 Consensus Statement, audiologists Jerger and Musiek (2000, p. 469) asserted that:

> "*Auditory processing problems can occur independently or can co-exist with other, nonauditory disorders in the following combinations:*
>
> ***A.*** *A pure auditory processing disorder;*
>
> ***B.*** *An auditory processing disorder and a disorder or disorders in other modalities (i.e., multisensory);*
>
> ***C.*** *A disorder that initially appears to be nonauditory but is actually auditory;*
>
> ***D.*** *A disorder that initially appears to be auditory but is actually nonauditory*".

Now, as if all of this were not sufficiently ambiguous and bewildering, Jerger and Musiek went on to acknowledge that a diagnosis of APD will also be influenced by other disorders that impact auditory function, such as ADHD, language impairment, reading and learning disorders, ASD, and ID. It appears that this "Consensus Statement" was little more than a bet each way. So, why refer in 2017 to a Consensus Statement published in 2000 that we don't think produced diagnostic clarity? Because this statement has been influential with respect to research and clinical thinking on APD in the two decades since, in spite of which definitions have continued to be elusive moving targets.

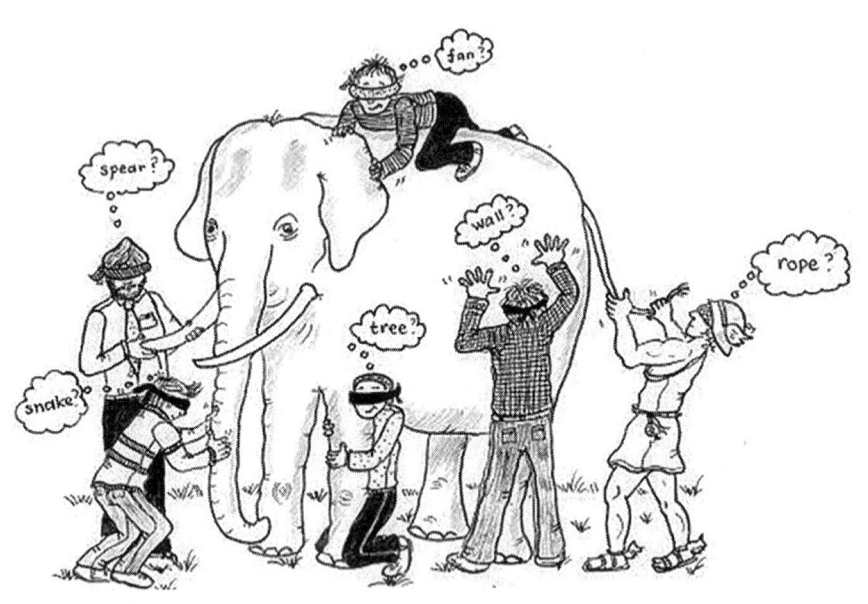

Helen Rippon

How do receptive language deficits, ADHD, and APD differ? SPOILER: IT MAY DEPEND WHO YOU ASK

A fictional (APD) elephant might help comprehension of the messy state of affairs surrounding auditory processing difficulties. This is because answers in response to the important question posed above may depend on who you ask. Audiologists as a group are probably more likely to refer to APD, while SLPs/SLTs as a group will tend to prefer language disorder; however, this is no clear-cut distinction. Educational and developmental psychologists are likely to bring in the ADHD dimension, teachers may refer to behaviour and/or reading difficulties, and of course all practitioners will be on the alert for features of ASD. Enter John Godfrey Saxe (b. 1816 d. 1887) with his poem *The Blind Men and the Elephant* (accessible via Google). It is about six blind men attempting to discern "by feel" the nature of the creature before them. The upshot, of course, is that they all make dogmatic (but incorrect) assessments based on the particular part of the elephant to which they have access. The one who can feel the tail proclaims that the elephant is like a rope; the one who can feel the tusk says the elephant is like a spear, and so on, as Helen's illustration depicts. This sense of different practitioners all being *partly* correct in relation to children diagnosed with APD is well summarized by Kamhi who observed that "If all processing deficits were distinct clinical categories, the list of disorders would be interminable" (2011b, p. 269). Kamhi brought unusual candour to the debate on APD versus language disorder when he posed, and answered, a question that is front and centre for clinicians, and no less relevant to parents and teachers:

> *"So, why did auditory, attentional, and sensory integration problems become distinct clinical entities?*
> *A number of factors contributed to the creation of these distinct clinical entities, but the following three factors were particularly important: (a) Each disorder is associated with a distinct profession and practitioner (audiologist, psychologist, occupational therapist); (b) a certified, licensed professional in the discipline is the only one qualified to administer the assessment battery and make the diagnosis; and (c) the label for the disorder is not stigmatizing and is easy to understand, remember, and communicate to others (i.e., a good meme...)."*
> Kamhi, 2011b, p. 269

When Kamhi referred to these disorders becoming "distinct clinical entities", he was referring only to the way they are thought about and presented by researchers (and to a lesser extent, clinicians) – not to an objectively verifiable diagnostic framework that works well for parents and teachers. Fey et al. (2012, p. 388) summed up the frustrating and unsatisfactory state of affairs regarding terminology thus: "The only consistency in nomenclature is that it continues to be inconsistent". We cannot detect significant progress towards consensus on this important question in the five years since Fey et al. expressed this view. This is hugely frustrating and unsatisfactory for parents who, understandably, take to the Internet to gain clarity to help make decisions that are in the best interests of their children regarding diagnosis and intervention.

Corresponding to the messy diagnostic landscape, the intervention terrain is equally ill-defined, with no shortage of quick-fix programmes developed by folk who are either blind to, or selectively ignorant of, the muddled state of the diagnostic research.

Interventions for APD

Historical context is always important, and it is notable that when APD took off as a diagnostic label in the 1980s, it coincided with rapid development of information and communication technology (ICT). For the first time, personal computers (PCs) were accessible to the mass market. PCs were greeted eagerly by educational and clinical software designers, excited by the potential of computer programs (software) to hasten progress for children with developmental disabilities and adults with acquired brain injuries. Their main approach was to break complex tasks, such as attention and listening comprehension, down to granular, graded elements in games, puzzles and other "educational" formats, to be practised and refined before moving to more complex levels. Hectic software development work proceeded exponentially, and in a disorganized way. Rather than researchers designing software, including CD-ROM-based packages, step-by-step, and exposing them to careful laboratory-based assessment before their roll-out in well-controlled field studies, there was a free-for-all

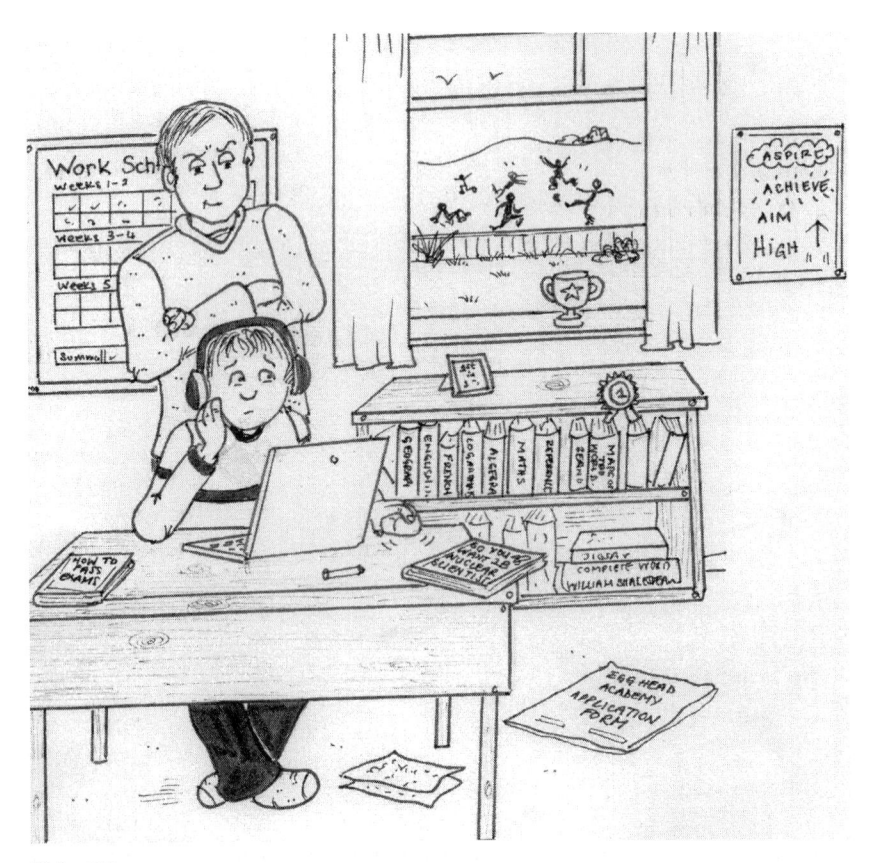

Helen Rippon

grab for the rehabilitation and child development dollar, without much regard for whether the programs and packages actually worked.

Decades on, we have the benefit of systematic reviews of a large body of research (albeit of varying quality) and current guidelines that *do not* support reliance on repetitive computerized programs to improve everyday attentional skills after brain injury (see Sloan & Ponsford, 2013). There is a lack of evidence of generalization of improvements on the computer tasks to everyday tasks that require attentional skills, e.g., driving a car, or following conversation in noise (Ponsford et al., 2014). The story is similar with respect to the use of software for children diagnosed with APD.

Some of the key players in the APD treatment field include "Auditory Integration Training" approaches such as the Tomatis® Method, the Berard Method, The Listening Program, and Samonas™ Sound Therapy; and interventions such as Earobics®. We summarize the features of these approaches, and then examine the findings of systematic reviews of research evidence regarding their claims for effectiveness. Some other auditory integration therapies are marketed both for their purported listening benefits and for their benefits for low reading skills, for example Fast ForWord® and Interactive Metronome®, and they are discussed in Chapter 9.

The **Tomatis® Method** (www.tomatis.com and www.solisten.com.au) takes its name from its developer, Alfred Tomatis, an Ear, Nose and Throat specialist who worked with patients ranging from factory workers to opera singers, and emphasized the (obvious) connection between listening and the development of receptive and expressive language, motor control, learning and motivation. Dr Tomatis opined that the voice can only produce what the ear can hear, a "principle" that became known as the "Tomatis Effect", and this was said to account for the underlying difficulty responsible for poor auditory processing, reduced language comprehension, and related problems. He argued that "the ear" of affected individuals needed "re-programming" using the Electronic Ear, a nifty device he developed aimed at strengthening and improving the function of the middle ear. Among other things, the function of the Electronic Ear is to filter out unhelpful lower frequencies (pitches), magnify higher frequency sounds, and to make money.

Developed by and named after a French physician who had worked with Tomatis, Dr Guy Berard, the **Berard Method** (www.drguyberard.com) uses Auditory Integration Training to target difficulties associated with a range of behavioural and learning problems (e.g., autism, depression, hyperactivity and learning disorders), via a "re-education" of the hearing process. The program comprises 10 hours of listening to electronically modified music via headphones, with filters dampening peak frequencies, during two 2.5 hour sessions per day, for 10 weeks. Intervention must be delivered by clinicians trained in the Berard Method, using one of two approved devices, the Earducator™ or the Audiokinetron (no, we are not making these names up, and your giggling is not helping). "Audio tests" are conducted prior to, at the midpoint, and following the end of the intervention, and booster sessions are not permitted.

Earobics® (www.earobics.com) is a computer-based tutorial programme that, as the name suggests, comprises "exercises" aimed to improve skills in auditory attention and discrimination, sound segmentation, phonological awareness, auditory memory, and phonemic synthesis – skills needed for auditory-verbal comprehension, and effective reading. Earobics® was developed and is marketed by Cognitive Concepts. It comes with three levels of complexity, to be practised in the child's home.

Samonas™ Sound Therapy (http://developmentallistening.org) was developed by Ingo Steinbach, a German sound engineer. It is a CD-based programme which can be self-guided or administered by a professional who has undergone Samonas™ training. It comprises more than 40 specialized recordings, stratified for intensity; these are mainly of classical music, but also of some nature sounds. Dr Steinbach developed an envelope-shaped modulator that enhances the upper frequency range of the music, so that for certain periods of intense filtering, the listener almost exclusively hears these upper frequency sounds, with the aim of increasing their ability to attend to the upper ranges of the speech frequency spectrum.

The Listening Program® (http://a.advancedbrain.com/tlp/the_listening_program.jsp) was developed by Advanced Brain Technologies and is a music-based auditory stimulation approach that, according to company promotional material, "trains the brain" to help improve the auditory skills needed for effective listening, learning and communicating. The programme is CD-based and includes classical music by Mozart, Vivaldi, Corelli, Bach and others, mixed with nature sounds and all intended to improve spatial awareness and listening skills. It is mainly intended for home use and for implementation in places like schools and healthcare centres. According to its developers, it is especially effective for correcting auditory processing problems and for improving short-term auditory memory, and the capacity to listen against background noise. Its core programme is typically administered five days per week for 15 to 30 minutes each day. The intervention lasts from eight to 16 weeks, and learners might complete a second or third cycle to ensure maximum benefit.

Johansen Individualized Auditory Stimulation (JIAS) was developed by Dr Kjeld V. Johansen, Director of the Baltic Dyslexia Research Lab in Denmark. Like the programmes described above, it is based on the unsubstantiated notion that "inefficient" auditory processing underlies many children's language and reading difficulties, not to mention autism, low self-esteem, memory difficulties, and dyspraxia. The essence of JIAS intervention is the provision of a customized music CD (based on analysis of the child's audiogram[1]) which the child must listen to via headphones for 10 minutes daily for at least 12 weeks. Links to so-called evidence for this intervention on the JIAS website (www.johansenias.com/research.aspx) lead to examples of unusually weak, non-peer-reviewed "studies" from which no substantiations of efficacy or effectiveness can be drawn.

Common features

These programmes share some common features, notably the controlled delivery of auditory signals, whether speech or non-speech, and repeated practice under laboratory conditions on listening tasks of graded complexity. Some programmes provide intervention on a fairly open-ended basis, while others are time-limited; some are done only in a clinical environment and others can be done at home or at school. All involve a financial commitment from parents as well as an important *opportunity-cost*, i.e., a sacrifice of precious time and motivation that could be expended on other, perhaps low- or no-tech, but more efficacious approaches that directly strengthen everyday important skills. Many of these programmes also carry the important red flag of claiming effectiveness for a disconcertingly wide range of developmental disorders. We consider these questions more closely below.

Do the programmes work?

There is certainly some face value in the notion of taking apart a complex task such as auditory processing, breaking it into small segments, and attempting to build up processing capacity via repeated practice of increasingly complex sub-skills (analogous to some approaches to the treatment of attentional

---

1 An audiogram is a graphic representation that plots the thresholds at which different sound frequencies (pitches) can be detected by a patient, with both ears assessed individually. It should be derived from an assessment conducted in a sound-proof booth, by a qualified audiologist. See also page 170 regarding routine hearing assessments.

disorders, outlined in Chapter 3). Doing this via auditory signals that have been modified and simplified also makes a certain intuitive sense, and we have no reason to doubt the authenticity of the motivation behind the work of scientifically trained personnel such as Tomatis, Berard, Steinbach and Johansen. Unfortunately, however, there are many false dawns in interventions for children with developmental disorders, and the research evidence amassed in recent years suggests that auditory integration therapies belong on the pile of interesting, tried, tested, but not overly helpful approaches.

There is a newer product from the Tomatis® stable called Solisten® with country-specific web presences dotted around the world, e.g., www.solisten.com.au, where the promotional statements are quite representative of the claims to be found on all the AIT sites. Each Solisten® site contains glib statements such as, "The human ear can be compared to a dynamo which provides the brain with energy and thus requires stimulation", that are just that: glib statements, with no scientific merit regardless of the fact that they appear under a tab labelled "science". And pronouncements such as "If you change the way the ear works, you affect all the body's major organs" are simply laughable. For starters, auditory processing has more to do with the workings of the brain than the ear, notwithstanding which we can see no plausible reasons why changes in the way the ear works would impact, for example, on the gall bladder, the kidneys, or the liver. This is just nonsense.

While individual studies of auditory integration therapies suggest promising results, many of them have fundamentally flawed methodologies, and probably should never have been published in the first place (refer back to pages 4–5 for consideration of reasons why some low-quality research manages to see the light of day in peer-reviewed journals). As McArthur observed, "Such studies should not be published because they are too often used by commercial marketing departments and ill-informed reporters as 'scientific proof' for a training program" (2009, p. 143). Naturally, commercial websites promoting APD interventions will mention these studies but they will not indicate methodological flaws such as small, biased samples, lack of consideration of transfer of improved scores on test measures to real-world tasks, little or no follow-up to determine whether any gains made hold over time, and the lack of a no-treatment control group (or of a control group that receives some other standard therapy). The badging of satisfied client testimonials as "evidence" is another common feature of these approaches and should ring alarm bells for parents and teachers.

In their Cochrane Review of auditory approaches for children with ASD, Sinha, Silove, Wheeler and Williams (2006) concluded that: "There is no evidence that auditory integration therapy or other sound therapies are effective as treatments for autism spectrum disorders" (2011, p. 2). This is particularly significant knowing that a key feature of a Cochrane Review is the *removal* of low quality, methodologically weak studies *before* analysis occurs and conclusions are drawn. Sinha et al. echo the American Speech-Language-Hearing Association (2004) *Auditory Integration Training Technical Report* which concluded that:

> "Despite approximately one decade of practice in this country, this method has not met scientific standards for efficacy and safety that would justify its inclusion as a mainstream treatment for these disorders. The American Academy of Audiology (1993), ASHA (1994), the American Academy of Pediatrics (1998), and the Educational Audiology Association (1997) all concur that AIT should be considered an experimental procedure."
> www.asha.org/policy/TR2004-00260

We therefore consider it particularly unhelpful for parents to receive advice such as: "Adding to the controversy is that many therapists aren't knowledgeable about the various forms of listening therapy or cite a lack of peer-reviewed research as a reason for parents to avoid some of them", from www.kidsenabled.org/articles/intervention/power-sound-therapy-worth-listening. While we agree with the first part of this statement, we cannot endorse the reprehensible second part, that casually dismisses the scientific method.

We also note the conclusion of Murphy and Schochat, following their systematic review of studies of auditory integration training, that: "Most of the papers that investigated the use of software demonstrated that this approach can be an effective form of training for improving auditory temporal processing…However, whether this learning generalizes to language skills remains controversial" (2013, p. 1369). This is like saying that training learner drivers in computerized driving simulators produces improved reaction times on the simulation tasks, but such gains do not necessarily translate into improved (vital) on-road driving skills, in which conditions are more complex and unpredictable.

For parents and teachers, the equivalent of "on-road" performance is what matters most for children rather than their scores on over-simplified and sometimes contrived computer-based tasks that are completed under laboratory conditions. So our concern with programmes such as Tomatis®, Samonas™, Berard AIT and JIAS is not so much that they have been developed, but that their promotion continues long after the gains associated with them have been shown, through empirical scientific reviews, to be marginal at best. It is not ethical to promote, let alone charge for, interventions that look like they *should* do some good when they clearly do not.

Can musical training help auditory processing and language skills?

In order to learn to read, children must be able to attend to the acoustic properties of speech at both micro and macro levels. At the micro level, phonological awareness (PA) and its subcomponent phonemic awareness are important (see page 225) so that attention can be paid to auditory information that occurs below the level of the syllable, e.g., being able to hear that "slip" has one more sound in it than "sip", or recognizing that adding voice to a consonant changes word meaning (e.g., "big" vs. "pig"). At the macro level, children need to attend to the prosodic (melody, intonation and loudness) aspects of speech in order to process its pitch, rhythm, timing, and associated meaning (Gordon, Fedh, & McCandliss, 2015; Patel, 2011). Shared acoustic properties of speech and music, and the brain's ability to analyze and synthesize these, form the basis of research on a possible role for musical training to support children's reading skills. Patel (2011) proposed a theoretical framework termed the *OPERA hypothesis*, reflecting and extending the argument that "…music-driven adaptive plasticity in speech processing networks occurs because five essential conditions are met" (p. 1). This hypothesis is outlined as follows (Patel, 2011, pp. 1–2):

> **O**verlap: there is overlap in the brain networks that process an acoustic feature used in both speech and music, **P**recision: music places higher demands on these networks than does speech, in terms of the precision of processing, **E**motion: the musical activities that engage this network elicit strong positive emotion, **R**epetition: the musical activities that engage this network are frequently repeated, and **A**ttention: the musical activities that engage this network are associated with focused attention.

Research on the acoustic properties of speech as an important (though not exclusive) basis for the transition to literacy has led researchers to ask (a) are there associations between musical ability and reading skill, and (b) can music be employed as a therapeutic medium to strengthen early reading skills?

In response to question (a), there is a large body of mainly cross-sectional research that shows *associations* between musical ability and reading skill (e.g., François, Grau-Sánchez, Duarte, & Rodriguez-Fornells, 2015; Hornickel & Kraus, 2013; Kraus et al., 2014a, b; Tierney & Kraus, 2013). However, cross-sectional research always throws up the chicken-and-egg question: does enhanced musical ability lead to improved reading skills, do improved reading skills enhance musical ability, or are there underlying factors (e.g., hereditary predispositions) that account for intrinsic variability in both?

Researchers who have explored question (b) through meta-analysis (Gordon et al., 2015), systematic reviews (Cogo-Moreira et al., 2012; Murphy & Schochat, 2013) and commentaries (Evans et al., 2014) are unable to endorse musical training as a tool for enhancing children's reading skills. This is largely because of the dearth of well-controlled studies that employ clinically meaningful outcome measures and follow children up over sufficient periods of time to see whether any apparent initial gains are maintained. Reviewers also note that where gains have been reported, they are typically modest.

We think musical training is intrinsically valuable for a range of fundamental and largely self-evident reasons: it can be enjoyable, contributing to social, cultural, and psychological connections across the lifespan. For *some* children, it *may* also contribute to improved language and literacy skills, but we do not endorse music lessons with language and literacy improvements as primary aims. Expose your child to music: listening, playing, and performing in as many ways as your time and budget (and your child's motivation and enjoyment) will allow, but if you seek to improve his or her language and literacy skills, select approaches that address these directly.

What can the parent of a child who diagnosed with an APD do?

We cannot go past Richard's conclusion that, "Despite more than 50 years of research and clinical practice, definitive diagnosis and treatment have not emerged from evidence-based systematic reviews. The inadequate research base in APD suggests that we should stop using the term and evaluate parameters of language performance that are deficient" (2011, p. 300).

This position echoes the conclusions of a review by Fey et al. (2011), and was more recently affirmed by the authors of a 2016 systematic review (de Wit et al., 2016), who concluded that the listening difficulties observed in children diagnosed with APD may reflect underlying cognitive, language, and/

or attention problems rather than being accounted for by a discrete auditory processing deficit.

As to the question of what to do *instead of* APD computer-based training, we leave the final word in this chapter to Dr Alan Kamhi, a professor at the University of North Carolina, cited on page 207, who provided the following sensible, plain-language synthesis of the current state of play around APDs and their management for practising SLPs/SLTs (2011b, p. 270). We think parents and teachers can also take much away from this. The emphasis is ours:

- Do not assume that a child who has been diagnosed with APD needs to be treated any differently than children who have been diagnosed with language and learning disabilities;
- **Do not provide auditory intervention** for a child who has been diagnosed with APD. Our systematic review found no evidence that auditory interventions provided any unique benefit to auditory, language, or academic outcomes… Language interventions are just as effective as auditory interventions in improving a child's auditory abilities;
- **Perform a comprehensive assessment** of the child's speech, language, and literacy abilities just as you would do with any other student who was referred for an evaluation;
- **Consider non-auditory reasons for listening and comprehension difficulties**, such as limitations in working memory, attention, motivation, language and conceptual knowledge, and inferencing abilities;
- Target **speech, language, literacy, and knowledge-based** goals in therapy;
- **Avoid goals that target processing skills** like auditory discrimination, auditory sequencing, phonological memory, working memory, or rapid serial naming. There is no compelling evidence that targeting these skills significantly improves a child's language or reading ability;
- Recognize that acquiring the language, conceptual knowledge, and reasoning skills necessary to talk, understand, read, write, and reason well is **challenging even for typical learners**. Learning these skills will, therefore, be particularly challenging for students with language and learning disabilities;

- Keep searching for more effective and efficient ways to improve children's language and reading abilities, but **be wary of interventions that promise quick fixes;**
- Most important of all: Devote most of your time and effort **teaching students the knowledge and skills that will help them talk, understand, read, write, and reason better.**

We could not have said it any better ourselves.

9 Reading

Few areas of child development occupy as contested a space as that claimed by reading instruction. This is a great shame, because reading is the foundation for early educational success and indeed for the ability to flourish across the lifespan. If you cannot read easily and fluently after three years of school, you will struggle to master the increasingly complex demands of school texts (across the whole curriculum), and you will probably come to an early conclusion that you and education are incompatible. Along the way, you may start acting up, so that your teachers and parents describe you as a child with a "behaviour problem" (they might use slightly fancier language such as Conduct Disorder or say you have "Behaviours of Concern", but they are all essentially the same). In this chapter, we review current thinking about reading, reading instruction, and optimal ways of helping poor readers. In so doing, we consider some popular, widely-employed approaches that do not withstand scrutiny through the evidence lens, as well as those that do have robust theory and evidence to support them.

What do we know about reading?

Language is a symbol system for representing information, experiences, and ideas. Reading, in turn, is a form of language, providing another way of representing information, experiences, and ideas. Broadly, language consists of *vocabulary* (words and their various shades of meaning), *syntax* (the rules of *grammar* that we use to link words so that they make sense when we talk), *morphology* (the smallest units of meaning, or our understanding of word components such as prefixes and suffixes, that change the meaning of the word while maintaining their base: trust, trusts, trusted, trusting, trustworthy, trustworthiness, trusty, mistrust, distrust, distrusting, mistrusted, untrustworthy, etc.), *phonology* (the rules governing which sounds are used in a given language and how they are organized into patterns of sound contrasts), and *pragmatics* (culturally determined, "understood", and implicit rules about how we use language in different contexts). All components of language need to develop in roughly the same sequence and at or close to the expected rate in order for communicative competence to be achieved.

Humans have used spoken language for about a million years, and it is a fundamental attribute that differentiates us from our primate relatives. Reading and writing, however, became a reality only five to six thousand years ago: a mere blink of an eye in evolutionary terms (see Snow, 2016). This means that reading is a comparatively "new" skill for humans. It caught on because we could see social and cultural advantages in sharing information, both with each other and with future generations. As a human invention, reading differs from spoken language. Spoken language is innate, not "taught", and parents and others foster its development, whereas reading is *not* innate and *must* be taught as what Gough and Hillinger (1980) called a "biologically unnatural act". Thinking about learning to read as something that *doesn't* come naturally, helps our understanding of the learning needs of all children, and the particular support needs of children who find it difficult to conquer literacy in the early school years.

The common feature of written and spoken language is that they are both symbol systems, or learned codes. Literacy is a powerful and sophisticated by-product of spoken language. There are, however, some important differences.

How do reading and writing differ from listening and speaking?

Language is innate and literacy has to be learned via years of specific classroom instruction and much exposure to books and other types of text, but the essential differences between the two are more wide-ranging than that. Notably, written communication is often more structured and formal in certain genres (e.g., contracts, agreements, reports and letters), and abbreviated and informal in others (e.g., email, lists, memos, text messages, and tweets), so while it is reminiscent of spoken language, it is not its mirror. Spoken language typically occurs in the context of an interaction of some sort, most commonly in conversation. Conversation comprises a lot of stopping and starting, interruptions, overlapping utterances, repetitions, and fillers ("um", "er", and if you are much younger than us, "like"), and pauses, hesitations, and false starts. By the time written language has been edited and proofread, it is more-or-less free of these messy human errors, and so appears much more formal and "tidy".

What skills do children need to become proficient readers?

Historically, reading was seen as predominantly a visual task and the reasons it could be misconstrued in this simplistic way are obvious. Sure, under typical circumstances, children are *looking* at text on a page and their eyes are scanning across it, but that is only a part of the reading process. The so-called "simple view of reading" (Hoover & Gough, 1990) is accepted by many reading academics and practitioners and encompasses the notion that reading consists of two key skill-sets: decoding the text and understanding it. As the following analogy with learning a foreign language demonstrates, both processes are essential to successful reading. If, years ago, you studied a foreign language such as French but have not spoken it since, you may still be able to decode a page of French text, in that you can read it aloud (albeit maybe not with a very Parisian or Québécoise accent, but that's another story). However, if you have forgotten much of your French vocabulary, you will not be able to *understand* the text, even though you can convert it into speech. When children are learning to read, they need to do these two things too – they need to *decode* text and *understand* the text they have decoded. It's as simple and as complicated as that.

In order to decode, children must understand that there is a system of linkages between what is written on the page and the spoken word. Sometimes this is referred to as acquiring the *Alphabetic Principle* – the notion that sounds (phones) and letters/letter combinations (graphemes) go together in rule-governed ways, even though some of the rules are more obvious and easier to learn than others. Strictly speaking, a phoneme is not something you can hear, as it is the "underlying" representation of a sound, that you "think" in your mind. A phone, meanwhile, is the spoken, audible "surface form" that linguists also call "phonetic realizations". In literacy research and practice circles, however, it is common for SLPs/SLTs and teachers to refer to "phones" as "phonemes", meaning "speech sounds", despite the anguished cries of clinical linguists.

Recognizing the confusion that arises over all the similar-sounding "phon words", such as phone, phoneme, phonological, phonetic, phonemic, and "phonics", Scarborough and Brady (2002) wrote a helpful, well-explained glossary. *Phonological awareness* (PA) is the ability to attend to, identify and manipulate a variety of sounds within the speech stream. It implies conscious knowledge, at any age, of the sound-structure of spoken words, from syllables to phonemes. *Phonemic awareness* (or *phoneme awareness*) is one aspect of PA, related to consciousness of the smallest speech units: the consonant and vowel *phonemes*. As a sub-type of PA, phonemic awareness relates to an individual's cognizance of the phonemes in a given word. The skills it covers are: identification of word onsets (e.g., knowing *chains* begins with /tʃ/);

phoneme isolation and segmentation (knowing that *chains* can be broken down into the sequence of phonemes identified as /tʃ/, /eɪ/, /n/ and /z/); and phoneme manipulation (e.g., knowing: /tʃ/, /eɪ/, /n/ and /z/ is *chains*, and /k/, /eɪ/, /n/ and /z/ is *canes*; that adding /ɹ/ after /k/ in *canes* results in *cranes*, and that removing /n/ from *cranes* makes *craze*). Were it not so fascinating, all of this could drive you crazy! Figure 9.1 shows the relationship between phones and phonemes, and graphemes and letters. The Alphabetic Principle is acquired through exposure to *phonics-based instruction* but, as explained below, the extent to which children are exposed to this kind of teaching in an explicit and systematic way is highly variable in most education systems in the industrialized world.

Once our emergent readers have decoded (read) the text on the page or the screen, the next task is for them to *understand* it. Comprehension draws on children's existing language-store and their knowledge of the world, as well as their ability to form, and mentally test, inferences about information that is implied but not directly stated. Inferencing is a skill that becomes

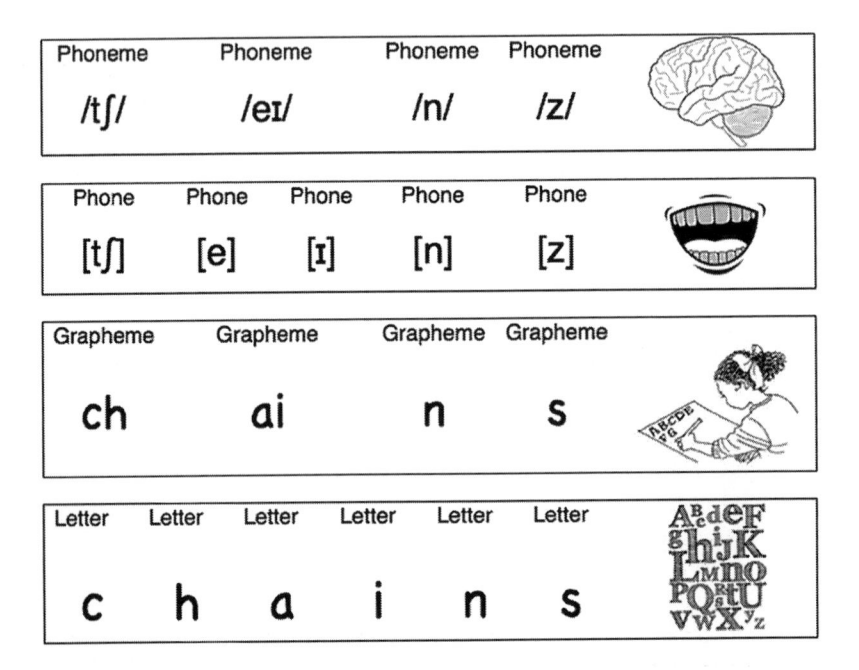

Figure 9.1 Phonemes, phones, graphemes and letters in the word "chains".

more important as children move up through school grades and must read texts that are less and less literal, more abstract and conceptually demanding. In this endeavour, they need to be proficient decoders in order to be able to focus their energies on extracting increasingly abstract meaning from the text.

Is English *really* such a difficult language for early readers?

The history of English tells us that it is a language that has cheerfully appropriated words from many other languages, as a result of invasions (not so cheerful, actually), trade, and migration over many centuries. Because of these borrowings, or "loan words", English does not have a completely *transparent orthography*, meaning that there is not a 1:1 correspondence between sounds and letters. Examples of transparent orthographies include Italian and Spanish; once you know the rules about how sounds and letters connect, you can decode just about anything (remembering, though, that decoding and understanding are not one and the same). Languages with transparent orthographies are easier to learn in the early stages, but that does not allow us to sidestep the comprehension issue.

English has 26 alphabet letters, which between them represent 44 sounds (phones) including consonants and vowels. *Digraphs*, or combinations of consonant-letters such as "sh", "th", "ch", represent some phones, while others come from *diphthongs*, which are combinations of two vowels, such as the "ay-ee" sound in "A" – say it slowly, and you'll hear separate "ay" and "ee" sounds. Still others come from foreign pronunciations that English has acquired, e.g., the /ʒ/ at the end of "rouge". There is a direct linkage between sounds and letters in about 50% of English words and a further 36% break only one sound-letter rule (usually via a vowel); 10% can be spelled correctly if word structure (morphology) and derivation (etymology) are taken into account, and fewer than 4% are truly irregular (Moats, 2010). So people who say that, "English is not a regular language" perpetuate the myth that English has poor sound-letter correspondences.

The "five big ideas" of reading instruction

There are two quite distinct world views on reading instruction, and the ideological battleground between the two continues as an expensive, resource-sucking exercise in pitting ideology against science. Irrespective, however, of the approach taken to reading instruction, there is broad agreement on these so-called "big ideas": vocabulary, comprehension, fluency, phonemic awareness and phonics-based instruction (see Buckingham, Wheldall, & Beaman-Wheldall, 2013, and 1 to 5 below).

1 Vocabulary

Vocabulary refers to our mental word store, or lexicon. We all need a rich collection of nouns, verbs, adjectives, adverbs, conjunctions and prepositions to combine into unique utterances in our interactions with each other. A toddler may learn that the family pet, a canine with four legs and a tail (or the remains of one), is called a "dog". Initially, our toddler may over-generalize this term to other four-legged canine pets, such as cats, but will be promptly provided with a more precise label by a caregiver, thus expanding her vocabulary to now take in "cat". Similarly, as they grow, young children will learn that there are more specific terms for referring to dogs – some are Labradors, some are Poodles and some are Boxers, and so on. A growing vocabulary provides the toolkit for expressing and understanding increasingly nuanced shades of meaning. By the final years of secondary school, for example, a student will need to understand why a protagonist in a novel felt *humiliated* by another's actions and, in turn, how this emotion differs from other feeling states such as angered or embarrassed.

2 Comprehension

We have already touched on comprehension, above – the idea that, as readers, we need to understand what we are reading by drawing on our knowledge of vocabulary, as well as our everyday knowledge about the world and how it works. Early readers frequently need assistance to make sense of what they are reading. In many cases, such assistance comes in the form of pictures alongside text, but these are gradually withdrawn in the middle primary years, and at that time the difficulties of children who are "behind" as readers may become more noticeable to parents and teachers. Sometimes comprehension problems reflect an underlying language disorder (explained in Chapter 7), which may or may not have been identified previously.

3 Fluency

Reading is more meaningful and enjoyable when a child is able to link words together in such a way that their relationships with each other in the sentence reflect the writer's meaning. Written text, like speech, has a certain "melodic flow" to it, and this relies on words being connected to each other rather than being read as separate entities. Beginning readers typically lack fluency, reading instead in a stilted, faltering manner. As skill and confidence develop, so too does the ability to make the words flow into each other. In turn, this boosts comprehension and enhances the child's enjoyment of the reading process.

4 Phonemic awareness

Phonemic awareness is an aspect of phonological awareness (PA) and is the ability to detect the presence and location of different sounds in a word. If we take the word "ship", for example, a child with phonemic awareness can detect an initial "sh" sound, followed by the "i" vowel and the final "p". Skills such as segmenting (taking words apart to isolate their component sounds) and blending (putting sounds together to make new words) are strong predictors of early reading success. Furthermore, they are strengthened by phonics-based reading instruction.

5 Phonics-based instruction

Phonics – elaborated in further detail below – is a teaching technique that draws heavily on correspondences between sounds and letters, whether regular or irregular. Not all phonics instruction is the same, though. The two key forms of phonics are *systematic synthetic phonics* and *analytic phonics*.

It may have occurred to you that there is a paradox here. Reading and writing are *separate skills from spoken language*, and yet they are *completely reliant on oral language skills* for their emergence and ongoing development. It has even been said that "literacy is parasitic on spoken language" (Liberman, 1971); however, when we consider that the relationship between parasites and their hosts is not mutually beneficial, it is probably preferable to think of oral language and literacy as being inseparable best friends. We recommend the aptly named Five-from-Five (www.fivefromfive.org.au) initiative for further evidence-based and open-access information about these five key literacy concepts and how they can be embedded in classroom practice from the time of school entry. Five-from-Five has a resource page especially for parents (www.fivefromfive.org.au/parent-resources-alphabet-letter-sounds), with information about early reading development and suggested activities for parents and children to enjoy together.

Phonics vs. Whole Language instruction: Why "versus"?

In simple terms, it can be argued that there have been two main schools of thought in the last 4–5 decades about how reading should be taught.

Phonics-based instruction

Until the 1970s, in most industrialized countries the dominant approach was *phonics* – i.e., instruction that was based on linking sounds and letters, starting with those connections that are regular ("transparent") and gradually progressing to the less regular. In systematic phonics-based instruction, teachers start with a few consonants, for example, "s", "t", "p" and a few vowels, e.g., "a", "i" and "o", and teach children how they correspond and what happens when they are manipulated in some way, e.g., if you start with "s", "i" and "t", and blend the sounds to make the word "sit", you can then take away the "s", replace it with a "p" and blend the sounds again to form a whole new word. As children progress, they are introduced to letter combinations that at first glance appear irregular, e.g., the "-igh" found in many common English words (high, nigh, sigh; night, fight, right, might, sight, etc.), but are in most cases, rule-governed and can be understood via basic interrogation of their origins.

The aim of systematic phonics-based instruction is to arm children with the essential skills of decoding so that they can tackle new words, which they will increasingly have to do as they progress through primary school and beyond. Research tells us that when skilled early readers encounter a novel word, they use *decoding* skills rather than skimming ahead in the hope of working it out, or trying to guess from a picture (Foorman, Francis, Fletcher, Schatschneider, & Mehta, 1998). Good phonics instruction equips young children with essential decoding skills that are necessary, but not sufficient, to get them on the road to becoming proficient readers.

Phonics-based teaching is also important for mastery of spelling. Children who learn, and can apply, rules of sound-letter correspondences have greater success at producing their own texts using at least near-correct spelling. Phonics-instruction proponents are not afraid of correcting spelling mistakes (while always praising the child's efforts, of course), because spelling is a skill that requires practice and feedback. Letting children make and practise errors via their own "invented" spelling misses valuable "teachable moments" for them to learn and consolidate their grasp of a spelling pattern or rule (Moats, 2009).

Whole Language-based instruction

In contrast to phonics-based instruction, Whole Language (WL) instruction starts from the scientifically *unsupported* premise that reading and writing are biologically natural acts, "just like" talking and listening. The argument here goes something like this: Children do not receive specific instruction in learning to talk, but rather they just "pick it up" from being spoken to and interacting with those who care for them. Therefore, they do not need specific instruction in learning to read either: they will just "pick it up" by being immersed in text. WL instructors, usually qualified teachers, employ a range of strategies that encourage children to either remember whole words, or to guess at unfamiliar words by using context cues, either from the text itself or from accompanying pictures. Instead of decoding, WL proponents – some of whom are high profile children's authors (e.g., Fox, n.d.; Jennings, 2004), but not necessarily literacy experts *per se* – argue that the key skills of early readers are "prediction" and "meaning-making" If schoolchildren are being encouraged to deal with unfamiliar words by following a three-step approach of using context, grammatical structure, and finally sounding out the first letter of the problematic word, they are being taught to read in a WL classroom. This is sometimes referred to as the "Three-Cueing Approach" (or "Searchlights" or Multi-cueing) to early reading. In these approaches, the use of phonics-based decoding may be actively discouraged, or implemented only as a last resort. Even then, it usually does not go much beyond the first one or two letters of the word, at which point the child is again encouraged to guess. This approach (often called "analytic" phonics) is contrary to the scientific evidence on what works for the vast majority of children, and conflicts fundamentally with the recommendations arising from national inquiries in Australia, the UK and US into the teaching of reading (see below). It is also a cautionary reminder that when teachers say they are "doing phonics", this does not necessarily mean they are teaching in accordance with the best scientific evidence on how this should be done to the greatest advantage for all learners.

Let's look at the arguments underlying WL instruction. First up, while children do not go to preschool or school to learn to speak and understand language, they do receive a great deal of "specific instruction" in the form of intensive interactions with carers who, from their infant's early weeks, pare back their own language (sometimes referred to as "motherese", "parentese", or more officially, "child directed language") to the simplest and most exaggerated elements, with pauses that give babies time to respond. Parents provide endless modelling, repetitions, expansions, verbal and nonverbal responses, praise, and other forms of positive reinforcement (smiles, laughter, clapping, exaggerated facial expressions, "yay!"), and corrective feedback and guidance from early infancy and throughout toddlerhood and the preschool years. So it is not true to simply say that children acquire language "naturally". Sure, it is a natural, innate skill, but it is also a skill that is heavily shaped by experience and interactions with others, over many years.

The second part of the WL argument, that children can learn to read and write almost via osmosis in a text-rich environment, has failed to garner support despite decades of cognitive psychology, linguistics, SLP/SLT and education research. In fact, the research literature comes down heavily in favour of the importance of early *systematic synthetic phonics* instruction, and so too have the outcomes of the three (to date) national inquiries into the teaching of reading: one each in the USA (the National Reading Panel, in 2000), Australia (National Inquiry into the Teaching of Literacy; Rowe, 2005), and the UK (the Independent Review of the Teaching of Early Reading; Rose, 2006). Although these reviews all support calls by WL proponents for children to be exposed to high-quality and engaging texts, without exception they reject the view that there is anything "natural" about learning to read. While some children learn to read and write much more easily and seamlessly than others, most will require specific and prolonged instruction to fully master the intricacies and nuances of the (written) English language. For that reason, teachers and teacher training need to cater to the needs of *all* children, not just those whose genetic make-up and/or social circumstances give them a head start.

Balanced Literacy (Balanced Instruction)

So you would be forgiven, dear reader, in the face of such contested territory, for thinking the entrance of a sensible-sounding player like Balanced Literacy might save the day for early readers. There was some undoubted authenticity in attempts to bring the reading wars to a close by striking a compromise and adopting the best from both worlds. Balanced Literacy (aka Balanced Instruction) is, at best, a well-intentioned and cleverly titled piece of marketing and at worst a mishmash of ideas that is impossible to subject to scientifically rigorous research. What Teacher 'A' interprets as Balanced Literacy will likely be different from the interpretations of Teacher 'B', or Teacher 'C'. Imagine this scenario in a medical context. If three doctors had different interpretations of the same treatment approach, we would be unhappy as patients, and scientists would be unable to group them together for research purposes. In essence,

Balanced Literacy is a strategic manoeuvre by WL advocates to acknowledge, albeit reluctantly, the incontrovertible evidence about the importance of early phonics instruction. Parents must be mindful, however, that it does not necessarily position *systematic synthetic phonics* as a starting point, as per the recommendations of those three national inquiries mentioned above. We see no compelling reason, therefore, to view Balanced Literacy as anything other than a market-savvy re-badging of WL instruction, with a homeopathic tincture of phonics thrown in as a sop.

A word about sight words

Some words occur frequently, and beginning readers must be able to rapidly and easily read and understand them. Ultimately, of course, we want nearly every word readers encounter to be recognizable by sight, rather than laboriously and individually decoded. Recognizing words by sight (particularly words with weak phoneme-grapheme links) has a number of benefits: it reduces the hesitations and unduly long pauses experienced by beginning readers, and thereby increases fluency and comprehension, leaving room for decoding skills to be applied to unfamiliar words. Unfortunately, sight words (sometimes referred to as "Dolch Words", after Dr William Dolch (b. 1889 d. 1961) who compiled a list of 220 commonly-occurring "service words", excluding nouns, and a separate list of 95 nouns) are often taught unsystematically in schools, without due consideration of the fact that some are as easily decodable as the so-called "regular" words (e.g., "from", "that"), while others are not (e.g., "does", "could", "through"). Asking beginning readers to simply memorize lists of unfamiliar words without any grounding in the Alphabetic Principle (see pages 221–222) is not an efficient use of a young child's time or mental resources, and can create frustration for children, teachers and parents. We support the teaching of sight words alongside systematic synthetic phonics instruction, but not as a virtually meaningless and unnecessarily onerous visual memory task. Questions on the teaching of sight words to beginning readers are explored by Dr Anne Castles, a Distinguished Professor at Macquarie University, in the Read Oxford blog (www.readoxford.org) and by Melbourne Speech Pathologist, Alison Clarke, who blogs at Spelfabet (www.spelfabet.com.au).

Is "dyslexia" a helpful term for reading difficulties?

If you have a child who is having trouble learning to read, you will have encountered the term dyslexia in your search for "answers". Interpreted literally, dyslexia means, "problems with words" (dys: impaired; lexia: words). As a function of its use in academic, clinical-education, and media circles, in recent decades it has come to mean impaired reading. Some organizations have their own particular definitions of dyslexia, most emphasizing some combination of reading and writing (spelling and composition) difficulties, which may or may not co-occur with other school-related difficulties, e.g., problems with verbal expression more broadly and difficulties with mathematics. It is usually implied, if not openly stated, that the presence of dyslexia reflects a brain-based dysfunction of some sort.

On the face of it, "dyslexia" is a medical-sounding diagnostic label that is applied after careful assessment by a properly credentialed professional, applying rigorously developed criteria. The first part is certainly true; it *is* a medical-sounding label, but it falls down badly with respect to having a tight definition that distinguishes children with so-called "dyslexia" from those with other reading difficulties. We fully understand that having a diagnostic label (especially one that has been conferred by a professional such as an educational psychologist) can bring both relief and a sense of validation to parents desperately seeking to turn around their child's poor progress and, in some instances, to attain funding. Unfortunately, however, "dyslexia" is dismally unclear as a diagnostic category – what one practitioner calls dyslexia, another will call specific learning disability (SLD), or even simply a reading disorder. This means that when researchers study so-called "dyslexic" children they are simply studying children with reading difficulties of varying origins and degrees of severity, not a homogeneous group. A further argument against the use of the term dyslexia is that it does not point to special interventions for children so labelled. The evidence-based interventions for low-progress readers do not change as a function of whether or not a dyslexia diagnosis has been made.

In our view, the persisting international and interdisciplinary confusion about this term means that it has run its course, and is no longer a useful way of identifying, classifying and, most importantly, *helping* all children with reading difficulties. Many children have reading difficulties of unknown origin, and at least a proportion of them are "instructional casualties"; that is, they have been in classrooms where early reading teaching was suboptimal and they missed out on key initial reading skills such as decoding (see Dr Reid Lyon's interview on the *Children of the Code* website). Should we call these children "dyslexic"? They have reading problems that will cause them to lag behind their peers and probably exit school prematurely with few marketable employment skills. Why should such children be viewed as "less special" than those whose families can afford to spend hundreds, if not thousands, on professional assessments and reports that happen to conclude with a diagnosis of dyslexia?

Those who argue against the use of the term dyslexia (e.g., see Elliott & Grigorenko, 2014) do not claim or imply that children with reading difficulties do not exist, or that their battles with the written word are unimportant. On the contrary, those who challenge the use of this term call insistently for *better* early reading instruction and *better* early identification of and intervention for children with reading difficulties. Reading difficulties need to be thoroughly addressed in *all children*, irrespective of the suspected underlying cause and of whether it is labelled dyslexia. Some of the interventions we discuss below are marketed specifically at parents of children with dyslexia but, for simplicity, we treat dyslexia as being synonymous with reading difficulties.

Specific approaches to helping low- or slow-progress readers

As SLPs, our professional lives have straddled both health and education. This has given us a close look at how both paradigms view, access, critique, and ultimately employ or reject research findings. In health, there has been a strong shift in recent years towards the application of evidence-based decision-making in clinical scenarios. As patients, or patients' partners, parents, or children, we all reap the benefits of these endeavours. Do medical practitioners always get it right? No, of course not, but at least in industrialized nations we can reasonably expect that there is an evidence-informed line of thinking behind decisions about our healthcare. We can interrogate that thinking, can request second opinions, and in many cases we can check the evidence for ourselves (e.g., through reviews published by the Cochrane Collaboration at www.cochrane.org). Education as a field, however, is in a less unified position on its evidence journey, and some sociologists argue it is a completely different journey, in which conventional conceptualizations of evidence are not relevant and should yield to postmodern notions of democracy and "different discourses" with their different "meanings of evidence" (see Biesta, 2007). This creates a messy landscape and one in which almost anything goes, as summarized by Dr Louisa Moats:

> *"Unfortunately, lack of rigor and respect for evidence in reading education are reinforced by the passivity of education leaders who feel that any idea that can muster a vigorous advocate is legitimate and deserves to be aired."*
>
> Moats, 2000, p. 12

Evidence in this context, then, refers to authoritative (ideally peer-reviewed), sources that contain independent and scientifically-derived data and interpretations. It does not, for example, refer to an ePortfolio or to an education student's or teacher's personal log of professional development. There has been undoubted progress on this front in the last seventeen years, but a worrying degree of debate persists in education circles about the extent to which teaching should be informed by empirically-derived principles. While education policymakers and practitioners debate in one room, down the hall in the classroom and in the clinic room, snake-oil merchants, some more heavily disguised than others, have set up shop. Let's look at some of their wares, bearing in mind that it would be impossible here to provide a comprehensive review of *all* interventions on offer. We will cover some popularly-adopted programmes in the hope that you will see what to look for, and will be able to apply similar filters as critical, educated consumers.

Reading Recovery

Readers may be surprised to see Reading Recovery™ (RR) included here. It is widely used in schools throughout Australia, Canada, Ireland, New Zealand (where it originated), the UK and the US. So if everyone's using it, it must be a good thing, right? Alas, no, the picture is not so rosy.

RR[1] is the registered trademark of a reading intervention approach that was developed by Dame Marie Clay (b. 1926 d. 2007) in the 1970s (see Clay, 1993), in an effort to help the poorest-performing children (up to 20%) in a class at the end of the first year of school to catch up with their more able peers. Specially-trained RR teachers take lowest-progress readers aside for individual sessions of about 30 minutes' duration over 12 to 20 weeks. RR is purported to be an individualized approach, with the teacher tailoring remediation to the learner's needs. A key tool of the approach is the Running Record; a sheet that contains all the words a child needs to read when tackling a particular book. While the child reads aloud, the RR teacher records the errors (called "mis-cues") that are made. In theory, these mis-cues provide diagnostic clues as to the child's intervention needs.

Superficially, RR is an intervention that should instil confidence in parents as a safety-net at the end of the first year of school. However, while it has the

---

1 Readers may also encounter *Switch On Reading*, which is a derivative of RR usually delivered by teaching assistants in the UK.

seal of approval from various education departments worldwide, it has not fared so well when subjected to research scrutiny.

Regrettably, many of the published studies on RR have been of low quality with respect to methodological rigour, but this has not stopped education decision-makers, some with poor research literacy (see pages 309–310), from endorsing its adoption and implementation, both for teachers' professional development (PD) and as an intervention method for children who show early signs of falling behind in reading. Careful perusal of studies of RR reveals serious and unacceptable methodological problems, including biased samples, lack of longitudinal follow-up, and selective discontinuation of students so that they are not included in outcome data.

RR is a product of the Whole Language reading instruction enterprise and this raises immediate red flags for all the reasons outlined earlier in this chapter. Because it is WL-based, little emphasis is placed on phonics-based decoding skills – the very skills that the authors of a large open-access meta-analysis (Galuschka, Ise, Krick, & Schulte-Körne, 2014) showed to be the most effective remediation technique for readers who are trailing their peers. RR has been described as a "wait-to-fail" approach, which assumes that up to one in five children will not achieve adequately in the context of standard instruction. Why would any school, or any teacher, employ a teaching technique that has such a high failure rate as a built-in assumption? Consider, too, the term "recovery". This implies that something lost needs to be regained, or rallying after illness or accident. What exactly is a child in a RR session "recovering", or "recovering from"?

Unhappily, the few rigorous, long-term studies of children who have undergone RR (e.g., Tunmer, Chapman, Greaney, Prochnow, & Arrow 2013) show that, for the most disadvantaged learners, apparent initial gains are not maintained over time. This means that our unfortunate low-progress readers have received a temporary cosmetic "patch" over their difficulties, but as the academic demands of text increase, these children tend to fall further and further behind their peers. This was also borne out in an evaluation in New South Wales that showed that initial improvements by low-progress readers are not sustained across the primary years (Bradford & Wan, 2015).

In our experience, RR can have something akin to an evangelical fervour attached to it in schools. Sometimes RR teachers *believe* (Gruber, Lowery, Seung, & Deal, 2003) in and advocate for its efficacy so trenchantly that they are unwilling to engage with discussion and debate about the equivocal, and at times frankly negative, data about it arising from the research literature. We know that all teachers working with children who have reading difficulties are there to do their best, but good intentions on their own are not enough to give all children access to the ability to read. Rather tellingly, research shows that even teachers who profess a commitment to RR express reservations about its actual effectiveness for low-progress readers when they are specifically probed about this (Serry, Rose, & Liamputtong, 2014).

Another concern about RR is its cost. We understand why parents might argue that, if an intervention works, cost should be no barrier to its implementation. However, the two problems here are that it is not at all clear that RR actually *does* work for the lowest-progress readers, and it is extremely expensive, at approximately $AUD3000 per year per student in Australia (New South Wales Department of Education and Training, 2016). Of course, some children do benefit from RR, as one would hope from any intervention that is provided 1:1 for 30 minutes a day, five days a week for up to five months! But here we must ask the cost-benefit question: is this the best investment of the limited education dollar? We think not.

Arrowsmith Program™

This Canadian programme, with current affiliates in Australia, Korea, Malaysia, New Zealand, Thailand and the US, was developed by Barbara Arrowsmith Young (b. 1951) who claims to have overcome her own significant learning difficulties by devising and repeatedly practising a series of remedial exercises that target specific underlying deficits that interfere with reading and other aspects of academic success (Brainex Corporation, 2015a). The for-profit programme requires 3–4 years of engagement (replacing normal schooling) and makes brave claims about what it can do for children with specific learning difficulties. If you want to see creative use of neuroscience-infused language, then the Arrowsmith Program is for you.

Readers will have gathered that we are inveterate writers on academic, research and professional topics, across several genres (articles, books, intervention resources, manuals) and platforms, including the Internet. Sometimes when we search the World Wide Web for information, our own words stare us in the face: whether they be in a webpage, a blog entry, or a contribution to an open Listserv™ or discussion group. Without giving the not-for-profit speech-language-therapy dot com (Bowen, 1998) and The Snow Report (Snow, 2013) sneaky plugs, we find that some of the things we want to say here, we have already said – as well as we are able – in html documents.

This applies to the sections on the Arrowsmith Program below, which is an adaptation of an original 2015 blog post in www.pamelasnow.blogspot.com.

The Arrowsmith website makes liberal use of terms that are designed to instil confidence (and a touch of awe) in parents, for example:

- cognitive
- neuro
- brain-based
- neuronal
- synaptic
- neural sciences
- cognitive-curricular research
- brain imaging
- targeted cognitive exercises
- neuroplasticity

We take issue with the claims made by the Arrowsmith Program™ on two key grounds: first, its scientific rationale is wanting; and second, it is unsupported by *any* juried research evidence.

While consumers are meant to be bedazzled by Arrowsmith's neuroscience jargon, it is a thin veneer that does not bear up under scrutiny. Yes, neuroscientists have a broad knowledge of the function of different regions of the brain, in many cases derived from detailed study of adults with brain lesions. Interventionists are not, however, in a position to plug children in to specific exercises that selectively enhance the function of particular brain regions which they happen to think (rightly or wrongly) are important for a particular skill. Advances in neuroimaging in recent years are exciting for sure; however, there is growing unease in neuroscience circles that we get ahead of ourselves in thinking we understand what some of these pretty pictures actually mean (McCabe & Castel, 2008). In reality, there is so much room for experimenter manipulation of the images that their usefulness in everyday clinical and educational settings is dubious at best. As a parent, what is more important to you – that your child acquires reading skills that are closer to those of her classroom peers, or that an image of her brain (apparently) shows enhanced growth in a particular region after a period of particular cognitive exercises? We know what we would be wanting for our children and grandchildren.

It is some 30 years since the inception of the Arrowsmith Program™, but there is still no independent, peer-reviewed research about its efficacy. A search (July 2016) of the Google Scholar, ProQuest Central, ProQuest Social Sciences Premium Collection, Web of Science, and Education Resource Information Center (ERIC) databases yielded zero papers with the term "Arrowsmith Program" in the title. This is in spite of the fact that the Arrowsmith website refers to "peer reviewed research" (Brainex Corporation, 2015b). Some links point to images of conference posters; however, these do not constitute peer-reviewed publications. Academic conferences may well have scientific committees who assess submissions and determine whether an abstract is to be accepted, and if so, in what format (short course, platform paper, poster, seminar, or workshop); however, this process (a) is not the same as having a full paper peer-reviewed by a journal and (b) is constrained by conference organizers needing to maximize registrations, so that accepting an abstract, even for a poster presentation, assures another backside on a seat. How can parents, who are not in the conference politics game themselves, be expected to have a nuanced knowledge of how research communication works?

Instead of peer-reviewed literature, the Arrowsmith Program™ is heavily reliant on small-scale studies (e.g., sample sizes of 5, 7, 15), in-house reports, and testimonials from satisfied clients. Testimonials are always red flags in the intervention space, because of their inherent cherry-picking bias and the absence of stories from *dis*-satisfied clients. If a school-based intervention occurs over a 3–4 year period, in the context of low staff:student ratios, we should expect significant gains. What we do not know (without properly conducted, robust research trials) is how much those alleged gains can be attributed to "active ingredients" in a specific programme versus the intensity of the attention, practice, and no-doubt enhanced motivation that students feel in such intervention settings. We also do not know how many children did not benefit from the programme, or may even have experienced negative consequences as a result of their participation in it.

While the Arrowsmith website suggests that there is much research in process, this is cold comfort for parents who are expected to fork out *tens of thousands* in hard cash if they enrol their child in it. If a programme has been around for three decades and its developers cannot go to the marketplace with established evidence-based credentials, we say buyer look elsewhere.

Cellfield ™

This computer-based approach to remediating reading difficulties was developed in Australia by a team comprising a lawyer, an engineer, an IT specialist, and someone with an MBA; not your typical reading intervention line-up, but let's plough on. Like the Arrowsmith Program™, Cellfield™ draws heavily on the language of neuroscience to build its rationale, in particular referring to brain plasticity and the science of neuroimaging. Considering our reservations about the term "dyslexia" (see pages 229–231), you will understand why we are unsettled by statements like this: "Brain imaging research has shown consistent differences in how dyslexic brains are wired compared to normal readers" (Cellfield Pty Ltd., 2015). We also know there is a range of views on person-first terminology in the disability field but, notwithstanding this, we dislike terms like the term "dyslexic brain" with their connotation that the brain of someone with dyslexia is unambiguously different from those of people who do not have reading difficulties. Conclusions based on neuroimaging should be drawn cautiously; these images allow researchers to *hypothesize* about active regions of the brain during reading, but we cannot be fully certain about what it means when a particular region does or does not "light up" during a scan. Further, brain scans are *not clinical tools* in the treatment of reading difficulties. A cynic might even opine that they are research toys. We suspect that, in a few years' time, commentators will look back on the zealous enthusiasm for neuroimaging in the first two decades of the 21st century and roll their eyes.

Dyslexia is not an "all or nothing" phenomenon, so this talk of the brain's wiring is a patronizing over-simplification, and implies that remediation is a simple matter of *re*-wiring. It is not possible, using even the most powerful neuroimaging techniques, to observe the "wiring" of the brain (its microscopic neural networks). All we can observe is whether a given child has learned something, and thankfully we do not need expensive, inconvenient, intrusive, and potentially scary (for a child) neuroimaging to do that. We agree with the developers of Cellfield™ that reading difficulties can have many underlying causes, and we also agree with their proposition that reading is a skill that needs to be specifically taught. However, their reasoning becomes fuzzy when on the one hand, they argue that there are many underlying causes of dyslexia, and on the other they emphasize its visual basis. Which is it – many or one?

Canny parents see red flags, hear alarm bells, smell a rat, suspect something fishy, and detect snake oil, when those behind an approach claim it will remediate difficulties across a wide range of functions. This is the case with Cellfield™ which, on the basis of one methodologically limited study (Prideaux, Marsh, & Caplygin, 2005), claims benefits across cognition, attention, working memory, and auditory, visual, and spatial processing (among others). We applaud the fact that this peer-reviewed study exists, but it is now over a decade old, and it stands alone as a weak and uncontrolled source of evidence for the programme's efficacy. It is also notable that the Cellfield™ website directly addresses reservations about its efficacy which were raised in a Macquarie University Special Education Centre (MUSEC) Briefing (page 302), though we do not believe the website adequately answers the concerns in the MUSEC Briefing. Further, it is not correct to say that MUSEC Briefings are the equivalent of an opinion-piece in a newspaper. They are compiled and updated periodically by research-savvy academics, well able to distil the current state of play for parents and teachers.

Fast ForWord®

Fast ForWord® (FFW) is a series of computer-based intervention programmes developed by Dr Paula Tallal and colleagues in the late 1990s, intended to improve oral language and literacy skills in children with language learning difficulties. The theory underlying the FFW software is that children's language and reading difficulties can reflect impairments in rapid auditory temporal processing skills; where "rapid temporal processing" is the brain's capacity to handle rapidly presented auditory or visual stimuli. Following from this, its academic developers argued that targeted training can produce lasting improvements in underlying neural systems that support language and reading, with concomitant improvements in children's language and reading skills (Merzenich, Jenkins, Johnston, Schreiner, Miller, & Tallal, 1996).

After the publication of two small-scale, methodologically weak studies in the mid-1990s (Merzenich et al., 1996; Tallal et al., 1996), the corporation Scientific Learning® was established by Merzenich, Tallal and two collaborators. Today, FFW products comprise game software ordered thematically into language, literacy and reading modules, spanning both primary (elementary) and secondary school years. These games, with names that are appealing to children and teenagers, are organized across many difficulty levels, depending on the student's starting point. The key feature of FFW programmes is their slowing down and amplification of auditory (heard) information so that it is more easily processed and understood by the learner.

Despite the publication of studies that show no benefit of FFW, plus a major review to the same effect (Strong, Torgerson, Torgerson, & Hulme, 2011), it is now in widespread use internationally, and the Scientific Learning® website (www.scilearnglobal.com) contains bold claims for language and literacy gains of one to two grade levels after only 8–12 weeks' training. In June 2016, the same site included, and probably still does, the assertion that "Fast ForWord does what **no other intervention** can do: it starts with cognitive skills like memory, attention and processing speed and works from the bottom up, using the principles of neuroplasticity. Fast ForWord aims to remediate the underlying difficulties that keep struggling readers and English language learners from making progress" (www.scilearn.com/products/fast-forword).

The theory underlying FFW has empirical support, as many children with language and literacy difficulties have evident difficulties processing spoken language and display poor PA, including poor phonemic awareness skills. A strong theory, attractively packaged software, and clever marketing do not, however, necessarily make for an effective intervention. Strong et al.'s (2011) meta-analysis of methodologically-sound peer-reviewed studies of FFW found no evidence that it "…is effective as a treatment for children's reading or expressive or receptive vocabulary weaknesses. In contrast, evidence suggests that conventional forms of therapy can effect modest but reliable improvements in these skills" (p. 233). So in spite of FFW's popularity and widespread use, the lesson here is that engagement in nice-looking computer-based language and literacy programmes may well be enjoyable to students, but this only creates an *illusion* of progress in the eyes of parents and teachers, who know that unless gains are transferred to real-world tasks, beyond virtual computer games, time and money would be better spent elsewhere.

Interactive Metronome®

Interactive Metronome® (IM) is an approach that has grown out of the same line of thinking that underpins FFW, i.e., that children with language and reading difficulties have an underlying impairment in rapid auditory processing. Although that may have been its initial impetus, IM has rapidly morphed into a "treatment for everything", as evidenced by the US version of their website stating that it is "…an assessment and treatment tool used by therapists and other professionals who work with pediatric and adult patients with neurological conditions that affect cognitive and motor functioning" (Interactive Metronome, n.d.). So that pretty much encompasses the full A–Z of brain-based disorders, from ADHD to Zellweger syndrome, across the lifespan. A veritable one-stop shop!

Resembling Arrowsmith and FFW, IM is a computer-based intervention that draws heavily on "neurospeak" to convince OTs, parents, physiotherapists, teachers and SLPs/SLTs of its scientific respectability. Terms such as brain-based, neurosensory, neuroplasticity, and neuromotor abound. During the treatment, learners listen to a computer-generated, repeated metronome beat via headphones and are required to match clapping and/or tapping motions to the beat presentation while using a hand or foot trigger. Immediate auditory feedback is provided on the accuracy of response rhythm and timing.

It is hard to argue with some of the basic assertions of the approach, e.g., "Motor planning and sequencing are central to human activity—from the coordinated movements needed to walk or climb stairs, to the order of words in a sentence to provide meaning" (Listen and Learn Centre, 2014). When deconstructed, however, this is as profound as saying "A cardiac rhythm and lung function are central to human activity". Further, the fact that these functions are basic to human existence does not in itself constitute a rationale for a particular intervention. That's just woolly thinking.

The "IM Science and Research" link on the IM website lists an assortment of sources, ranging from peer-reviewed papers, to conference posters, a doctoral dissertation and ostentatiously-named "white papers". "White papers" has an official ring to it, suggesting a government briefing document. In this case, however, it is simply code for "in-house" or otherwise non-peer-reviewed publications. It is also notable that few of the links on this page refer to studies of children with reading difficulties. On the other hand, studies about golf swing accuracy, soccer performance, recovery after brain injury or stroke, hand function, and balance in aging adults are all listed. True, there is the odd study specifically examining reading abilities using the IM approach, including one by Ritter, Colson and Park (2013) suggesting some reading benefits, notwithstanding some methodological weaknesses. The body of "scientific research" that is offered as a substantiation for IM is, however, incoherent. Given this, it is unfortunate that it is an approach that has entered allied health and education practice, as the science is definitely not in for this approach.

Coloured Lenses/"Irlen® Syndrome"

"Irlen Syndrome" (with "syndrome" capitalized à la Irlen) is a crafty example of disease mongering: the process of creating a new disorder and simultaneously marketing its treatment. Moynihan and Henry have outed disease mongering by Big Pharma[2], defining it as "…the opportunistic exploitation of both a widespread anxiety about frailty and a faith in scientific advance and 'innovation'—a powerful economic, scientific, and social norm" (2006, p. 425). A key feature of disease mongering is taking normal everyday behaviours and experiences, and re-packaging them as some form of pathology. In this case, normal phenomena that all readers, of all ages experience from time to time (e.g., rubbing your eyes while reading, taking a break during reading, preferring not to read in bright light) are re-cast as signs of so-called Irlen® Syndrome (also known as Meares-Irlen Syndrome, Scotopic Sensitivity Syndrome (SSS) and Visual Stress).

Irlen® Syndrome, first described in the 1980s by US psychologist Helen Irlen, was an instant sensation in the popular media. The key proposition is that nearly half of children with reading difficulties have visual-perceptual difficulties that cause text on the page to seem as though it is "moving" and/or be hard to clearly discern from the background. The answer for people with this syndrome lies in the purchase and use of coloured overlays or spectacle lenses, but not just *any* coloured overlays or lenses from the local office supplier or optometrist. No, these need to be prescribed by an Irlen® practitioner, specially manufactured, and purchased on a bespoke basis. Kerching!

The Irlen® Self-Test (www.irlen.com/get-tested/short-self-test) has to be one of the easiest tests in the world to "fail", which is hardly surprising given that it is an entry point to sourcing practitioners and services. If you answer yes to only *three* of 14 questions, then you might be experiencing symptoms of Irlen® Syndrome. Then again, given the complete lack of specificity behind questions such as "Do you find it harder to read the longer you read?", you might also be getting bored, hungry, or distracted by noise around you (rest assured, someone else in the bazaar will be able to assist you with these other "disorders").

There is no mainstream academic acceptance of the notion that visual-perceptual disorders such as those described by Irlen® are the basis of reading disorders, and the disorder "Irlen® Syndrome" retains its status as a controversial and contested entity. Being featured on *Sixty Minutes* does not change this fact, and neither does the little ®. Hence you need look no further than the American Academy of Pediatrics' position on Irlen® Syndrome and coloured lenses/overlays: "There is no scientific evidence to support the use of eye exercises, vision therapy, tinted lenses or filters to directly or indirectly treat learning

---

[2] The term Big Pharma is used to refer collectively to the global pharmaceutical industry.

disabilities, and such therapies are not recommended or endorsed. There is no valid evidence that children participating in vision therapy are more responsive to educational instruction than children who do not participate" (July, 2009).

Similarly, other forms of Behavioural Optometry lack a suitable evidence base. While it may be demonstrable under research conditions that eye movements (saccades) of children with reading problems differ from those of typically-developing peers, research does not demonstrate (a) to what extent such differences actually contribute to reading difficulties, or (b) whether any such difficulties are a *cause* of reading difficulties, or an incidental *consequence*. There is widespread agreement among reading academics that, in the overwhelming majority of cases, the problems underlying reading difficulties lie in the *language* system and not the *vision* system. For this reason, our advice is that approaches that emphasize visual remediation miss the mark and waste potentially valuable intervention time and money. Notwithstanding this, an assessment of visual acuity by an appropriately qualified practitioner is always advisable (e.g., to ascertain the need for glasses), particularly where learning concerns are present. Such practitioners will not waste time or jeopardize their professionalism to advocate Behavioural Optometry, the Chiropractic-Homeopathy Neural Organization Technique, Dynamic Vector Therapy, Dyslexia Apps, the Dyslexia Font, Dyslexie (see pages 248–249), strange notions of the "gift" of dyslexia, or Irlen® Lenses.

Orton-Gillingham

Named for its early developers in the 1930s and 1940s, Drs Samuel Orton (a child neurologist) and Anna Gillingham (an education academic), the Orton-Gillingham (OG) approach to the treatment of dyslexia has been adapted many times, and is found under a range of related names, including (but not only) the Spalding Method, Alphabetic Phonics, the Wilson Reading System, Writing Road to Reading, Language Tool Kit, and the Slingerland Approach. OG is described by the Academy of Orton Gillingham (www.ortonacademy.org, the US parent-company), and the Institute for Multisensory Language Education (IMLE; the OG auspicing body in Australia) as being: language based, multisensory, structured, sequential and cumulative, cognitive, and flexible. By "language-based", the folk at OG mean that they explicitly acknowledge the language basis (e.g., phonemic awareness, vocabulary, syntax, morphology, etc.) of reading difficulties in children. Multisensory refers to the purposeful use of visual, auditory and kinaesthetic stimuli. According to the IMLE website (undated) multisensory stimulation is used to "…enhance memory storage and retrieval by providing multiple 'triggers' for memory. This last part is critical. We believe that the best way to 'build pathways to connect speech with print' is to simultaneously use multiple channels of sensory input". The "structured, sequential and cumulative" aspects of the programme refer to the need to introduce various elements in a particular order, after specified levels of mastery have been achieved. This call for order is offset somewhat by the simultaneous requirement of flexibility on the part of the teacher, meaning that it can sometimes be necessary to go back to an easier level and reinforce prior learning. In the context of OG, "cognitive" refers to the fact that students are explicitly taught about the history and structure of the English language.

OG is an intensive, 1:1 approach that must be delivered by specially-trained OG teachers. It has many features that align well with current consensus about the basis of reading difficulties, most notably its emphasis on language-literacy links, and on systematic synthetic phonics teaching, as well as specific instruction about the structure and derivation of words in the English language. However, some reading researchers (e.g., Nicholson, 2011), have expressed concern that OG practitioners over-emphasize direct teaching of phonics rules, rather than allowing developing readers to infer at least some of these themselves through the experience of reading. Dr Orton's original hypothesis – that a lack of cerebral dominance in "dyslexics" means language is processed across both hemispheres, and causes unhelpful mirror images to be perceived by the child – has definitely not stood the test of time.

We consider that there are several sensible, research-informed elements in the OG programme; however, we agree with Elliott and Grigorenko (2014) that "Despite the enthusiasm for multisensory approaches held by many specialist dyslexia teachers … the theoretical grounds and scientific rationale for their use are questionable" (p. 150). Ironically, this view echoes the position taken by key *advocates* of multisensory approaches, Farrell and Sherman, who stated in 2011 that, "The appeal of multisensory instruction endures even though it has been poorly defined and is not well validated in existing intervention studies" (p. 39). Unfortunately, this amounts to, "We keep doing it because we think it works, even though there's little to no science behind it". A study by Labat, Ecalle, Baldy and Magnan (2014) lends some support to multisensory instruction; however, as it is not required for typically developing children, *without* reading difficulties, a more convincing case (based on replicated research findings) as to why multisensory instruction should be beneficial to children *with* reading difficulties must be built. Unfortunately, there is a strong likelihood that activities such as writing letters on a roughened surface, feeling movements of the articulators, using one's body to form letters ("body spelling"), or acting out meaning in a pantomime have nothing more than face validity for teachers, and no intrinsic learning value (alongside an accrued opportunity cost) for students. Studies that parse out the role of multisensory input from the other linguistically-based, and well-supported elements are thus needed. We note too that it is somewhat more challenging to assess the efficacy of the OG approach than many other interventions because, as noted above, it has morphed into so many other related product names, with the "original" OG people at www.ortonacademy.org distancing themselves from some, and it cannot be assumed that each of these delivers the same intervention. For this reason, the evidence-base for OG is equivocal; some studies show benefits across some reading skills, while others either do not or show benefits across different skills (see Ritchie & Goeke, 2006), so further research is needed. Beware the re-branding trick too. Currently, multisensory instruction is promoted to Australian teachers via the much more scientific-sounding, but no more evidence-based, "kinaesthetic scaffolding" (pli.education.tas.gov.au/programs/For-School-Teachers/Pages/Get-It-Right-For-Dyslexia-%E2%80%93-Get-It-Right-For-All.aspx). Its promotion via a state department of education testifies to the uphill struggle endured by campaigners for evidence-based practice in education.

Finally, we need to address the assertion made by Margaret Byrd Rawson (b. 1899 d. 2001), a past President of the USA-based International Dyslexia Association (formerly known as the Orton-Gillingham Society) on the IMLE website that, "Dyslexic students need a different approach to learning language from that employed in most classrooms". We agree with this statement inasmuch as many classrooms employ instruction approaches that are not solidly based on current evidence, as per the three national inquiries into the teaching of literacy mentioned earlier (page 228). However, there is no evidence that children with reading difficulties need *different* approaches from those recommended by the national inquires; they just need *more* exposure, and need this to be provided over a longer period.

Lindamood-Bell® Programs

In the years following World War II, US SLP Patricia Lindamood (b. 1923 d. 2006), who was working in schools, was struck both by the extent of reading difficulties in children across a range of cognitive ability levels, and the haphazard and inadequate approaches schools took to addressing the needs of such children. With her linguist husband, Charles H. Lindamood, and kindergarten teacher Nanci Bell, Lindamood went on to establish, in 1986, what would become one of the USA's largest education corporations: Lindamood-Bell®, which now has over fifty sites across the USA, Canada, the UK and Australia. Lindamood-Bell® programmes include Visualizing and Verbalizing, Seeing Stars, and Lindamood Phoneme Sequencing® (LiPS®, formerly known as the Auditory Discrimination in Depth® program). These programmes emphasize phonemic awareness, but go beyond the auditory channel to take in oro-motor feedback, explicit instruction, and use of visual imagery regarding how sounds are formed in the mouth. The Lindamood-Bell® programmes align with Paivio's Dual Coding Theory (Paivio, 1986; Sadoski & Paivio, 2004). Paivio asserted that cognitive processes such as reading require interaction between a verbal system and a nonverbal system, with both involving various sensory modalities, in particular visual, auditory, and haptic (touch). The sub-components of reading (decoding and comprehension) are explained via representation and processing within and between these two mental systems. According to Nanci Bell, students have reading difficulties because of weak *symbol imagery* and/or weak *concept imagery* (www.lindamoodbell.com), and in combination these two weaknesses are said to account for the full suite of reading difficulties that children experience. We note, however, that these imaginative terms are not derived from cognitive science literature on normal reading and reading difficulties, and can typically only be found in relation to the Lindamood-Bell® programmes. Programmes such as LiPS® are designed for implementation across whole-class, small group, and 1:1 levels, and emphasize mouth actions that produce different sounds. Like OG (above), we recognize sensible, evidence-based components in these programmes (e.g., explicit emphasis on phonemic and morphologic awareness); however, we have the same reservations here regarding the multisensory components (e.g., finger-tracing of letters, tracing letters in the air) which have not undergone sufficiently robust scientific examination with respect to the unique contribution they make to reported success with these programmes (e.g., Krafnick, Flowers, Napoliello, & Eden, 2011). Currently, there is only modest empirical support for these approaches, as per the What Works Clearinghouse Report (2015, p. 1) which concluded, "The WWC considers the extent of evidence for LiPS® on the reading achievement of elementary students to be small for two outcome domains—comprehension and alphabetics. There were no studies that met WWC design standards in the two other domains, so this intervention report does not report on the effectiveness of LiPS® for those domains". We are aware that many SLPs /SLTs and teachers who are Lindamood-Bell® proponents are wedded to its multisensory approach; however, we would like to see more research that systematically teases apart the elements of these programmes and identifies which aspects are essential and which may not be paying their way.

Other approaches to reading intervention

In this chapter, we have sought to provide clarity on current thinking about how children learn to read, and how best to assist *all* children through the application of evidence in early years' classrooms. We have also profiled some well-known but controversial approaches to reading intervention, hoping to debunk popular mythology surrounding their claims – both about the origins of reading difficulties and about optimal ways of responding to these. It is impossible to deal comprehensively with *all* controversial interventions here, but there are several others that deserve a few words.

In Chapter 11, we discuss some strategies parents can apply when appraising the market place with respect to interventions. The bottom line here is that *there are no miracle cures* and when glossy for-profit outfits – whose products are usually marked ®, ®, ™, and sometimes ©, so watch out for telltale symbols and superscripts – promise these, go right ahead and click the little "X" on the top right-hand corner of your browser. Beware, too, of reading method inventors who claim to "hold the key", to be "leaders" who can "unlock your child's potential" and include self-tests and diagnostic questionnaires on their sites, or who promote their particular programme as "the best", "widely implemented", or "research based" with *no signs that the said research has been peer reviewed*. RIP IT UP Reading© (www.ripitupreading.com.au) is one such example.

Others, such as the Davis® Dyslexia The Gift™ Program (DDA®: www.dyslexia.com) draw on personal experience (the so-called "gift" of dyslexia) and underpowered research studies that frequently compare their own intervention with *no intervention at all* (i.e., business as usual in the classroom). Something should always be better than nothing, and such studies do not deserve, in our view, to survive the peer-review process. If a hundred or so schools have fallen for neurosciencey hype and adopted a whizz-bang reading programme with slim credentials, it is not a good reason for your school to emulate them.

Some approaches to reading intervention are yoked to frontiers in neuroscience that are so distant on the horizon as to make the interventions themselves almost farcical in their struggle to gain a theoretical foothold. For example, there is the so-called "Crispiani Method" or Cognitive Treatment – Clinical Education; CO-CLI-TE (see Crispiani & Palmieri, 2015) which draws on emerging neuroscience evidence for a role of the cerebellum in cognitive functions such as language (see Justus & Ivry, 2001, and Mariën et al., 2014). The cerebellum is in Figure 5.1 (page 114) and, as you can see, it is located under the cerebral hemispheres in the posterior part of the brain. The cerebellum has long been known to have a central role in the execution of skilled, smooth, coordinated movements (the disruption of which is referred to as *ataxia*), but in more recent times neuroscientists have identified a number of nonmotor language functions of this structure. This is interesting in terms of our need to understand how the brain works, but is not information that even comes close at the present time to plausibly translating into therapeutic reading interventions focusing on motor skill, speed, and coordination like those (loosely) described by Crispiani and Palmieri.

In computing, a web application (web app) is a client–server software application (App) in which the "client" (user interface) runs in a web browser such as Chrome, Firefox or Safari, while mobile apps are designed to run on mobile devices such as smartphones and tablet computers. The market brims with web and mobile apps, such as ABC Reading Eggs (www.readingeggs.com.au) and Spellodrome (au.spellodrome.com). Such programmes have variable levels of theoretical robustness and adherence to developmental principles. ABC Reading Eggs, for example, includes activities that are likely to be engaging and fun for early learners. In some cases, however, it misses the mark on emergent reading skills, e.g., by having a recorded voice-over say a word when a child clicks on it to link it to a picture, in what is *meant* to be a reading task but becomes a hybrid reading-auditory comprehension task. In some cases, incorrect responses are not followed up with repetition of the stimulus and an opportunity to learn from the error. Tasks such as having a child use a mouse to join dots to form letters are irrelevant to the actual process of learning to write. These activities are in no way a substitute for rigorous classroom practice that follows a developmental sequence and applies established learning theory in the process.

Steiner Education/Waldorf Education

Some education philosophies, such as Steiner Education (also called Waldorf Education) warrant attention in this context because of their implications for reading instruction. Steiner Education's adoption of Whole Language-based approaches to teaching reading is exemplified by statements such as "…just as a child miraculously learns to speak her native language by the age of three without lessons, worksheets or a dictionary, so will a child naturally learn to read when she has a positive relationship with the spoken and written word" (Baldwin, 2011). There is a commendably strong emphasis on early oral language skills in Steiner schools, but the secondary place of phonics instruction in its early reading teaching means it is an approach we cannot endorse.

Complementary and Alternative Medicine (CAM)

Although in widespread use in the community and attractively marketed to parents, we see *no place at all* for homeopathy and/or chiropractic approaches in treating children with reading disorders. As noted in Chapter 2, homeopathy has been discredited. It is *not* an efficacious therapeutic model (for *anything*, let alone the treatment of reading difficulties). Its disreputable travelling companion, chiropractic, is at best a controversial treatment for spinal disorders, and at worst an approach that is potentially harmful in the treatment of children (Vohra, Johnstone, Kramer, & Humphreys, 2007) and babies. There is not so much as a tenuous link between current consensus among reading scientists about the linguistic (and in particular phonological) basis of reading disorders and the pseudoscience underpinning these approaches. Parents would do well to avoid expensive, time-wasting, and potentially harmful blind alleys such as these. And please, don't get us started on cranial osteopathy, craniosacral therapy, "dyslexia diets", and naturopathy and their "roles" in managing reading difficulties.

Does the use of a special font help?

In 2008, Dutch artist, Christian Boer, developed a so-called "dyslexia-friendly" font *Dyslexie* which can be downloaded free from www.dyslexiefont.com. Boer identifies as dyslexic himself and developed this font to address what he saw as a key feature of the disorder: difficulty differentiating between similar-looking letters, e.g., "b" and "d". Like many interventions for reading difficulties, this one was rolled out ahead of any scientific investigation. A study by Marinus et al. (2016) concluded that any benefits of the font reflect the spacing between letters rather than their shape. So wider spacing (a c h i e v a b l e w i t h a g r a p h i c a l w o r d - p r o c e s s i n g p r o g r a m s u c h a s W o r d) may be helpful for instructional and practice (homework) purposes but, ultimately, children need to acquire reading and writing (typing) skills that can be transferred to a range of fonts.

Handwriting

The advent of computers (desktops, laptops, and more recently tablets such as the iPad) has been transformational in government, industry, and education. A visit to almost any classroom will reveal children of all ages huddled over computers, either individually or in small groups. You will still see children with "old-fashioned" technology (pens and pencils) in their hands, but it is probably fair to say that in the course of their school years, modern students will spend more time producing text at a keyboard than they will via pen and paper. We will not enter here into cultural arguments about the importance of preserving handwriting as a high-level human skill (though we believe these are meritorious). However, we do note that the physical act of manipulating a pen or pencil in order to form a letter, while thinking about and saying its sound, is beneficial to the acquisition of sound-letter links and also of spelling rules, in ways that working at a keyboard are not (Kiefer, Schuler, Mayer, Trumpp, Hille, & Sachse, 2015; Longcamp, Zerbato-Poudou, & Velay, 2005; Santangelo & Graham, 2015). Children who are able to automatize these skills have the advantage of being able to free-up working memory to accommodate the demands of higher-order cognitive and language skills needed for text composition (Medwell & Wray, 2007). This does not mean that in the 21st century children should not acquire keyboard skills; they need them, and they should. However, these should not be seen as a "new for old" proposition that is educationally superior to a skill that we predict will continue to be relevant well into the next century.

So, what *does* work for children with reading difficulties?

The circumstances of each child will differ, depending on their age, related (co-morbid) disabilities that exist alongside their reading difficulties, and the extent to which secondary complicating factors, such as anxiety and avoidance, are further interfering with their ability to keep up with educational demands. Each education jurisdiction also differs with respect to the threshold that must be reached for specialist assessments and intervention services to be provided. As these are generally far from adequate, the void that is created inevitably leads parents to the Internet and a confusing maze of both snake oil and good oil approaches.

In the meta-analysis of randomized controlled trials examining the efficacy of intervention approaches for children with reading difficulties mentioned earlier, Galuschka et al. (2014) concluded that phonics instruction was "…the only approach whose efficacy on reading and spelling performance in children and adolescents with reading disabilities is statistically confirmed". Of course, this does *not* mean that the only thing that children with reading difficulties need is phonics-based interventions. Many will need interventions that target their comprehension, which will mean addressing general knowledge and underlying difficulties with vocabulary and syntax. In the secondary years, comprehension difficulties may sit above the level of literal sentence processing, requiring the reader to draw inferences at a text level. Unless decoding problems persist, phonics-based instruction will not be useful here. Galuschka et al.'s findings do, however, affirm the language basis of reading difficulties and the need for these to be specifically addressed via evidence-based interventions. In general, we suggest adopting interventions that focus on specific sub-skills, where there is an obvious link between practice tasks and meaningful skills your child needs to acquire (e.g., improved spelling). An example of an approach that appears to apply evidence-based principles, but without having been empirically assessed in its own right, is Toe-by-Toe (www.toe-by-toe.co.uk). This approach has an explicit focus on highly-structured synthetic phonics instruction, decoding of nonsense words, and syllable division, the likes of which, if regularly employed in early years' classrooms, might reduce the need for 1:1 intervention, though its reference to "multisensory" instruction arouses the same concerns as those we have articulated above regarding OG and Lindamood-Bell®. It is unfortunate and perplexing that, instead of being a standard component of early years classroom practice, programmes such as this are typically only resorted to as interventions for children and adults (including prisoners) with reading difficulties.

Irrespective of the nature and extent of empirical research that underlies a particular approach, interventionists should be able to explain to you, your child, and other interested professionals the rationale behind it or any of its procedures or activities (e.g., App-based games), using commonsense language, without recourse to opaque neurobabble. If a provider says they are working on your child's spelling, it should not look to you as though they are working on hand-eye coordination, or the ability to perform a tummy rub with closed eyes while standing on one leg.

Along the way, you will encounter various classroom methodologies that are not *interventions* (or "intervention approaches") per se, but rather are *procedures* and *activities* that are used in an effort to support students' learning and provide variety and motivation in the classroom. Approaches, procedures and activities that explicitly link sounds and letters are important for beginning readers, but as children progress the emphasis must shift to comprehension and fluency. Some teachers employ Choral Reading or Echo Reading activities (both described on the Reading Rockets website (www.readingrockets.org)). According to Dr Louisa Moats (personal communication, 1 May 2016):

> "Choral reading and echo reading should simply be viewed as two of several ways to engage a group of kids in reading a text together. I would add to that list alternate oral reading (teacher reads some, students read some), and structured partner reading … time spent reading text of appropriate difficulty is one of three critical aspects of instruction. ….
> I would disagree with anyone who tries to present choral reading or echo reading as a primary instructional strategy. These are merely ways to vary reading in class and practice application of the reading skills that have been taught. The text, in the beginning stages, should be decodable. As time goes on, it should be within the students' instructional range. They should be well prepared to read it and know the purpose of the reading. Good comprehension instruction must be employed."

MultiLit

Making up Lost Time in Literacy (MultiLit; www.multilit.com) is an evidence-based programme of reading interventions that was developed in the mid-1990s by a team of reading and special education experts, led by Dr Kevin Wheldall, an Emeritus Professor at Macquarie University, in Sydney, Australia. The MultiLit portfolio includes programmes aimed at preschool-aged children (MiniLit), as well as low- or slow-progress readers from Grade 3 to adulthood (MacqLit). In 2017, a series of 60 decodable beginning readers will be released (InitiaLit), to assist beginning readers to consolidate early phonics skills while reading age-appropriate and engaging texts. Reflecting the recommendations of the three national inquiries into the teaching of literacy (see page 228), MultiLit programmes emphasize efficient decoding, as well as comprehension, fluency, and competent spelling. The evidence-base supporting the MultiLit approach is impressive and easily accessed. In addition to providing graduated resources to assist with all aspects of reading and spelling, the MultiLit team offers training for practising teachers, individualized and small-group interventions, and makes services available to children via online tutoring. We recommend and endorse the MultiLit platform for any low-progress reader, irrespective of the nature or basis of their reading difficulties. We also recommend MultiLit as a means whereby teachers can up-skill themselves on evidence-based reading instruction and remediation. Parents, teachers, and clinicians can all feel confident with this one.

Effective and efficient literacy intervention

Targeting the aspects of literacy learning that actually promote attainment of gains, means children, young people, parents, teachers, and therapists do not have their precious time wasted on hollow fad-based promises that have no scientific foundation in either theory or practice. In general, we advocate approaches that emphasize early phonemic awareness and other aspects of phonological awareness, and endorse systematic synthetic phonics as a starting point, while simultaneously building on success by promoting vocabulary, comprehension, and fluency. For this reason, children with reading difficulties should, ideally, be assessed by professionals who have a solid theoretical and clinical grasp of the linguistic basis of learning to read. SLPs/SLTs are among those, alongside specialist literacy coaches, many of whom have education backgrounds. There are pitfalls to avoid when it comes to coaching and tutoring schemes, and these are discussed in Chapter 8. Parents, however, should probe for detail about the rationale behind a practitioner's approach, while not being blinded by the bright lights of neurosciency-sounding buzzwords, as we discuss further in Chapter 11. If a miracle cure for reading were available, rest assured, we would all know about it.

As with all human miseries (and have no doubt, being unable to read properly is a misery), prevention is better than cure. The scientific literature and our clinical experience affirm that some children have a tough time learning to read and/or in keeping up with reading demands across the grade levels, because they have not been exposed to optimal early instruction approaches: Reid Lyon's so-called "instructional casualties" (Lyon, n.d.) mentioned on page

239. Teachers do the best that they can, with the approaches that they have been taught; however, in many industrialized nations, these approaches are not in line with recommendations arising from the three important national inquiries into the teaching of literacy (see page 228).

If, in the first two years of school, your child's teacher discourages parents from explicitly linking sounds and letters, and encourages children to guess an unfamiliar word by looking at pictures and using context, rather than decoding, then your child is not in a classroom where the recommendations of the three national literacy inquiries are ordained. Evidence-based classrooms use explicit, first-line teaching of systematic synthetic phonics (sometimes also referred to as direct instruction), and provide graded, decodable texts[3] to beginning readers. Knowing this might equip parents to initiate a discussion with their child's teacher or school principal. We would encourage such proactive approaches, but caution that they will not always be warmly welcomed.

Stop Press!! Children can learn new things

Many, though not all, reading interventions make explicit or thinly-veiled promises to "change your child's brain". These are overblown at best, and completely misleading at worst. Getting up in the morning and eating breakfast "changes your child's brain", in the same way that reading this book changes your brain. Do the benefits of *your* reading this book, or for that matter, *our* writing it, lie in changes in our brains, or changes to our understanding and thinking? We'll leave the final word on this to Dorothy Bishop (who wrote the Foreword). She observed that, "Essentially, saying the brain is plastic and not fixed boils down to saying that children can learn new things—hardly a remarkable finding" (2013, p. 248). We suppose that Professor Bishop's brain changed from irritated to calm(er) once she got *that* off her chest.

---

3 There are many examples of decodable texts, including the Fitzroy Readers series (www.fitzprog.com.au), Pocket Rockets (see www.spelfabet.com.au/2015/04/cheap-decodable-books-pocket-rockets), Dandelion Readers (www.phonicbooks.co.uk/dandelion-readers/units-1-10-2-1), and Hooked On Phonics (www.hookedonphonics.com).

10 Diets, supplements and nutrition: What's on the menu?

Our debatable degustation menu in Chapter 10 is huge, with side orders of dietary supplements, to be washed down with scepticism, and lashings and lashings of lemonade (Blyton, 1951[1]), alongside healthy nutritious fare: the core business of dietitians, and not food guru wannabes.

Who's who in the food game?

The Dietitians Association of Australia (www.daa.asn.au) explains, on its website, the legal distinction between a dietitian (or dietician) and a nutritionist. In addition to, or as part of, their qualification in human nutrition, a dietitian has completed studies incorporating theory and supervised professional practice in clinical nutrition, medical nutrition therapy, and food service management. So, in Australia, all dietitians are nutritionists but a nutritionist without a dietetics qualification is prohibited, by law, from taking on the specialized role of a dietitian, and from using the title. The British Dietetics Association (www.bda.uk.com), draws the same distinction: "Dietitians are the only nutrition professionals to be regulated by law, and are governed by an ethical code to ensure that they always work to the highest standard" (BDA, 2014).

As in the UK, legislation in Australia, Canada, Ireland, New Zealand, South Africa, and the US protects the title "dietitian". In those countries, "nutritionist" and "food scientist" are non-accredited titles that *may* pertain to people who have university qualifications in nutrition, so the need for consumers – no pun intended – to check credentials is strong.

---

1 Enid Blyton's *Famous Five*: Julian, Dick, Anne, George (who detested being called Georgina), and Timmy the dog, were famous for their wartime and post-WW2 adventures (1942–1963), and for the large range of food they enjoyed. In a period when British children were well but austerely fed, there is an authenticity about their diet of hams, new potatoes all gleaming with melted butter and scattered with parsley, onions, jam tarts, hard-boiled eggs, potted meat, porridge, drop scones, bacon, crusty bread, creamy milk, buns, cucumber sandwiches, carrots, fruit cake, homemade salad-cream, tomatoes, humbugs, handfuls of radishes, toffee, cream cheese, plums, mustard and cress, ginger cake, crisp dewy cool fresh lettuces, ginger beer, and most lavishly, lashings and lashings of (homemade) lemonade.

Food gurus

Scientists, by virtue of their science degrees, whose expertise is in food, may work in the nutrition sector, in edutainment, journalism, manufacturing, marketing, media, pharmaceutical, public health promotion, research, or retail pursuits. Because the titles are unprotected in law, *anyone* can assume the titles "food scientist" and "nutritionist".

These designations are liberally applied to individuals in the media, retail, and CAM who have *no* dietetic studies under their belts. They are variously well-informed and misinformed about food and healthy eating, as chefs, cooks, epicures, farmers, foodies[2], gardeners, gastronomes, gourmets, kitchenware salespersons, "home cooks", and niche farmers; and as people who have taken brief courses in nutrition, sometimes as part of a larger field of study such as beauty therapy, child care, physical education or nursing. CAM or "integrative medicine" practitioners, with no dietetics background, regularly expound on nutrition, supplements, and all things "food is medicine[3]" (Augustine, Swift, Harris, Anderson, & Hand, 2015). Conspicuous non-dietitians, from Paleo-Food-Is-Medicine-Pete-Evans (Australian chef, TV personality and food writer), to Gwyneth Paltrow (US actress, singer, and food writer), to Gillian McKeith (British TV presenter and food writer), are associated with eating advice, the term "nutritionist", and variations of it: "clinical nutritionist", "diet guru", "food warrior", "nutrition expert", and "macrobiotic counsellor", to characterize their roles.

Coincidentally, and in a remarkably short period, Victoria Beckham, Miley Cyrus, Lady Gaga, Elisabeth Hasselbeck, Jasmine and Melissa Hemsley, Miranda Kerr, and Gwyneth Paltrow have publicly celebrated the joys of going "gluten free" (GF): to become a nicer person (Paltrow, in a book), for nice skin, physical and mental health, and "because gluten is crapppp" (Cyrus), to improve gut health (clean eating wellness evangelists Hemsley and Hemsley), to "alleviate" autism (Hasselbeck, in a book), and to lose weight (Beckham, Gaga, and Kerr). It seems almost as though there is a marketing-someone, involved in the-GF-way-is-the-healthy-way PR arm of the giant GF-food industry, writing cheques in return for celebrity backing. Almost.

---

2 A foodie (or foody) is a person with a particular interest in food. A gourmet, gastronome or epicure is a connoisseur of good food and drink – a person with a discerning palate.

3 CAM practitioners regularly quote Hippocrates: "Let food be thy medicine and medicine be thy food." Hippocrates also said, "Primum non nocerum" (First do no harm).

Hello, I'm the Doctor

Gillian McKeith (www.gillianmckeith.com), says she is "the internationally acclaimed Holistic Nutritionist and presenter of *You Are What You Eat* hit Channel 4 (BBC) series that took the nation by storm". The storm began in 2004, but the climate changed thanks to an exposé by Ben Goldacre (who blogs at www.badscience.net), for her phony scholarship and concocted doctoral credentials (Goldacre, 2008, pp. 112–135). Dr Goldacre, a physician with two Honorary Doctorates from British universities, was outraged by "the mumbo-jumbo she dresses up as scientific fact" (Goldacre, 2007), and dangers inherent in her recommendations for crash-diets, detox-diets, colonic irrigation, and blue-green algae. Prolific as a "top selling health author", Ms McKeith is a member of the American Association of Nutritional Consultants. As it does not screen applicants' credentials before certifying them, Dr Goldacre successfully registered his Dead Cat Hettie (who tweets beyond the grave as @catnutritionist) for the same accreditation.

> **Pseudoscience alert**
>
> *""I always think of the tongue as being like a window to the organs. The extreme tip correlates to the heart; the bit slightly behind is the lungs. The right side shows what the gallbladder is up to and the left side the liver. The middle indicates the condition of your stomach and spleen, the back the kidneys, intestines and womb."*
> "You Are What You Eat", McKeith (2004, p. 33)
> 2 million copies sold within 2 years of publication

Channel 4 axed her show in 2007, and she had to stop calling herself "doctor", but Ms McKeith still tells the gullible and the incredulous what ails them; recommending intervention via a beady-eyed squiz at their numbers one and two, pimples if any, and Mr Tongue. In 2016, she materialized on *Celebrity Big Brother 17*, as a "therapist", there to "detox" the contestants, inspecting and critiquing the stools of four of them, so preserving her "Dr Poo" persona. Funds permitting, we too can become "doctors" of clinical nutrition, by taking a correspondence course from a non-accredited institute. In Ms McKeith's case, the shonky party was the American Holistic College of Nutrition (Goldacre, 2007) later called the Clayton College of Natural Health (CCNH[4]) in Birmingham, Alabama until it ceased business in July 2010. But who would want to consult, or be, a Clayton's college graduate? The bottom line is, care must be taken in choosing a "diet professional", and in choosing what to watch and believe on TV, hear and believe on radio, and read and believe *everywhere*, including on the Internet and in retail pharmacies.

Retail pharmacy and CAM

Web searches for "pharmacists + homeopathic products", "pharmacies + non-evidence based merchandise", and "pharmacists + complementary medicine" return hundreds of articles in which medical practitioners and AHPs, consumer affairs journalists and savvy health care consumers call for more accountability within retail pharmacy. Stressing that pharmacists are healthcare professionals, they criticize those who sell and promote CAM, and their evident abrogation of a duty of care to customers. The Pharmaceutical Society of Australia (PSA) makes clear in its 2015 position statement (www.psa.org.au/download/policies/position-statement-complementary-medicines.pdf) that a pharmacist's duty of care includes awareness of the available clinical evidence to support marketing claims for the contents of *all* the bottles, boxes, jars, packets, and sachets that crowd pharmacy, chemist shop and drugstore shelves. The statement says, "PSA does not support the sale of homeopathy products in pharmacy" (p. 1) and that: "In the event that a consumer chooses to use a product with limited evidence, the pharmacist must advise the consumer on the risks of rejecting or delaying treatments for which there is good evidence for safety and effectiveness. PSA strongly encourages all consumers considering taking complementary medicines to first consult their pharmacist for sound, evidence-based advice" (p. 3). In our experience in various countries, many pharmacists and their staff do not restrict themselves to issuing sound, evidence-based advice, and the guidance they offer on the "properties" and "benefits" of arnica, echinacea, Garcinia cambogia, ginkgo, St John's Wort, and the rest, resembles the recommendations made in health food shops by proprietors and staff with no pharmacology training, eager for sales. In a 2005 Australian study, Naidu, Wilkinson and Simpson found that pharmacists took a positive view of CAM, believing that

---

4   In November 2010, a class-action suit was filed on behalf of over 5000 litigants who had enrolled in CCNH and submitted most or all of their tuition fees in advance. They alleged that CCNH refused to refund tens of millions of tuition dollars for undelivered programmes. "A Clayton's___" is an expression, derived from "Claytons – the drink you have when you're not having a drink" to describe something that is largely illusory; a poor substitute or imitation.

such products enhanced their customers' image of pharmacy, while increasing customer numbers and annual sales – reflecting a blatant conflict of interests.

Swallowing

Swallowing is a reflex that is as vital to life as breathing. Each of us swallows 900 or more times per 24 hours: around three times per hour during sleep, once per minute during waking hours (Afkari, 2007), and more often at mealtimes (Afkari, 2007; Lear, Flanagan, & Moorrees, 1965). Children tend to swallow more frequently than adults (Lear et al., 1965).

People with normal swallows are only conscious of their swallowing when they have an earache, tonsillitis or a sore throat severe enough to make swallowing painful or difficult, or when something "goes down the wrong way". With every swallow we unconsciously hold our breath momentarily, to ensure that the food or drink goes down the oesophagus to the stomach rather than via the larynx, down the trachea, and via the bronchial tree into the lungs. Twenty-six muscles and many nerves are used in swallowing, and the timing must be precise and reliable in order for it to be efficient and trouble free.

As a complex biomechanical process, swallowing has three phases, oral, pharyngeal, and oesophageal. In the **oral phase**, often split into "oral preparatory" and "oral" stages, food is chewed and mixed with saliva to form a bolus, a soft, slippery "ball", which the tongue then moves to the back of the mouth. Individuals with impairments of the oral phase may have difficulty forming a seal with their lips around a fork, chopsticks or spoon, chewing solid consistencies, forming a bolus, or moving it back, ready for the pharyngeal phase. In the **pharyngeal phase**, the vocal cords close to prevent food and liquid from entering the airway; the larynx rises, and the epiglottis, a flap of cartilage behind the root of the tongue, is lowered to cover it, affording even more protection to the airway. If the pharyngeal phase is impaired, mouth contents can move into the throat before the swallow reflex is triggered. If this happens, the food and liquid touch the vocal cords or even penetrate them, moving them into the lungs. This can result in coughing spasms before, during or shortly after swallowing, shortness of breath, choking sensations, and altered voice quality. Finally, in the **oesophageal phase**, the bolus moves to the oesophagus – the muscular tube or "food pipe" – that contracts to propel the bolus into the stomach. If this phase is impaired, the affected individual might belch, gulp, vomit, or experience heartburn, abdominal pain or wind.

A typically developing (TD) newborn drinks from breast or bottle, using expert little mouth muscles to suck; holding the nipple at the back of the mouth so that the well-aimed squirt of milk triggers the swallow reflex. Some new mothers and babies need help from a lactation consultant, SLP/SLT, baby health nurse, or even a grandmother with the necessary smarts (in what seems to be mainly "women's business") to get started. Around 87% of full-term babies latch on effortlessly and proceed with feeding with few hiccups (Mercado-Deane et al., 2001).

The World Health Organization (2003) recommends that babies be introduced to their first solid foods ("first solids") from age 6 months, to complement their feeds and to help meet their changing nutritional needs. In the industrialized world, there are two schools of thought on how this should happen, and the topic is remarkably divisive. Cichero (2016) reports the recent phenomenon in which baby-led weaning and spoon feeding are seen as mutually exclusive options. In the baby-led weaning corner, babies direct and control the weaning process, are offered soft foods to hand-hold and safely chew, and are allowed to "decide" what, how much, and how quickly to eat. In the "traditional" spoon-feeding corner, first solids are fed *to* the baby in a hierarchy from runny through to chewable foods. Noting anecdotal, impassioned blog and online-discussion-support for baby-led weaning, e.g., www.babyledweaning.com/forum, considered by Rapley (2011), Cichero advocates well-designed research into first solids' introduction, and suggests *combining* the methods, with vital supervision of infants to avoid choking. Weighing the advantages of both, she explains (p. 72) that, "Spoon-feeding provides an opportunity for infants to develop oral skills necessary for safe management of solids and may facilitate intake of iron-rich foods at weaning, whilst baby-led weaning promotes greater participation in family meals and exposure to family foods".

Irrespective of how first solids are introduced, babies gradually learn to move food from front to back in the mouth, to elicit the swallowing reflex. They learn to chew – inexpertly at first – to combine food with saliva. The chewing action and salivary enzymes cause the food to break down into tiny pieces, forming an easily-swallowed bolus. For infants with dysphagia, sucking, chewing, and swallowing are problematic, and these problems can persist, particularly if early intervention is not available or accessed.

Dysphagia

SLPs/SLTs are the only professionals expressly qualified to assess and treat communication and swallowing difficulties (dysphagia) across the lifespan.

Dysphagia involves any problem with the swallowing stages outlined above: forming a lip seal, sucking and drinking (via breast, bottle, cup, spout or straw), chewing and eating, and swallowing while protecting the airway. Depending on the age of the individual and the presenting picture, SLPs/SLTs may counsel on approaches to infant feeding, recommend changes to the textures and consistencies of foods or drinks, and provide techniques and exercises that promote safe and comfortable swallowing while still optimizing the enjoyment of food. When dysphagia is severe, the SLP/SLT may advise on tube-feeding that channels food and drink directly to the stomach. Tubes can be nasal tubes: nasogastric, naso-duodenal or naso-jejunal; gastric tubes or G-tubes including percutaneous endoscopic gastrostomy (PEG) and long tubes; gastro-jejunal tubes; and jejunal tubes. These are inserted by paediatric surgeons in close consultation with the treating SLP/SLT.

Mercado-Deane et al. (2001) found that 26% of preterm babies have dysphagia, which is twice the reported incidence among full-term infants. Other at-risk infants are those: who suffered perinatal stroke, or vocal cord paralysis; born with heart defects, foetal alcohol spectrum disorder (FASD), or genetic disorders such as Down or Prader Willi syndrome; with anatomic differences affecting the head, neck and face (e.g., cleft lip and palate); and with difficulties with oral-motor function (e.g., cerebral palsy). Those with Autism Spectrum Disorders (ASD), acquired brain injuries, progressive neurological disorders, and Food Protein-Induced Enterocolitis syndrome (FPIES) are also at risk.

Among the early signs of dysphagia may be mealtime choking, coughing, or gagging, unusually slow eating (taking over 30 minutes to finish a meal), eyes tearing-up or watering during a meal, "pocketing" (food remaining in the mouth after a meal), swallowing without chewing, and effortful swallowing. Oesophageal reflux, nasopharyngeal reflux, nasal regurgitation, or vomiting may also occur. Reflux occurs when the oesophagus valves let stomach contents (food, drink and gastric acid: hydrochloric acid, potassium chloride and sodium chloride) regurgitate, as far up the digestive tract as the throat, and even into the mouth or nose.

Dysphagia encompasses difficulties with: *eating* food; *drinking* liquid; *chewing* food; *sucking* ices, confectionary, nipples, straws and teats; *swallowing* saliva, liquids, food and medications; and maintaining the necessary *lip seal* that prevents food or saliva escaping through the lips. Some individuals with dysphagia have problems protecting the trachea, so food and drink "go down the wrong way". Potentially, this can cause choking and, in many cases, can lead to chronic lung disease via recurrent aspiration, chest infections, and pneumonia.

For those with dysphagia, the physiological aspects of eating and drinking can be painful, stressful and complicated. They can suffer embarrassment when eating in front of people beyond, or even within, the immediate family. They must also withstand the bother of – and sometimes, personal comments and insensitive advice about – needing to adhere to a modified diet, or to assume certain postures while eating or drinking, or to deal with persistent drooling. Such factors can seed feelings of loneliness and anxiety, and a downward spiral to social isolation and depression for them and for those close to them: emotionally and practically tough situations.

Problematic eating behaviour

Aside from, or in conjunction with dysphagia, problematic eating behaviour poses substantial challenges for affected children, their families, and professionals who work with them (Thoyre et al., 2014). The behaviours can include "selective eating": refusing certain foods or all food, gagging while eating or in anticipation of eating, avoiding certain textures, "mouth stuffing" (over-filling the mouth), or insisting that food is offered in a certain way.

Jack, of Weather King repute (see pages 62–65), with an ASD diagnosis, enjoyed a balanced diet comprising the five core food groups[5], small amounts of unsaturated fats, oils and spreads, one litre of water a day, no soft drinks, and fast foods and "unhealthy snacks" as rare treats. He had no difficulty with food temperatures or tastes. *But*, if his place setting was "wrong", or if textures he would accept independently were combined, he reacted with angry tears, weeping to the point of vomiting, and would be "off his food" for up to a week.

At 8 years of age, Jack needed precise mealtime conditions. He had to sit on a chair at a table (any chair and table, anywhere, luckily), an orderly thicket of short, sharp upwards-pointing IKEA pencils and a small notebook in his shirt pocket at all times, wearing his hat. Placed directly ahead of him would be a *Bunnykins* melamine plate and mug, like those he had used as a 2-year-old, on a natural bamboo placemat, and to the right, on an identical placemat, a "Tree Toys" *Bunnykins* ABC Building Blocks spoon and fork – a setting of six items. Duplicates stayed at school, at his grandparents' houses,

---

5 The five core food groups: (1) vegetables and legumes; (2) fruit; (3) grain (cereal) foods; (4) lean meats and poultry, fish, eggs, tofu, nuts and seeds, and legumes/beans; (5) milk, yoghurt, cheese and/or their alternatives.

and in his parents' cars for use when the family ate out. In their shed was a box of replacements – just in case. Food had to be arranged discretely on his plate, and he sobbingly rejected textured foods mixed with smooth foods: breakfast cereals with milk, and jellies, juices, soups or spreads with "bits" in them were out. Jack would consume almost anything, but the setup *had* to be his way.

Gluten and casein

There is no such thing as a gluten (or casein) "allergy", but there is such a thing as coeliac disease (CD). As the most common autoimmune condition, CD is unevenly distributed globally, affecting from 0.5% to almost 2.0% of people across the world's population (Gujral, Freeman, & Thomson, 2012), and rising (Kenrick & Day, 2014). It is a lifelong and debilitating illness that produces an inflammatory response to gluten, damaging the gut wall, resulting in malabsorption of nutrients by the small intestine, bloating, diarrhoea, gas, pain, and weight loss.

Currently, the only treatment for CD is a permanent gluten-free (GF) diet. Far from being a "lifestyle choice" or food fad, the diet should be instigated following medical confirmation of CD, normally by a gastroenterologist, with guidance from a dietitian with expertise in the area (Kenrick & Day, 2014). Despite endorsements from Victoria Beckham, Miley Cyrus (who declares having "allergies" to gluten and casein), Lady Gaga, Hemsley and Hemsley, Elisabeth Hasselbeck, Miranda Kerr, and Gwyneth Paltrow, the diet has doubtful benefits for the nearly 98% of people *without* the condition. Nevertheless, the most popular, but scientifically unproven, intervention for ASD is the GF *and* casein-free (GFCF) diet (Buie, 2013), with an associated jihad against grains and sugar, aided and abetted by celebrity endorsement and an undeniable global GF-food marketing push.

A GF or GFCF diet is sometimes adopted in the belief that a child with ASD has coeliac disease, irritable bowel syndrome (IBS), or an as-yet unconfirmed condition called "gluten sensitivity" or "non-celiac gluten sensitivity" (NCGS) that popped into someone's head in the 1980s (Verdu, Armstrong, & Murray, 2009). The diagnosis of NCGS in adults and children is controversial (Vriezinga, Schweizer, Koning, & Mearin, 2015), with some researchers suggesting that gluten may not be the problem but rather malabsorption of certain sugars, namely FODMAPs: fermentable, oligo-, di-, monosaccharides, and polyols (Biesiekierski et al., 2013). FODMAPs are in disreputable farty-foods like beans, onion and broccoli, and also in milk, apples, wheat, high-fructose corn syrup, and more.

The casein-free (CF), GF, and GFCF diets have a new competitor for consumer moolah in the ASD food fad field: the Low-FODMAP diet. For years, ASD advocacy groups, families and clinicians have fallen for sharp advertising of the GFCF diet, with scientific-sounding phrases: "evolving paradigm", "promising research trend", "new understandings", "latest discoveries" – but soon, the Low-FODMAP diet may become the new black, despite no demonstrable link as yet, between FODMAPs and ASD.

Dysphagia, problematic eating behaviour, and teamwork

Anyone with dysphagia and/or problematic eating behaviour is at risk for inadequate nutrition – hence the importance of cooperation between families, SLPs/SLTs and dietitians. In paediatric dysphagia, SLPs/SLTs and dietitians work collaboratively in teams that *will* include the child's family and, within reason, the child if they are old enough and able to have a say in what, where, how, and with whom they will eat. Teams may also include aides, behaviour analysts, lactation consultants, medical practitioners, food preparation staff, food service supervisors, mealtime volunteers who patiently implement secure feeding practices (Edwards & Marlise Martin, 2011), nurses, OTs, physiotherapists, psychologists, and teachers.

Management by SLPs/SLTs starts with expert screening (Delaney, 2015) and assessment (Thoyre et al., 2014). The SLP/SLT then implements techniques and interventions such as setting the stage for successful oral feeding (SOFFI), a programme for medically fragile neonatal intensive care unit infants (Horner et al., 2014), bottle selection (Ross & Fuhrman, 2015), the Pre-Chaining and Food Chaining© Therapy programmes (Fraker & Walbert, 2011), or school-based interventions (Homer & Carbajal, 2015). The treatment of dysphagia will involve the best combination for the client's needs of medical, surgical, or behavioural interventions, postural and positioning techniques, and dietary modifications, while accounting for social, cultural or belief-based food rules and traditions, nutritional requirements, and where practicable and low-risk, personal preferences.

Ankyloglossia (tongue-tie)

On *rare* occasions, an SLP/SLT may recommend **lingual frenectomy** because of the *carefully assessed* negative impact of ankyloglossia (short lingual fraenum) on a child's speech. It is only in unusually severe cases of tongue-tie that speech is ever affected, however, and it is more likely that an SLP/SLT would recommend frenectomy, involving tissue resection under general anaesthetic, in the interests of oral health (e.g., if tongue movements were sufficiently restricted to prevent "sweeping" food debris). SLPs/SLTs are less likely to be consulted on the need for **lingual frenotomy** ("tongue clipping"), a procedure performed under local anaesthetic, on neonates with tongue-tie, to enable them to latch and suckle. Lingual frenotomy is a well-tolerated surgical procedure (Aras, Göregen, Güngörmüş, & Akgül, 2010) and considered by many to be beneficial (O'Callahan, Macary, & Clemente, 2013; Steehler, Steehler, & Harley, 2012; Toner, Giordano, & Handler, 2014) in remediating mother-and-baby difficulties with breastfeeding (Buryk, Bloom, & Shope, 2011; Hogan, Westcott, & Griffiths, 2005) and bottle-feeding (Hogan et al., 2005).

Perusal of two Facebook groups reveal that "tethered oral issues" are more than a niche interest for SLPs/SLTs, and that those involved are guided more by advertising, anecdotes, non-peer reviewed CPD and the entrenched views of popular gurus in the field than by empirical evidence. The Australasian Society for Tongue and Lip Ties is "a dynamic group of multidisciplinary health care professionals supporting optimal outcomes in families and individuals affected by Tongue and Lip Ties through integrating and sharing of up to date clinical experience, research and resources". The Coalition of Speech-Language Pathologists for Tethered Oral Tissues "is a SLP professionals only group for collaborating, learning, and advocating for best practices in tethered oral tissues...a place to band together and dispel the many myths of tethered oral tissues and provide opportunities for learning in this unique area". In both groups, regular contributors guilelessly (or disingenuously) explain how their practices have been informed by non-evidence based approaches to tongue-tie, including: Beckman Oral Motor, bodywork, chiropractic, craniosacral therapy, Feldenkrais, kinesiotaping, Mr Tongue, Myofascial Release, NS-OME/NS-OMT, osteopathy, PROMPT©, TalkTools®, and Therapeutic Speech Massage (www.tsmus.info) from Russian reflexology practitioner Dr Elena Dyakova.

Turning to the juried literature, we find that ankyloglossia has no standardized definition, is over-diagnosed in babies by a range of non-experts, including chiropractors (for example www.silverbackchiropractic.com/tongue-tie-in-infants), dentists and naturopaths, and well-baby, early childhood health, and infant welfare nurses; and opinions vary as to its clinical significance and optimal management (Brinkman, Reilly, & Meara, 2004; Eschler, Klein, & Overby, 2010; Messner & Lalakea, 2000).

Nutrition

It is hard to compensate later in life for poor early nutrition, and everyone's diet must satisfy specific nutritional requirements for daily physical activity, healthy weight maintenance and optimal development. Infants', children's and adolescents' food and drink intakes must be nutritionally adequate in supporting typical growth and development, including oral health. Knowing this, WHO, government departments, and dietitians' associations internationally provide accessible (online or in print), multilingual, culturally appropriate, and usually "budget aware" dietary guidelines for individuals across the lifespan.

Reliable guidance on eating plans is readily available, augmenting the *necessary* advice of dietitians and doctors (e.g., cardiologists, endocrinologists, gastroenterologists, paediatricians, and specialist physicians), for children and young people with allergies, anaemia, anorexia nervosa, childhood obesity, coeliac disease, Crohn's disease, FPIES, failure to thrive, food intolerance, malnutrition, phenylketonuria, Prader Willi syndrome, or Type 1 diabetes. Their scientifically-based eating plans differ from the "special diets" for children with developmental difficulties that proliferate in CAM, "holistic health", "integrative medicine" and "food guru" spheres. We discuss these below, but first an answer (of sorts) to THAT QUESTION!

Can your child's diet boost her intelligence?

Louise Fulton Keats says it can. She is a "club expert" at the (duopolistic Australian supermarket chain) Woolworths Baby & Toddlers Club (www.woolworthsbabyandtoddlerclub.com.au), a food and nutrition writer and cookbook author, showcased at www.louisefultonkeats.com. A qualified lawyer, Ms Keats is a Le Cordon Bleu Australia graduate and, according to her web bio, "has postgraduate nutrition qualifications from Deakin University, one of the world's leading universities in the field of nutrition and dietetics": so, not a dietitian.

Scientists say

She writes (Keats, n.d.), without citing said scientists, "Scientists have identified five dietary factors that are important when it comes to brain function", explaining the benefits of omega-3 fats, iron, iodine, breakfast and an overall nutritious diet. She continues, without detailing the two studies mentioned;

"One study by the MRC Epidemiology Resource Centre at the University of Southampton found that children who had eaten higher amounts of fruits, vegetables and home-cooked meals during infancy (i.e., 6–12 months) had a higher IQ at four years old. Another found that children who had eaten a healthy diet (with more rice, salad, fruits and pasta) at three years old had a higher IQ when tested at eight years old, compared with children eating lots of processed foods with a high fat and sugar content". Even without access to the studies, we hazard that factors other than diet were at play, to account for the well-fed 4- and 8-year-olds' superior IQs. Health science students typically learn in research methods that correlation does not mean causation, but simply that something else is going on. They learn to ask pertinent questions in these situations: Did the brighter children's parents perchance interact more with their offspring, have higher IQs, more advanced levels of education, better housing, higher socio-economic status, and more spondoolicks for food and "opportunities" than the comparison group parents? We also guess that, should we ever identify the studies, we would find that the researchers emphasized and discussed these significant confounding factors. But that will not help Woolworths sell rice, pasta, fruit and vegetables.

Brain foods

Phil McGraw (www.drphil.com) says you can increase your child's intellectual *performance*, putting his faith in "brain foods for brainpower" to nourish young minds. Dr Phil has a BA in psychology, an MA in experimental psychology, and in 1979 earned a PhD in clinical psychology, exploring a psychological intervention for people with rheumatoid arthritis. He stopped practising psychology in 1990 but kept his Texas licence-to-practice current until 2006. Although untrained in dietetics, he has written several weight-loss books, and is unstinting with half-baked advice on children's nutrition. Without mentioning dairy foods, he recommends: citrus for memory and performance; green, orange, purple and yellow fruits and vegetables to protect the brain against damage and prevent mental fatigue; wholegrain and iron-fortified cereals for sharp mental performance; eggs for memory building; fish for brain building fats; and lean meats for learning and memory. For Dr Phil, it is not all about brain foods. On a page that offers the opportunity to "test your child's IQ", and to "click here for a CD on enhancing your child's IQ", he advises: creating an empowering internal dialogue, doing controlled breathing exercises and mental gymnastics, increasing opportunities for verbal interactions as a family, encouraging repetitive reading, creating a stimulating environment, introducing music and rhythm, and staying physically active (McGraw, n.d.).

A difficult game

Brainy Child (www.brainy-child.com) has an article by its owner, Andrew Loh, called *How to Improve Your Child's IQ: Learning the Basics*. He says, "Raising or improving your child's IQ is a difficult game as it involves manipulating your child's brain functions with a series of revolutionary techniques and methods." In a site crammed with "Brain Foods for Kids" and "Over 100 Recipes to Boost Your Child's Intelligence", Mr Loh signs numerous articles as "Publisher & Editor, BrainyZine" without revealing his qualifications. He has a lot of time for pseudoscientific tactics that we discourage: brain balancing, brain-based learning, Brain Gym®, Glen Doman™, right brain learning, learning styles, and Shichida™. So, we sidestepped the revolution, hoping our discerning readers will do likewise.

What does IQ mean?

Technically, Intelligence Quotient (IQ) refers to a numerical value derived from a standardized test of intellectual functioning such as the Wechsler Intelligence Scale for Children® (WISC) and the Kaufman Brief Intelligence Test (K-BIT). All IQ tests have a mean (average) of 100. Because IQ is "normally distributed" within a population, when tested, 50% of people will have IQs below 100 and 50% will have IQs above. It is common to describe IQs between 70 and 100 as "average" and those between 100 and 130 as "above average". IQ tests have a standard deviation (a statistically-derived measure of variability around the mean) of 15. Hence 70 is a score two standard deviations below the mean and 130 is two standard deviations above. Until the release of the classification tome DSM-5 (American Psychiatric Association, 2013), the term "mental retardation" was used in the US to refer to people with IQs below 70, whereas Australia, the UK and Europe, and New Zealand have used the more enlightened "intellectual disability" (ID) for some time. Thankfully, ID replaces "mental retardation" in the DSM-5. In Britain, "learning disability" is often used to refer to people who in other countries would be said to have an ID. In Australia, *learning disability* typically denotes children and adults with average or above-average IQs who struggle significantly with literacy and numeracy (without requiring special schooling). It is confusing to parents and frustrating to clinicians and researchers that these international inconsistencies persist, despite the influence of diagnostic frameworks like the DSM and the International Classification of Diseases: ICD (WHO, 2016).

IQ tests characteristically cover conceptual, problem solving, and "executive" skills in two broad domains: verbal (concerning language) and nonverbal (concerning visuo-spatial skills). Correspondingly, they yield three scores: Verbal IQ, Nonverbal ("Performance") IQ, and a Full-Scale IQ that is derived from the first two. The scores are of interest, as are any significant discrepancies (as determined by reference to the test scoring manual) between the Verbal and Nonverbal components. Inevitably, IQ tests are subject to the vagaries of human "off" and "on" days. Children who feel tired, distressed, unwell, or "anti", perform significantly less well than they would on a day when everything is more favourable. Accordingly, there is a margin of error around an IQ score; it is not precise. This can be problematic if IQ scores are used as arbitrary cut-offs to establish eligibility for services. IQ tests are "restricted", so should only be sold to, owned by, administered, scored and interpreted by registered psychologists. Unfortunately, just as there may be child factors on the day, the skill and experience of the practitioner comes into play too, introducing even *more* variability into an inexact "science".

IQ tests derive from the early 20th-century desire to identify which children would need special support in school. In response to the question "What does IQ mean?", it is tempting to respond tongues-in-cheeks with, "IQ is what IQ tests measure", because in a sense that is true. IQ tests "tap" functions that many people in western industrialized nations think are important for academic, social, and life success – the abilities to think conceptually, reason and problem solve, demonstrate mastery of language, and perform well under time pressure. In addition to individual factors "on the day", these skills are heavily influenced by cultural context and life experience, so scores must be viewed alongside important psychosocial information.

In some cases, the administration of such measures is unfair and ridiculous. Consider, for example, a 5-year-old Aboriginal child living in a remote community in Australia's far north. This child may be flourishing in all respects, developing proficiency in multiple languages, but unacquainted with the learning experiences that assist performance on standardized IQ tests. We delude ourselves if we fancy that IQ tests tell the full story of a child's abilities or capacity for academic achievement. So, it is pleasing that the DSM-5 does not define ID as a score below a certain arbitrary point. Rather, it considers the conceptual and social domains alongside essential observational and interview data about the individual's *adaptive* functioning: their ability to look after themselves and manage in a practical sense in the (hopefully *their*) real world.

Harvard University Developmental Psychologist, Howard Gardner, challenged the narrow way in which intelligence came to be framed as a single number. In 1983, Dr Gardner proposed a Theory of Multiple Intelligences (MI), incorporating aptitudes in: linguistic, logic-mathematical, musical, spatial, bodily/kinesthetic, interpersonal, intrapersonal, and naturalistic domains. His influential 1983 book was updated and re-released in 2011 – testament to his theory's enduring impact. MI is a conspicuous "idea" in education that has a certain face appeal, even if the science underpinning it is debatable (and debatable it is). On the credit side, Dr Gardner's theory has probably helped schools to identify and value student skill-sets that lie outside traditional, often narrowly-defined, achievement metrics. Detractors argue that MI so permeates pedagogy that it represents a "dumbing down" of education. In 2003, reflecting on two decades of the influence of his theory on education policy and practice, Dr Gardner stated:

> "I have come to realize that once one releases an idea—a 'meme'[6]—into the world, one cannot completely control its behavior—anymore than one can control those products of our genes called children. Put succinctly, MI has and will have a life of its own, over and above what I might wish for it, my most widely known intellectual offspring."

Reading between the lines, we think that Dr Gardner is none too pleased with the often-uncritical application of MI theory. The genie, however, is well and truly out of the bottle.

Oral health

The World Health Organization (2012) defines oral health as "a state of being free from chronic mouth and facial pain, oral and throat cancer, oral sores, birth defects such as cleft lip and palate, periodontal (gum) disease, tooth decay and tooth loss, and other diseases and disorders that affect the oral cavity". Poor oral health may disturb quality of life and a person's ability to eat, drink, sleep, and function painlessly. Oral health and disease, including dysphagia,

---

6 Meme: an idea, behaviour, or style that spreads from person to person within a culture. See Kamhi (2004) for discussion.

are powerful in their own right and for their relationship to wellbeing and participation in society without physical or social discomfort.

In the US, the Centers for Disease Control and Prevention (CDC) determined that dental caries (decay) is five times more common than asthma, and seven times more common than hay fever in children, and that over 40% of children have dental caries by the time they reach kindergarten age (Dye, Xianfen, & Beltrán-Aguilar, 2012). More recently, the CDC stated that approximately 23% of children aged 2–5 years had dental caries in primary teeth. Untreated tooth decay in primary teeth among children aged 2–8 was twice as high for Hispanic and non-Hispanic black children compared with non-Hispanic white children. Among those aged 6–11, 27% of Hispanic children had dental caries in permanent teeth compared with nearly 18% of non-Hispanic white and Asian children. About three in five adolescents aged 12–19 had experienced dental caries in permanent teeth, and 15% had untreated tooth decay (Dye, Thornton-Evans, Li, & Iafolla, 2015).

The magnitude of the problem of poor oral health, in the US and worldwide, cannot be overstated. In Australia, in 2013–2014, of a population of 23.13 million inhabitants, nearly 31,000 children aged 0–14 underwent emergency dental extractions *involving a general anesthetic* in hospital (Australian Institute of Health and Welfare, 2016). Children with decay in deciduous teeth are at much greater risk for cavities in their adult teeth, and again, in Australia, around 45% of children aged 12 have decay in their adult teeth (Russell, 2014).

Commenting that "for many children with developmental disabilities, their smile is their most effective way of interacting with the world," Norwood, Slayton, Liptak and Murphy (2013) speak to the specific oral health difficulties of children with special needs, including those in care. The helpful Norwood et al. article (pediatrics.aappublications.org/content/131/3/614) is openly accessible and covers such important topics as children who do not take food or fluids orally, and children with oral aversion, functional limitations in self-care, craniofacial anomalies, and chronic dental erosions secondary to maladaptive behaviours.

> *"Children with developmental disabilities, including conditions that affect behavior and cognition, often have limitations in their abilities to perform activities of daily living. They may have special health care needs as well. Examples include children with autism spectrum disorders, intellectual disability, cerebral palsy, craniofacial anomalies, and other*

health conditions. As a group, children with developmental disabilities are more likely to have unmet dental needs than are typically developing children and are considered to be at greater risk of developing dental disease. The reasons include frequent use of medicine high in sugar, dependence on a caregiver for regular oral hygiene, reduced clearance of foods from the oral cavity, impaired salivary function, preference for carbohydrate-rich foods, a liquid or puréed diet, and oral aversions."

Norwood, Slayton, Liptak, & Murphy 2013, p. 614.

Dental health dietary recommendations

All national dental and dietetics associations make explicit nutritional recommendations for oral health across the lifespan. For dental health they advise three serves daily of dairy foods such as milk, cheese and yogurt, because "dairy" provides at least 10 essential nutrients: protein, carbohydrate, vitamins (A, B12, and riboflavin); and minerals (calcium, phosphorus, magnesium, potassium and zinc), aiding in reducing tooth decay and protecting tooth enamel.

They emphasize that casein (a protein in dairy foods), when combined with calcium and phosphorus, creates a protective protein film over the enamel surface of the tooth, while the "strengthening minerals" calcium and phosphorus help repair teeth after acid attacks. Milks, flavoured or unflavoured, contain about 5% sugar from lactose. Lactose has low cariogenicity[7] compared to other sugars, contributing little or nothing to tooth decay. Artificially sweetened flavoured milks contain no added sugar (sucrose). It is helpful to know, too, that dietitians and other health professionals articulate a *strong* case for limiting serves of fruit juices, as they often contain similar sugar content and kilojoules (calories) to soft drinks and "fruit juice cordials" (squash) (see www.nutritionaustralia.org/national/resource/drinks-children).

Food for thought

Some of the words in the preceding paragraphs: *calcium, casein, cheese, dairy, lactose, magnesium, milk, minerals, phosphorus, potassium, protein, vitamins, yogurt,* and *zinc* appear in the sections below, in the context of irrational

---

7 Cariogenicity: Producing or promoting the development of tooth decay via cariogenic foods (or cariogenic bacteria).

diets that exclude foods necessary for general, dental and oral health, thereby jeopardising children's wellbeing, and adding to the uphill grind they and their families already experience. You will also find below the words *fruit* (dried and fresh), *legumes* (beans, chickpeas, lentils and peas), *mushrooms, potatoes* (bang goes the fibre!) and more, precluded from several of the diets.

Alternative medicine

> *"There is no such thing as alternative medicine; there are just treatments that work, and those that don't. Those that work will find their way into the standard armamentarium of medicine, while those that don't are destined to remain in the realm of quackery."*
>
> Edzard Ernst, 2015

Complementary and alternative medicine (CAM) includes: (1) biologically-based practices; (2) mind-body therapies; (3) manipulative and body-based practices; (4) energy therapies; and (5) traditional and holistic medical systems. The first one, biologically-based practices, is germane to our diets, supplements and nutrition topic, remembering that practitioners (or parents) will often combine them with the other four when working with children with developmental difficulties.

Many parents pursue CAM (Christon, Mackintosh, & Myers, 2013) alongside mainstream therapies and medical treatments (Matson, Adams, Williams, & Reiske, 2013), but they may keep this quiet. Other than parents forgetting to mention it, and health care professionals (HCP) failing to ask, there is a range of reasons why the reported 50% (Ernst, 1999), to over 70% (Adams et al., 2013; Christon et al., 2013), to 82% (Aburahma, Khader, Alzoubi, & Sawalha, 2010), to 88% (Valicenti-McDermott et al., 2014) of parents who use CAM with their children do not tell their HCP. It can be because they:

- Regard their CAM providers and preparations to be "complementary" and not "alternative";

- See their HCP as not interested in, or as resisting understanding, why they use CAM;

- Fear that their HCP will react negatively, humour them, or think them foolish;

- Do not think of the complementary medicines they take as "drugs" or "medicines";
- See their "ancient", "Ayurvedic", "biodynamic", "body and soul", "botanical", "herbal", "homeopathic" "holistic", "integrative", "natural", "organic", "pure", "traditional" or "whole" formulations as safe, and unlikely to trigger side effects or to interact problematically with prescription medicines, so disclosure is irrelevant;
- Believe that their HCPs know less than their (trusted) CAM advisers about the properties, benefits and risks of CAM.

Biologically-based practices

In the CAM category of biological interventions, herbal and other nutrient and non-nutrient substances are used. Examples of herbal (plant) remedies are arnica for bruises, echinacea for colds, ginkgo biloba and ginseng as memory aids, and cranberry for cystitis. Other nutrients or "nutraceuticals" might be fish oil (omega-3 fatty acids) to address a host of conditions including Childhood Apraxia of Speech (CAS) and ASD, and chondroitin sulfate (from shark and cow cartilage), which some say relieves pain and slows cartilage breakdown in osteoarthritis. Non-nutrients include vitamins like ascorbic acid (Vitamin C) for scurvy and colds, and folic acid (a B complex vitamin) during pregnancy; mineral supplements such as iron in pregnancy and for anaemia; and chemical compounds, for example injected or oral ethylenediaminetetraacetic acid (EDTA), and Epsom salts baths for ASD.

"Nutraceuticals", "functional foods" and dietary supplements

The term *nutraceutical* was coined in 1989 by Stephen L. DeFelice MD, a self-proclaimed Doctornaut for 40 years, founder and chair of the Foundation of Innovation Medicine (www.fimdefelice.org). It is defined as "any substance that is food or a part of food and provides medical or health benefits, including the prevention and treatment of disease". Usually, nutraceuticals consist of dietary supplements (vitamins, minerals, amino acids, and herbal substances) or *functional foods* (those containing or "fortified with" health-giving additives such as Vitamin D added to milk). Both terms vary with respect to their legal status around the world. For example, in Canada, a nutraceutical can be marketed as either a food or as a drug, and the terms nutraceutical and functional food have no legal distinction, and under US law "nutraceutical" has no legal meaning whereas "dietary supplement" has.

The US Food and Drug Administration (FDA) defines a *dietary supplement* as "a product taken by mouth that contains a 'dietary ingredient' intended to supplement the diet. The 'dietary ingredients' in these products may include: vitamins, minerals, herbs or other botanicals, amino acids, and substances such as enzymes, organ tissues, glandulars, and metabolites. Dietary supplements can also be extracts or concentrates, and may be found in many forms such as tablets, capsules, softgels, gelcaps, liquids, or powders" (Dietary Supplement Health and Education Act (DSHEA) of 1994: www.ods.od.nih.gov/About/DSHEA_Wording.aspx). Such products do not require FDA approval prior to marketing, but companies must register their manufacturing facilities with the FDA. With a handful of clearly-specified exceptions, in the US dietary supplements may only be marketed to support the structure or function of the body, but cannot claim to treat a disease or condition. Labels must include the words: "These statements have not been evaluated by the Food and Drug Administration. This product is not intended to diagnose, treat, cure, or prevent any disease."

Omega-3 fatty acid supplementation

Among the most popular nutraceuticals is a group of polyunsaturated fatty acids called omega-3 or "essential" fatty acids. These include eicosapentaenoic acid (EPA) and docosahexaenoic acid (DHA), available in fish and seafood, and alpha-linolenic acid (ALA) found in grains and seeds, including nuts. DHA and EPA are fundamental to neurodevelopment, and neurotransmitter function because they influence synaptic processes, and the mechanisms for releasing dopamine and serotonin as required. For health, omega-3s must be contained in the diet as food or in supplement form, since they cannot be synthesized in the human body.

Omega-3 deficiencies are thought to adversely affect mood, behaviour (e.g., aggression), and emotional states (e.g., anger). Exploring the relationship between omega-3 fatty acids and aggressive behaviour specifically, Gajos and Beaver (2016) performed a meta-analysis of 40 studies encompassing intervention and observational research designs. They found that omega-3s appear to have small to large effects on reducing aggression, with effect-sizes conditioned by how participants' aggressive behaviours were measured; whether by self-report or parent/teacher surveys for example. Gajos and Beaver saw promising signs that Omega-3 *supplements* (rather than upping the omega-3s in food intake) may reduce aggressive behaviours in both children and adults. Somewhat favourable results have also emerged from studies of the impact of omega-3 supplementation on ADHD (Gow, Hibbel, & Parletta, 2015) encouraging further research effort.

By contrast, the audacious and baseless claims made for omega-3s in treating CAS (e.g., Morris & Agin, 2009) are associated with no credible evidence, while the results of the Mankad et al. (2015) study failed to support high-dose supplementation of omega-3 fatty acids in young children with ASD. Among the miracle products to avoid, that are supposed to target CAS, are Deepak Chopra's NutriiVeda (www.chopra.com) endorsed by Lisa Geng's Cherab Foundation (www.cherab.org; see also www.pursuitofresearch.org); Mark Nottoli and Roy Bingham's Nourish Life SPEAK (www.speechnutrients.com) prosecuted by the Federal Trade Commission for deceptive advertising in 2015; and the bespoke "Speech Diet" that stay-at-home-mom Kate Welder (www.apraxiaspeaks.com) devised for her daughter and now promotes, along with her book, *Apraxia Explained*, and jumping therapy (or "rebounding") to improve speech, increase mental acuity, and remediate learning disabilities. Hard- and soft-bounce Rebounders are mini-trampolines. Spuriously, "when you are rebounding, you are moving and exercising every brain cell just as you are exercising each of the other body cells. Toxic heavy metals are leached out of these brain cells to free up the neurons to work more effectively. Rebounding has you work from the outside, from the nerve endings in toward the brain". Sorry? How do you assess that the toxins are *there*; and leached from the brain to *where*, precisely? Rebounding fans past and present include Rabbi Dr Gabriel Cousens (see page 287), Donna Gates (page 281), actor Bob Hope, President Ronald Reagan, motivational speaker Tony Robbins, and raw foodist, author, Flat Earth theorist, CAM promoter, and NutriBullet spokesperson, David Wolfe.

Chelation

The word *chelation* comes from the Greek for claw, and in English has come to mean "to grab" or "to bind". In chemistry, chelation is a type of bonding of ions and molecules to metal ions. "Chelation therapy" is a process whereby EDTA – a water-soluble synthetic chemical solution – is injected into the bloodstream with the aim of binding (removing) heavy metals and/or minerals. EDTA is also widely used in industry to remove lime scale and "hard water" deposits, the tough, dirty-white, chalky deposit found in kettles, hotwater boilers, and old pipes.

In medicine, chelation therapy is an *approved* treatment for *heavy metal poisoning* resulting from an accumulation of iron, mercury, arsenic, and lead. Mercury, arsenic and lead serve no function in the human body, and are toxic if present in sufficient amounts (Flora & Pachauri, 2010). Heavy metal poisoning is an *uncommon* diagnosis, and it can arise from industrial exposure, air or water pollution, foods and medicines, wrongly coated food vessels, or swallowing lead-based paints. It cannot arise from dental fillings, nasal sprays, or vaccines. Ever.

Certifiable mercury madness

Chelation is a costly, futile and potentially treacherous intervention for children with ASD (Davis et al., 2013). Chelation "therapy" (irony intended) is administered to children with ASD, orally or by injection one to 12 times weekly, in the erroneous belief, based on invalidated theory, that their ASD symptoms are associated with specific levels of metals in the body; notably mercury in the MMR vaccine[8], in nasal sprays, in mercury-contaminated fish, and in dental amalgams.

---

8 This belief arose from observations that (1) the volume of cases of ASD was *apparently* growing (actually, the criteria for ASD diagnoses were broadened) and (2) the number of recommended childhood vaccines was increasing. Some conflated the two, blaming thimerosal, a mercury-containing preservative in some vaccines, for causing autism. The theory was promulgated by the disgraced and discredited former surgeon and medical researcher, Andrew Jeremy Wakefield who was struck off the UK medical register in 2010. The theories, and all of Wakefield's assertions, published in *The Lancet* in 1998 and subsequently withdrawn, have been scientifically refuted (DeStefano, Price, & Weintraub, 2013). Undeterred, Wakefield, now based in the US, continues his anti-vaccination rabble-rousing activities as a martyr to the fraudulent cause. Thimerosal has not been used in vaccines specifically for children since 2001. It is still used in some flu vaccines (recommended annually for all children). Parents worried about thimerosal can request a flu vaccine without it. Most single-dose vials and pre-filled syringes of flu shot and the nasal spray flu vaccine do not contain a preservative because they are intended to be only used once.

> *"Perhaps the greatest concern in regards to the selection of chelation treatment for children ASD is the lack of construct validity. In some ways, chelation therapy represents the "cart before the horse" scenario in that the hypothesis supporting of the use of chelation treatment failed to be validated prior to the application of chelation. Chelation treatment aims to eliminate specific metals from the body. However, empirical evidence has yet to support the hypothesis that the core ASD symptoms are caused by the presence of such metals in the body. Because empirical evidence does not support the hypothesis that the core ASD symptoms are associated with specific levels of metals in the body, the use of chelation to remove metals from the body in order to ameliorate ASD symptoms could be seen as unfounded and illogical."*
>
> Davis et al., 2013, p. 54

Davis et al. refer to two surveys of parents of children with ASD in which 7.4% of 552 parents, and 8% of 74 parents said that their child had received chelation. This is sad and potentially disastrous, as there is no scientific basis for these useless, costly treatments, which expose individuals with ASD to risks – including the risk of dying (Beauchamp et al., 2006).

Amalgam Illness and the Cutler Chelation Protocol

Chemical engineer and anti-vaxxer[9] turned "health care consultant", Dr Andrew (Andy) Hall Cutler (www.noamalgam.com) concocted and then contracted (or, not that it matters, caught and then created) an ailment he called Amalgam Illness, caused by mercury in dental fillings. Using his brainchild, the Cutler Chelation Protocol, he healed himself. Lo and behold, he then "realized" that

---

9 Anti-vaxxer (informal): a person who is opposed to vaccination, typically a parent who, despite well-publicized and well-understood dangers, does not wish to vaccinate their child; or a person who is making money as an anti-vaccination speaker, writer or "personality". Celebrity anti-vaccination proponents include Jim Carrey, Robert F. Kennedy Jr., and Jenny McCarthy. President Donald Trump sends mixed messages: "I'm all for vaccinations, but I think when you add all of these vaccinations together and then two months later the baby is so different then lots of different things have happened. I really—I've known cases…I've seen people where they have a perfectly healthy child, and they go for the vaccinations and a month later the child is no longer healthy." www.rawstory.com/2012/04/trump-warns-fox-news-viewers-autism-caused-by-vaccines/. Dr Sherri Tenpenny, an osteopathic physician and anti-vax activist from Ohio, is one of the loudest voices in supporting misguided beliefs that vaccines cause autism, asthma, ADHD and autoimmune disorders.

Diets, supplements and nutrition: What's on the menu?

autism is mercury poisoning. In case you missed it: autism IS mercury poisoning. Next, he found out that Amalgam Illness and/or other heavy metal poisoning triggers *43 more* diverse human conditions, including: ALS (amyotrophic lateral sclerosis or Lou Gehrig's disease), Alzheimer's dementia, asthma, ADHD, chronic fatigue syndrome (CFS or myalgic encephalomyelitis: ME), fibromyalgia, hypothyroidism, infertility, insomnia, lupus, multiple sclerosis, panic attacks, Parkinson's disease, rheumatoid arthritis, and "yeast syndrome". Dr Cutler also claims that Amalgam Illness or heavy metal poisoning underpins anorexia nervosa, bipolar disorder (*and* "manic depression"!), borderline personality disorder, bulimia, depression, obsessive-compulsive disorder, psychosis, and schizophrenia; with apologies to our colleagues, family and friends with mental illness: mercury madness indeed.

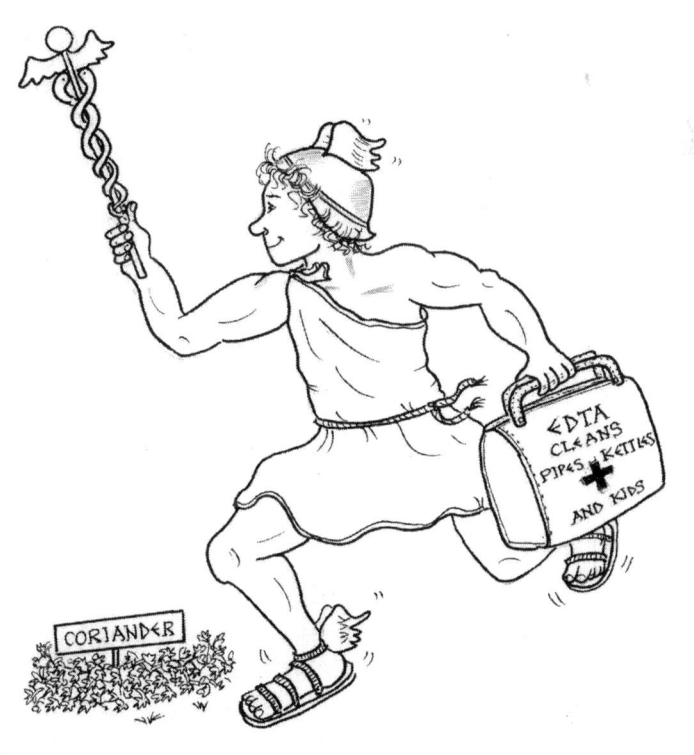

Helen Rippon

All this "science" is believed and applauded in a large, active, and open discussion group (www.groups.yahoo.com/neo/groups/autism-mercury/info), where: "most members are parents of children with autism, Aspergers (sic), ADD, ADHD, PDD, PDD-NOS, SID, oppositional defiance (sic) disorder, apraxia, speech disorders, and/or other related symptoms".

The "specially timed" Cutler Protocol for Amalgam Illness takes years to complete, and cannot be initiated until any dental amalgams containing mercury[10] are removed, and hair and urine tests have been completed. Dr Cutler's books, *Amalgam Illness Diagnosis and Treatment* and *Hair Test Interpretation: Finding Hidden Toxicities*, for sale on his website (alongside titles[11] by kindred authors), tell you how to do this. As laid out in the preceding section, mercury does not cause ASD and chelation is dangerous. Mercury is unattested as a causative factor in any of the diseases, conditions and syndromes that Dr Cutler lists.

If you suspect you or your child has mercury poisoning you will hasten to your doctor's office or a hospital ED, too focused on acute symptoms to stop for DIY hair and urine analysis, dentistry, or remedial coriander[12]. Symptoms include acute-onset disturbances of vision, hearing, speech, touch and coordination. The type and severity of symptoms depend on the exact toxin, the dose, and the method and duration of exposure, but it will not be due to dental amalgam.

Cascading diets

The Candida Diet or "candida cleanse diet", treats a made-up condition called "yeast syndrome". Aspiring to an "alkaline diet", it calls for avoiding so

---

10 Ironically, in this context, Mercury in Greek mythology is the god of financial gain, commerce, messages and communication (divination), travellers, boundaries, trickery and thieves.

11 "Biological Treatments for Autism and PDD" by William Shaw, PhD; "What Your Doctor May Not Tell You About Children's Vaccinations" by Stephanie Cave, MD; and "Nourishing Hope for Autism: Nutrition Intervention for Healing Our Children" by Julie Matthews, CNC (see footnote 13 on page 282 for an explanation of "CNC").

12 A Google search for "autism and coriander" scores some 72,000 results, linking to sites where providers and parents applaud coriander (cilantro), or cilantro and chlorella, for "cilantro detox", "mercury mobilization", "natural chelation", and "coriander as a heavy metal chelator". Chlorella is a genus of single-cell green algae belonging to the phylum Chlorophyta.

many foods that it makes for boring dining. Here are *some* of the no-no's: aged cheeses, coffee, alcohol, chocolate, dried and fresh fruit, cooking oils, fermented foods, gluten (pasta, white rice, corn, wheat, amaranth, buckwheat, oats, and barley), green olives, legumes, margarine, mushrooms, peanuts, pickles, potatoes, vinegar, all sugars, honeys and syrups, and foods containing yeast or mould: e.g., bread, muffins, cake, baked goods, cheese, and dried fruit. Numerous individuals labour under the misbelief that mould exacerbates ASD symptoms, and that a strictly regimented "alkaline diet", with or without probiotics (cha-ching!), will ameliorate them (Elder, 2008).

Body Ecology Diet (BED)

BED (www.bodyecology.com) is a variation of the Candida Diet. BED is sugar-free, gluten-free, casein-free, probiotic rich, and developed by "leading digestive health expert" and Rebounding (see page 276) aficionado Donna Gates, MEd, ABAAHP (Advanced Fellow with the American Academy of Anti-Aging Medicine – no, we did not invent ABAAHP, it is here: www.a4m.com). Ms Gates conceptualizes "most chronic diseases including autism" as a cascade. The cataract begins as a fungal infection in the gut. Pathogenic organisms then flood the intestines, inundating the rest of the body, and in the case of autism, infecting the brain. The solution is to follow the diet and drink Kefir, Ms Gates' lucrative formulation of goat or organic cows' milk (bring on the organic cows!), coconut water kefir, cultured vegetables such as raw sauerkraut, sea vegetables, organic eggs, fish, organic chicken, turkey, lean meat, sunflower and pumpkin seeds, salads and steamed vegetables, quinoa, amaranth grain, millet, buckwheat flour, coconut oil, and olive oil; or use her Kefir starter ("an absolute must after antibiotic use").

According to her fulsome web bio, "As a key figure in the autism movement, Donna works with top doctors in the field who view her diet as instrumental in changing the theory behind and treatment of the disorder. She founded Body Ecology Diet Recovering Our Kids (BEDROK), an active online community of over 2,000 parents, many of who (sic) have seen their children in "full recovery" www.bedrokcommunity.org". It is a nasty business that lures parents of children with ASD with "full recovery" claims. It should be warning enough that BEDROK turns out to be a lacklustre affair with minimal participation, but just the same, don't get caught!

Bioindividual Nutrition®

Susan Levin, CNC[13] (www.unlockyourchild.com), a nutritionist, family wellness coach, and mother of Ben "formerly" diagnosed with autism, swears by the Body Ecology Diet, in combination with home-schooling and the Son-Rise Program® (Levin, 2105). Ms Levin offers pricey programmes for families, based around a stupendously unscientific adaptation of the stupendously unscientific Body Ecology Diet, founded on the stupendously unscientific Candida Diet, which she has called Bioindividual Nutrition®, that we think is stupendously unscientific.

> **Pseudoscience alert**
>
> *"How did my son lose his autism diagnosis? We followed a roadmap to autism recovery with three main parts: Bioindividual Nutrition®, child-driven therapies, and ongoing biomedical support through supplements and detoxification. In my signature program, UnlockYourChild®, we will design a program perfect to support and help your child take major steps forward. I offer three programs, to support you in whatever capacity you need."*
>
> Susan Levin, CNC, www.unlockyourchild.com
> accessed 1 February 2016

Guts

Ms Levin is not the first to develop a variation of a variation of a variation of a diet that was pretty silly in the first place, and there are many diets similar to the Body Ecology, Candida and Bioindividual Nutrition® diets. Among them are the Specific Carbohydrate Diet (SCD), and the Gut and Psychology Syndrome (GAPS) and Gut and Physiology Syndrome (GAPS) diets.

---

13 The bogus CNC credential was awarded by the Society of Certified Nutritionists (SCN), established in1985 in the US, whose website appears to have vanished (but see www.americannutritionassociation. org, ANA). The SCN accepted, and the ANA accepts, individuals who have questionable nutrition qualifications as members, including: Certified Clinical Nutritionists (CCN), Certified Nutritionists (CN), and Certified Nutrition Consultants (CNC). Educated health information consumers regard SCN and ANA membership as a sign of poor judgement.

Specific Carbohydrate Diet (SCD)

The Specific Carbohydrate Diet (www.pecanbread.com), which "is very close to being a paleo type diet"[14], is based on "SCD Science". SCD Science explains why and how to starve gram-negative bacteria so that they leave the body, freeing the child with autism from being "a hostage to billions of pathogenic invaders that poison the gut and brain". The SCD is grain and lactose free, and is said to "treat" ASD, Crohn's disease, irritable bowel syndrome, and ulcerative colitis in children. Claiming that, "The latest research supports SCD as the best diet for Autism Spectrum Disorder!" susceptible parents are reeled in with statements like, "Children with Autism who are implementing SCD are demonstrating remarkable improvements in bowel function, language, eye contact, self-stimulatory behavior, anxiety, and mood".

The site contains reassurances that Epsom salts baths, activated charcoal capsules, green tea which "has an incredible ability to neutralize some of the harmful effects from bacterial toxins", chicken soup, bone broths, and 1/4 teaspoon baking soda with a pinch of salt in a glass of water will counter children's tendency to "hyperness, irritability, and whining" and other adverse reactions to the SCD.

> **Pseudoscience alert**
>
> *"The same toxins the gut pathogens have been giving off all along, which drive the kids into their world of autism... are all being released now, all at ONCE, as these bad guys bite the dust. Hopefully, you can think of it that way... it's not your child.... it's like your child's possessed by these bad guys who are DESPERATE to survive and are driving your child crazy. They WANT TO SURVIVE.... so they are sending your child messages to GO GET FOOD. Meaning, they want their Nutrigrain bars and their sugary cookies and all the other stuff that they've been thriving on all this time. They KNOW they will DIE if they don't get it.... so they are willing to go to desperate measures to influence their "host"... and break down your will to defeat them. This is a life or death struggle for them and they mean to win. You must make up your mind that your plan is to erradicate them from your child's body once and for all..... and determine you won't give in to them!"*
>
> KIDS & SCD www.pecanbread.com

---

14 Paleo diet: A diet based on foods presumed to have been eaten by early humans: primarily meat, fish, vegetables, and fruit, and excluding dairy or cereal products and processed food.

The reactions are listed as: "flu like symptoms, fever, extreme hunger, nausea, vomiting, dizziness, achy joints and back, diarrhea or constipation, strange skin rashes, runny nose and funny cough, headaches, behavior changes, irritability, tantrums, short temper and sleep disturbances". It is difficult to picture children with ASD, who are notoriously choosy eaters, willingly downing the broths, capsules, green tea, salt water, and soups.

GAPS and GAPS

GAPS (www.gaps.me) stands for **G**ut and **P**sychology **S**yndrome, a condition conceived by Natasha Campbell-McBride, MD, MMedSci (neurology), MMedSci (human nutrition) who trained as a medical doctor at Bashkir Medical University, Russia, later practising as a neurologist and then as a neurosurgeon in Russia (www.doctor-natasha.com/dr-natasha.php). She reports moving to the UK and completing a masters in Human Nutrition at the University of Sheffield, and in 2000 establishing the Cambridge Nutrition Clinic, which she runs. A passionate anti-vaccination advocate, Dr Campbell-McBride used the GAPS diet "to heal the gut lining, rebalance intestinal flora, and aid nutrient absorption" to reverse autism in her son, who is now "off the spectrum" (Campbell-McBride, 2010).

According to Dr Campbell-McBride, the gut and *psychology* diet can be confidently used to treat autism, ADD, ADHD, dyslexia, dyspraxia, depression and schizophrenia. It has expanded to include gut and *physiology* syndrome, to explain and treat, with the GAPS diet, "obsessive-compulsive disorders and other psychiatric conditions, and autoimmune conditions. These include but are not limited to: rheumatoid arthritis, lupus, coeliac disease, type I diabetes, multiple sclerosis, thyroid autoimmunity (Graves disease and Hashimoto's thyroiditis), psoriasis, chronic fatigue syndrome, fibromyalgia, food intolerances, and eczema". The diet permits no grains, sugar or starch, and is designed around "probiotics, healthy fats, and amino acids needed to heal and seal the gut wall".

It is hard to believe that Dr Campbell-McBride has bona fide medical or nutrition training, but she has steadfast followers, including Hemsley and Hemsley (www.hemsleyandhemsley.com), and the Web holds tales of ASD "cures", attributed to GAPS.

Gluten and casein

GFCF diets have a special place here as the earliest and most popular CAM food intervention for ASD. They originated in the 1960s when a physician, Dr F. Curtis Dohan, theorized that people with coeliac disease were more disposed to schizophrenia. Recall that gluten is a protein found in pasta and bread, and foods containing white rice, corn, wheat, and barley, and sometimes in oats if they are processed close to the other culprits. Studies of the effects of GF diets for people with schizophrenia failed to demonstrate significant symptomatic reductions (Lorenz, 1990, pp. 435–469). Dr Dohan's work, however, marks the genesis of the supposed link between nutrition and psychiatric and neurological illnesses.

In the 1970s, the suggestion of an *unproven* link between gluten, casein, autism and "leaky gut" emerged in the form of the "Opioid-Excess Theory". Casein is the main protein present in milk and, in coagulated form, in high protein milk products such as cheese, yoghurt and ice cream, but not cream and butter. It is also a common ingredient in processed foods.

The "Opioid-Excess Theory" contends that children on the spectrum are unable to break down the proteins in gluten (grain) and casein (dairy) causing opioid-like peptides (amino acids) to form. Children with ASD are also posited to have "leaky gut syndrome" (a theory supported by trifling evidence; Mulloy et al., 2010) due to which these peptides are able to escape the digestive tract, cross the intestinal membranes, enter the blood, and travel to the brain, causing the neurobehavioral symptoms of ASD. By applying the GFCF diet, free of gluten and casein, it was believed that you could diminish ASD symptoms.

Widely embraced by families (Adams et al., 2013; Levy & Hyman, 2015), some parents say that the GFCF diet has lessened their child's symptoms. Research, however, has uncovered little support for the GFCF diet and "leaky gut" theory, and no effects on social communication skills, sleep patterns or activity levels (Mulloy et al., 2010, p. 337):

> "...We must conclude that the published studies we located do not support the use of GFCF diets in the treatment of ASD. Additionally, the data from these studies do not support the Opioid-Excess Theory. Until conclusive evidence is found in support of GFCF diets, restrictive diets should only be implemented in the event a food allergy or intolerance is detected..."

It is possible that some children with ASD who have significant gastrointestinal (GI) problems like diarrhoea, constipation, bloating and intestinal motility disorders, may experience benefits from a GFCF or GF diet, especially if they, coincidentally, also have coeliac disease (gluten-sensitivity autoimmune disorder), which can cause behaviour difficulties. It is also possible that some children with ASD who are lactose (milk sugar) intolerant, suffering GI pain and discomfort and hence disturbed behaviour, and who go onto the GFCF or CF diet, will show improved behaviour because it excludes "dairy".

While the GFCF diet is not evidence-based, many parents pursue it, and more will want to try it. If you are tempted, or if your child is already on the diet and you have not already done so, we recommend you talk to your child's paediatrician *and* a registered (certified) dietitian.

Not only will the GFCF diet be more expensive, involve more food preparation, add a level of complexity to food shopping, and be harder to "sell" to your child than a regular diet, it may also place your child at risk for nutritional deficiencies. Eliminating dairy removes a critical source of *calcium* – we are thinking of strong teeth, bones and nails here; *protein* to build and repair tissue and produce enzymes, hormones and other body chemicals; and *vitamin D* that protects against infections, cancer, and diabetes and which is important in the smooth running of the immune system. Vetoing gluten means removing *B-group vitamins*, *iron* and *fibre*, so your paediatrician or GP may (probably first trying to deter you from taking the GF path) prescribe, and your dietitian will advocate, vitamin and mineral supplements to compensate, and possibly suggest a paediatric fibre preparation.

What about…?

The mass of dodgy diets, nutrition theories, supplements and interventions we found in searching for useful information to share is staggering. We know there are more, and that some readers will wonder, what about the non-evidence based: Defeat Autism Now DAN Diet (www.autism.com) designed by Dr Bernard Rimland; Sue and Howard Dengate's FAILSAFE (www.fedup.com.au); the Feingold diet (www.feingold.org), the toxic Miracle Mineral Solution (MMS) 28% sodium chlorite (bleach) "supplement" available online as an autism "cure", with the social media tagline, "Solving the puzzle one drop at a time"; Dr Kay Toomey's SOS Feeding Solutions (and her www.spdstar.org Feeding Therapy) which has minimal evidence to support implementation with children with developmental disorders, and then only in modified form (e.g., Benson, Parke, Gannon, & Muñoz, 2013); and so on? We have to stop somewhere, hoping that we have provided enough leads for you to know what to avoid and where to turn for trustworthy dietary guidance. We end this chapter on a spiritual note, followed by a few words about panaceas, placebos, and healthy nutrition ideology and dogma in dietetics.

Spiritual nutrition

A keen Rebounder, Rabbi Gabriel Cousens MD (www.treeoflifecenterus.com) writes that he "functions as a true and complete holistic physician, homeopath, psychiatrist, family therapist, Ayurvedic practitioner, Chinese herbalist, world leading diabetes researcher, ecological leader, spiritual master" and more. Dr Cousens is founder-director of the Tree of Life Rejuvenation Center in Patagonia, AZ. In the practice of Spiritual Nutrition, applying the Rainbow Diet, he is dedicated to blue-green algae: Aphanizomenon flos-aquae (AFA) also called "cyanobacterial blooms", or "cyanophyta" ("nutritional algae"). While he sees AFA as a super food with numerous uses, in voyaging through the algae he has met with setbacks.

> "I've had excellent results using the algae with children who've been autistic. One of the main characteristics of autism is the absence of verbal talking. These children only make grunting and other such noises. I remember one child case that began to talk in only one month after beginning using the AFA. Unfortunately, if you can believe this, the mother really didn't want the child to talk. She started complaining the child was talking too much, and made some excuse to stop giving the AFA to the child, which is very sad when you think about it."
>
> Rabbi Gabriel Cousens

For the record, no we don't believe it, and yes, we do think it sad, but not for the same reasons as the multitasking master of metaphysical mysteries.

Panaceas

A panacea is a cure-all for all known difficulties or diseases, and a sure sign of a specious intervention is a list of the myriad issues and conditions it addresses. Examples in this chapter are BED, the Cutler Chelation Protocol, Specific Carbohydrate Diet, and GAPS. Red flags also flutter when a panacea is claimed to cure a raft of known *and* made-up conditions like Amalgam Illness, Functional Disconnection syndrome, Gut and Psychology/Physiology Syndrome, Irlen® Syndrome, Multiple Chemical Sensitivity, Retained Neonatal Reflexes, Sensory Integration Disorder, or Wilson's Temperature syndrome. But why are some people convinced that certain non-evidence-based treatments work? Could the *placebo effect* be weaving its magic?

Placebo effect

"Placebo" means "I shall please" from the Latin, *placeō*, "I please" (Gensini, Conti, & Conti, 2005). It is defined (Quincy, 1787) as a remedy used more to please than to heal people. The term *placebo effect* does not refer to a "sugar pill" or *placebo* in a scientific study. The placebo effect refers to a pleasing perception of improvement that most people experience when they undergo treatment: they feel positive about getting better, are less aware of their symptoms, see progress in their child, and so on. The act of beginning a therapy (including medicines or diets) carries with it an optimism that things are on the mend; that the treatment will "please". In randomized controlled trials (the so-called gold standard of scientific inquiry), people – let's say people with depression – in the control condition receive either standard current treatment or an "inert" treatment, such as information sheets rather than active therapy or a sugar pill rather than an anti-depressant[15]. People in the active research arm receive the intervention of interest, e.g., a new diet, or a new form of cognitive behaviour therapy. It is common, however, for participants in *both arms* of such studies to perceive *at least some benefits*, at least in the short term. Placebo effects, the effects of human optimism and hope, and expectancy bias, account for a significant proportion of perceived improvement. Benedetti, Mayberg, Wagner, Stohler and Zubieta, say: "these placebo mechanisms have an important influence on the therapeutic outcome, and indeed they enhance the specific effect of a treatment" (2005, p. 10,391). Hence any new treatment must show itself to be *significantly better than placebo* (i.e., to value-add over and above the placebo effect) to cross the evidence line.

---

[15] This is done under the close review and monitoring of properly constituted Human Research Ethics Committees in Australia, and equivalent bodies internationally.

Ideology, dogma, and faith-based dietetics

An ideology is a set of opinions or beliefs held by an individual, a group such as a political party or religious denomination, or prevalently within a culture. Dogma is a principle, or principles, promulgated by an authority as inarguably true, while an article of faith is a firmly held belief (see Gruber et al., 2003, for discussion of "belief" in SLP/SLT).

Before embarking on *Making Sense of Interventions for Children with Developmental Disorders*, we allowed nutritional information that was unrelated to our work in dysphagia, ASD, voice, or oral health to be fed to us via popular print and electronic media. In examining the interesting but unfamiliar (to us) territory of evidence-based child nutrition, in peer-reviewed dietetics journals, we were struck by three things. First, the interlacing of ideological views into dietary advice that is supposed to be data-driven and scientific. Second, dogmatic adherence by some dietitians to out-of-date healthy eating advice, such as curbing total fat intake, long after the science has dismissed them as needless, ineffective, or detrimental. Third, the rise and rise of "ethical eating"[16] (not necessarily the equivalent of healthy eating) in the "new nutrition science" paradigm (Cannon & Leitzmann, 2016; Fardet & Rock, 2014) that sees traditional nutrition as reductionist, and needing to be reconceived in broader social and environmental contexts.

Untangling science from dogma, ideology, and marketing in mainstream print and popular media is difficult. When science, dogma, ideology and even *marketing* mix it in professional dietetics journals, it works against the case for helpful nutritional advice for parents of children with developmental disorders, and the professionals who work with them.

---

16 "Ethical eating" ("food ethics") enshrines the moral consequences of food choices, made by humans for themselves, and made for animals that are (e.g., cows, chickens), or produce (e.g., milk, eggs) food. Common concerns are cruelty to food animals, environmental consequences, exploitive labour practices unrepresentative of "fair trade" (or Fairtrade® a global movement that aims to secure stable prices, decent working conditions and empowerment of farmers and workers), food shortages for others, and the unintended deleterious effects of food policy.

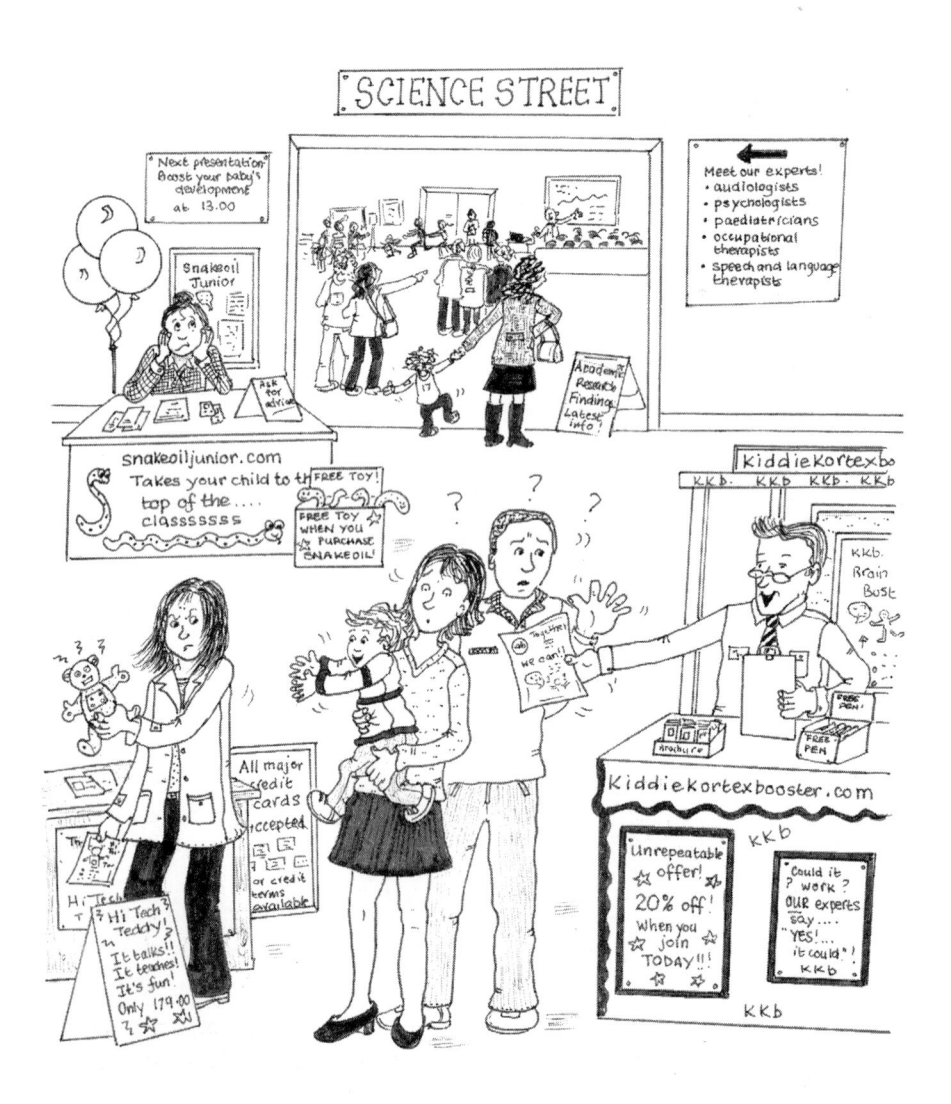

Helen Rippon

11 Parents navigating the marketplace

In writing this chapter, we picture parents and other family members dipping into the various sections of *Making Sense of Interventions for Children with Developmental Disorders* that are most relevant to their own child's situation – and then turning to this page. We sense the mixed feelings many have about the whole business of accessing appropriate help for him or her. And a business it is. The quest for appropriate treatment is similar to walking through a sparkling bazaar, with smiling vendors beckoning, making promises, eagerly admiring everyone's babies and children, eyeing-off purses and wallets, and urging parents or grandparents to sign up.

Beyond the bazaar, just past the soaring Pseudoscience Central complex, is Science Street, where comparatively dull-looking establishments are populated by mainstream professionals who do not thrive on the sell-sell-sell approach to getting clients through the door. Where Pseudoscience dons stilettoes or two-tone oxfords, flamboyant neckwear, and glittering tiaras or jaunty fedoras, science opts instead for sensible shoes, comfortable layers, and an umbrella; just in case. Pseudoscience is unencumbered by self-doubt, where science couches its propositions in conditional, cautious language, alert to the possibility of alternative explanations which do not necessarily align with popular thinking. Proponents in both camps may extol the virtues of an "open mind", but this means different things depending on who is issuing the advice. To scientists, it means that new evidence might prompt a revision of theory, and possibly of practice. To pseudoscientists, it means filling in knowledge gaps with "anecdata", magical thinking, social memes, and playing to parental anxiety. As Lilienfeld, Lyn and Lohr (2015, p. 5) remind us, however:

> "Keeping an open mind is a virtue but this mind cannot be so open that one's brains fall out".[1]

Most parents seeking the "right" intervention, or the "right combination" of interventions are wary of both the bazaar's fulsome promises (are the guarantees *too* good to be true?) and Science Street's conservatism and insistence on

---

1 Original source: NASA scientist James Oberg; see https://en.wikipedia.org/wiki/James_Oberg

systematically researched approaches to intervening with children with developmental disorders (are they *trying* to blind us with science and paralyze us with uncertainty?). Fortunately, in surveying the market in the information age, many parents have "consumer smarts" on their side, are alert to probable deceptions and dangers, and discerning about how their family's precious time and money will be spent.

So far, we have sought to show how academically-trained people scrutinize the claims made by individuals and organizations who promote themselves and their wares as "the answer" to children's difficulties. We set the bar moderately high, asking for more than testimonials from satisfied customers (the authenticity of which can be dubious anyway). You probably concluded quite quickly that there is not "one answer" relative to your child's needs and that, instead, there are different paths, associated with different costs and risks, and different potential benefits. We have put together a 7-point guide to thinking about the interventions presented here, those you encounter that we have been unable to cover, and those that have yet to hit the marketplace.

A 7-point safety-check

1. If something seems too good to be true, it probably is.

If there were a miracle cure for autism, ADHD, reading disorders, and so on, let's face it, we would all know by now. Miracle cures make for reality-escapes in movies but are not part of the real-life landscapes of parents or professionals. Improvements occur for a range of reasons and all the gains children make, even small ones, should be celebrated. But gains must be real and meaningful. As your child's advocate, your role is to ask penetrating questions and to maintain a position of respectful scepticism in the face of promises, made or implied, about benefits your child could derive once you sign up. Becoming faster or more accurate on a computer game or App might make your child feel good, but will it translate into meaningful, usable and needed skills? If you can't answer yes to this question, keep walking; soak up the bazaar's atmosphere, and then head for Science Street.

2. If a link to "research" leads only to unpublished, in-house reports, white papers, blog entries, and magazine articles, and not to peer-reviewed publications, be on the alert.

Similarly, if you find a little bit of what looks like *bona fide* research produced a decade (or longer) ago, step back slowly. Beware too of genuinely peer-reviewed research that is published in a low-ranking journal. A journal's status is not always obvious, parents and professionals can miss the subtleties, and the *Acme Journal of You-Beaut Child Performance* publisher is not going to *announce* that it lacks the high standing of other, more discerning and prestigious academic outlets. This is the subject of much ideological debate among academics, and is beyond our scope here, but one technique to try is to Google the journal's title to see if you can identify the organization that publishes it.

As if academic publishing were not already mysterious enough, it also dabbles in the dark arts, in the hands of predatory publishers. Their journals, whose names appear eerily similar to *bone fide* ones, are simply "fronts" for fly-by-night profiteers. The give-away for academics is that they receive cheesy emails extolling the virtues of their research (often described as being in a completely different field[2], but what the heck?) and inviting them to submit a paper to a special issue, whose closing date is typically next Thursday. As academics will attest, journal manuscripts take *months* to prepare, not days. With predatory journals, however, the manuscript review process is turned around virtually instantaneously (as opposed to the best-case scenario of 8–12 weeks normally assigned), and the editorial decision is *always* immediate acceptance without revisions (as opposed to the usual couple of pages of reviewer comments that need to be wrangled). And then there's the small matter of how much authors must pay for the privilege of having their work accepted in these sham publications.

This information about predatory journals is not intended as a cautionary tale for academics who pay for their work to be published. Indeed, we wish that *more* academics were positioned to meet the charges levied by reputable journals to make their papers "open access", i.e., readily available, in perpetuity for all; or better still, that scientific knowledge were not quarantined behind any pay-wall. We also understand the pressures on academics (particularly those in the early-to-mid career stages) to publish, and the difficulties that this can entail. However, it is a career-limiting rather than enhancing step to fall for the advances of predatory publishers. This landscape became easier to navigate from October 2012 when University of Colorado, Denver's professor Jeffrey Beall, created a regularly updated blog, "Scholarly Open Access",

---

2 As speech-language *pathologists*, we are regularly buttered up and praised by opportunistic, predatory publishers for our outstanding contributions to the field of *pathology*: blood banking, chemical pathology, haematology, laboratory medicine, and microbiology.

known as "Beall's List" (of predatory open access publishers). His site was "pulled" in January 2017, but is archived (to December 2016) at: https://web.archive.org/web/20170111172306/https://scholarlyoa.com/publishers/. If an intervention website lists supporting publications from a Beall's List journal, click the "X" at top right in your browser, with no further ado. We have both completed PhDs and so know first-hand the importance of formal research training and immersion in the scientific method. That said, we urge caution on findings that can *only* be located in PhD or other doctoral dissertations (theses), and that are not in the peer-reviewed literature. The examination rubric for a doctorate certainly incorporates originality, methodological rigour, and scholarly reasoning, but it is possible for a thesis to be passed even though the experimental work it describes could be difficult to publish. Increasingly, doctoral students are encouraged and supported to publish during their candidature and we think that is a good thing, as it will mean fewer AuD, DPhil, EdD and PhD (etc.) outcomes sitting forlornly in the no-mans' land of electronic databases and dusty library shelves where they can do next-to-nothing to influence knowledge or practice.

3. *Put your metaphorical sunglasses on so you are not blinded by the bright lights of (pseudo)neuroscience.*

The brain did not come into being in the last decade, and did not in the last decade become the body's organ of learning. It has always been the organ that allows us to process experiences via our many senses, learn, remember, plan and execute behaviour, communicate, and read and write – among numerous other functions. The so-called *Decade of the Brain* (1990–1999) designated by President George W. Bush has certainly made the brain a topic of everyday conversation in schools and clinics around the world. The extent to which anything meaningful has changed as a consequence, for *any* child is, however, dubious at best. Despite much excitement in neuroscience circles about technological advances such as functional magnetic resonance imaging (fMRI), this dizzying seduction has been tempered in recent times by reports of significant over-extrapolation from many fMRI studies (Oxenham, 2016). There is also evidence that when people are given "neurosciency" explanations of cognitive phenomena, no matter how cooked up and circular these may be, they find such explanations plausible and appealing (Fernandez-Duque, Evans, Christian, & Hodges, 2015). Science communicators therefore have a responsibility to communicate new "findings" with caution. Such advice is, of course, water off the news media's back when catchy headlines like "This is your brain while watching TV" translate so well into click-bait.

The bottom line here is that talk of "brain-based learning" is just silly – it is akin to referring to "lung-based breathing", "leg-based walking", or "stomach-based digestion". If you would not sign up for those, then you should not sign up for interventions that promise "brain-based learning" either. Many researchers in Twitter refer to "neuroflapdoodle" and "neurobollocks". There is a huge amount of it out there, aimed fairly and squarely at parents, with teachers and clinicians as collateral damage.

4. Many approaches work a little bit, or for a little while.

In Chapter 10 we discuss the placebo effect, and emphasize that this does not mean a "fake treatment" but rather refers to our (mainly charming) human tendency to impose an optimistic bias when it comes to anticipating outcomes in the face of challenges. In the 20th century, two important phenomena were described in the psychology literature that help to explain our unconscious positive expectancy biases: the Hawthorne Effect and the Rosenthal Effect. The Hawthorne Effect (named for the Western Electric Company's Hawthorne factory in Illinois, USA, where the study in question took place) is this: when under observation, particularly by people who look like "officials" or "experts", humans change their behaviour, and typically for the better (Roethlisberger & Dickson, 1939). In fact, the authors of the Hawthorne study found that the mere visible *presence* of experts improved the productivity of workers in the factory, at least for a while. More recently, social scientists have argued that the Hawthorne Effect actually refers to variables that researchers fail to adequately control in the design of a study, and hence they play havoc with accurate delineation of cause (intervention) and effect (outcome) (Wickström & Bendix, 2000). The Rosenthal Effect, on the other hand, refers to unconscious expectancy bias on the part of observers, whether they are scientists, practitioners, parents, or teachers. Sometimes also referred to as the Pygmalion Effect, this phenomenon arose out of an experiment in the 1960s (Rosenthal & Jacobson, 1968) that showed that teacher ratings of children's IQs were influenced by (false) information they were given about the likelihood that about 20% of them would be "intellectual bloomers". Whether as a result of these, or other sources of bias and optimism (see Chapter 10), even the most unlikely of interventions can produce an apparent honeymoon period in which some gains seem to be made, only to plateau or be lost soon after.

5. Use social media carefully.

Parents often find it useful to be part of Facebook groups, WhatsApp and Reddit communities, and email discussion lists that are concerned with a particular disorder (e.g., ASD) or issue (e.g., toilet training in children with ID), and there is no doubt that such groups, communities, and lists can foster support, reduce the sense of isolation and loneliness that some parents feel, and can provide new ideas about approaches that might be helpful. Be very careful, though, that you are not getting caught up in "group-think", the bandwagon effect (see page 316) or succumbing to peer-group pressure. We advise against signing up for an expensive bells'n'whistles programme just because someone else has and wants their decision validated by amassing disciples. You may or may not want to pose some of the questions we raise here in the wider group, but we hope you will consider them yourself.

We both use and enjoy the benefits of Twitter as a terrific medium for early exposure to new research, new ideas, new critiques of old ideas, and everything in between – including engagement and collaboration with other "Tweeps" (people in Twitter) whose interests coincide with our own, or who have different viewpoints and ideas that we like to consider. It also allows us to let off steam at times, and shake our sillies out. In Twitter, as in Facebook and on discussion lists, you can be a "lurker", one of the 90% of people in Twitter who soaks up and reflects upon other people's tweets, without tweeting, or rarely doing so. You do not have to request permission to follow a person or an organization (unless they have a locked account), or be "approved" by a moderator – just click on the "Follow" button and away you go (unless or until they "block" you for some reason!). We have been blocked by proponents of non-evidence-based interventions, including auditory integration training, Facilitated Communication, homeopathic vaccination, anti-vaccination, Whole-Language-based reading instruction, and non-speech oral motor exercises. If a person you follow tweets one too many cute kitten pictures or images of their culinary achievements, simply "Unfollow" or "Mute" them. Twitter also has clever algorithms that detect the kinds of twitter handles you might be interested in following, so keep an eye on the suggestions it makes for you.

6. *Use Google Scholar to access information from the peer-reviewed literature.*

One problem with modern academic publishing is that so much literature is pay walled. This means that it is only readily accessible to people who (a) work in universities, or (b) are willing to pay a hefty sum (around $AUD35 at the time of writing) per paper for access. When researching a particular disorder or intervention, you may need to access ten papers in order to land the one or two that are valuable to you. We know that this is unsatisfactory and lack immediate solutions. However, Google Scholar will at least usually give you access to the abstract (summary) of a paper, which should provide the general gist of the findings. Armed with the abstract, with a little more effort you may find that you can freely access the full text, e.g., from the "correspondence author", via the academic networking site ResearchGate.

The best way to use Google Scholar is to look for recent review papers, i.e., papers that survey the landscape on a particular topic and provide a (more or less) systematic and critical assessment of the state of play. Do this by entering something like the following into the search field: ["Make-My-Day Therapy" + Review]. If you are unable to find a review (this may mean that not enough research has been done to enable one), look for recent papers (published in the last 5–10 years). You can tailor a search by year range.

Once you find papers, click on "cited by" to see who has referred to the publication more recently, and follow your nose. Bear in mind, though, the old adage that "The proof of the pudding is in the eating", or that the real value of something can be judged only after it has been tried or tested. One study, in one region, in one country, with one group of children, does not constitute evidence that something does or does not work. Not nearly enough attention is paid to the science of replication and treatment fidelity before adopting so-called "findings" and applying them to everyday practice and, once interventions are let loose in the wilds of schools and clinic rooms, they can be impossible to rein back in.

Lilienfeld et al. (2015) remind us that the drive to be doing *something* is not licence to do *anything*. Interventions not only need to have benefit, they also need to not do harm, and one harm is opportunity cost. If you are expending time and money on Intervention X, that means you are less able to engage in Intervention Y. Intervention X may come with attractive packaging, marketing and testimonials, and Facebook followers, whereas Intervention Y (from Science Street) is more pedestrian, making modest claims, and aiming for small but achievable gains that are consolidated before moving on to a slightly higher level of complexity. Aesop's hare and tortoise remind everyone that sometimes the stronger bet can look unpromising at the start of the race. Your child has only so many waking hours that can reasonably be devoted to therapeutic and/or educational interventions, and you have only so much time and money to devote also. Less is sometimes more, and giving yourself, your child, and the rest of your family some downtime is likely to be a better investment in the long run than pursuit of spurious gains via poorly targeted, invariably expensive interventions.

7. Be wary of "flat-feet-to-halitosis" claims.

These are assertions that an intervention will have broad-ranging benefits across a whole range of disabilities and difficulty areas. When you buy a new outfit, you do not expect to be told that it is such a style classic that you can wear it in the office, at a pool party, when digging the garden, and while abseiling. You also do not want to hear that it will ride up with wear, down with wear, be cool in summer and warm in winter, and so on – because you know that one outfit can only do so much as part of your wardrobe. Similarly, one intervention can only do so much for any child. We are particularly wary of intervention approaches that claim equal effectiveness for a ridiculously wide range of disorders. There is no logical reason to expect that difficulties as diverse as disruptive behaviour, low reading skills, "stimming", and language processing problems (to name a few) should all respond *miraculously* to one *miraculous* approach. Australian special education experts Dr Kevin Wheldall and Dr Jennifer Stephenson of Macquarie University observed in the title of a paper they co-authored in 2008 about the discredited Dore or DDAT Program (see page 337) that *miracles* take a little longer.

Control groups *are* ethical (in ethically-approved research)

Educators sometimes claim that conducting school-based research that includes control groups is "unethical". As health professionals, we find this both puzzling and, well, unethical. No-one would expect a new drug or surgical treatment to be approved for implementation without *controlled*, ethically-approved investigations of their effectiveness, effects, and efficiency – the "three-Es" of treatment efficacy and quality assurance (Olswang, 1998, pp. 134–150)[3]. People in control groups, whether in schools or hospitals, are not left out in the cold, untreated. They are provided with current standard practice while the new, experimental intervention is trialled on the intervention group or "treatment group". In many cases, a cross-over design can be employed so that researchers swap the groups mid-way, and what was the control group now becomes the experimental group. People who say that the use of control groups in educational research is unethical simply do not understand modern research methods and the exacting ethical guidelines within which they operate.

---

3 Treatment *efficacy* refers to the extent to which an intervention works under the ideal, highly-controlled circumstances that occur in clinical trials. Treatment *effectiveness* studies establish whether a given treatment works in the real world. Treatment *effects* are the behavioural changes that occur, following treatment. In studies of treatment *efficiency*, researchers set out to determine whether one treatment method is better, and/or more economical than another.

Support and pressure from family and friends

Child rearing is challenging in the best of circumstances. Parents – whether parenting as a couple or as sole parents – who can rely on practical and emotional *support* from family and friends are fortunate indeed, and such support can make a material difference in getting through the sometimes tedious or stressful business of everyday life. Conversely, *pressure* from family and friends concerning your parenting is always unwelcome and rarely helpful. Probably, most people who "pressure" parents to investigate or adopt a particular approach do so out of a genuine concern for the wellbeing of that child, whether the child has a developmental disorder or whether the relative or friend sees the need for "hothousing" a child with typical development (see Chapter 2). So that might be a good meeting point on which to establish some common ground: thank them for their concern, and then say something like, "We all want the best for Abbie, Jack, Kim, Pattie, Robert-Louis and Tomás and so I've been doing some research, and this is what I've found. Perhaps you might be interested in doing some reading too?". We do not think you should have to *justify* your intervention decisions to family and friends but, in reality, we know you will sometimes feel a need to *defend* your approach. Invite your family and friends to understand and respect your thinking, to immerse themselves in their important role as aunt, uncle, grandparent, neighbour, etc., and to celebrate your child's gains, no matter how small. As a parent, you must be your child's best and strongest advocate, and this may sometimes mean having conversations that are awkward and uncomfortable, and accepting that not everyone's views can be accommodated all the time.

In our clinical experience, navigating intervention terrain often – and usually for practical, social or cultural reasons – falls to one parent, and this can leave the other parent "on the outer", creating situations where professionals and the "therapy parent" or "school parent" can form coalitions that can further exclude the "other" parent. Where a child has two parents (whether they are together, separated or divorced), we believe that both need to be as well-informed as possible about their child's strengths and needs, up-to-speed with what is going on regarding intervention, and physically and emotionally available to talk to and support each other. It is also essential to maintain clear boundaries around the couple relationship and around parent-child-sibling relationships, so that who is privy to personal discussions and decisions is regulated by the couple (with input from the child in some instances), in consultation with their professionals of choice, and not constantly overseen by intrusive friends, relatives and acquaintances.

The same reasoning applies to single parents, including those who do not have amicable relationships with the child's other parent. If, as a sole parent you establish boundaries around the people in your support system who actually are supportive – whether in person or online – keeping those who seem only interested in applying pressure at a manageable distance, it may make life easier. Remember too, that while your professionals are friendly and can feel familial, they are not really friends or family and that, with luck, their involvement in your child's life will be a passing thing.

In the context of conventional interventions, it is expected that therapy frequency and intensity is monitored and reviewed, taking into account progress, the child's motivation, and their family's capacity to engage. Periods of intense treatment may be recommended at certain developmental points, as may breaks from therapy, to give everyone a rest, allow consolidation of gains, and to make way for generalization of new skills. Clinicians come and go, and you and your child may feel stronger connections with some therapists than with others. Ultimately, an aim of therapy is to not need it any longer, but this conversation may not be a prominent feature of your interactions with snake-oil merchants, for whom your child's long-term dependence on treatment, and having *you* "there" as a devotee and possibly as an advocate for their wares, is intrinsic to their business model.

When your child's condition has no name

Throughout *Making Sense of Interventions for Children with Developmental Disorders* we refer to many developmental conditions that are identified via diagnostic processes, whether biomedical (blood tests, X-rays, MRIs), clinical assessment tools, or team-based assessments drawing together the expertise of a range of professionals. In some instances, there are a number of potential diagnoses under consideration, and these are listed and systematically tested for, slowly eliminating some while leaving others "on the table". This can all take time, and it is understandably stressful for parents to be without a diagnosis and wondering if they are wasting valuable intervention time. In a fortunately small number of cases, it can take years to arrive at a correct diagnosis and some parents find themselves dealing with the news that their child is one of a very small number globally with a particular disease, syndrome or condition. Such parents often traverse the full spectrum of medical and allied health specialists seeking "answers", and must deal with the loneliness and confusion of not being part of online support groups. Their children may become the focus of published case studies, in an effort to pave the way a little for the next family in the same predicament. It is to be hoped that the advent of the worldwide web has made life easier for such families, though we suspect this is a double-edged sword in terms of the unhelpful misinformation that is aimed at parents of children facing diagnostic uncertainty. Such parents require patience and persistence, sometimes, we are sad to say, in the face of our mainstream colleagues' unhelpful, dismissive, and even condescending "reassurance" that all is well.

My child's school has introduced a controversial programme

The 7-point safety check is all well and good when you are finding your own way in the marketplace, but what happens when you receive the news from your child's school saying that they have signed up for a programme that you believe has a weak or non-existent evidence base? Worse still, what if this programme is being rolled out for all children and will therefore reduce the class time available to conventional teaching? This will be tricky territory, but it can be navigated with the assistance of facts, in the form of peer-reviewed papers, position statements from professional bodies, respectful but assertive raising of concerns with school personnel and, if necessary, contact with the relevant educational authority (which may not apply in the case of independent schools).

This may turn out to be an unpopular move, but you know that anyway. You may also need to advocate for your child to complete standard classroom activities while the new-black educational programme is in action, conscious of the opportunity cost associated with unproven, time-wasting approaches. This can also be a problematic space for parents who are psychologists, SLPs/SLTs, medical practitioners, academics and similar troublesome types, who may be concerned about seeming to "pull rank" on schools and teachers, and other health professionals, if they query their intervention decisions. We say, put the awkwardness aside, because children are not in a position to give or withhold consent for what happens in the classroom or clinic room; they need informed adults to advocate on their behalf.

Keeping an "open mind" is OK as long as that is not code for "anything goes". An open mind should mean that evidence is appraised and decisions are made on the basis of current data. It does not mean you must avoid rocking the boat, simply because a well-meaning, kind, or influential person swears by a particular approach. Scepticism may be the most sensible response when an approach lacks a theoretical grounding that aligns with present-day scientific consensus. Historically, certain important ideas have begun this way (e.g., handwashing to reduce sepsis), but such examples are the exception and not the rule. Do not be afraid to ask questions, and to keep asking them if, after listening carefully to the answers, you consider them to be unsatisfactory. You may also find it useful to Google "MUSEC + briefings" to consult the Macquarie University Special Education Centre (MUSEC) Briefings, which are one-page intervention assessments written by special education experts. Teachers and school principals *should* be open to reading these and engaging in discussion about, and taking note of, their recommendations.

Articles in the popular press are particularly effective at creating a frenzy in school communities and in social media about the newest, shiny offering in the intervention bazaar. With notable exceptions, health and education journalists are not trained in the scientific method, and even if they were, they know that their editors are not looking for dry copy written in the conservative language of scientists: the results *appear to show*; findings *suggest*; it is *possible* that *some* children *may* benefit. No, what sells newsprint and makes good clickbait is sensational, feel-good stories, and tantalizing headlines: BREAKING: *Leading herbalist unlocks forces of quantum dolphin neuroscience and organic quinoa to halt Mystery Condition in local tots.*

Resolve to resist exploitative providers

We have endeavoured in *Making Sense of Interventions for Children's Developmental Disorders* to map a complex terrain; to mark out the highways and by-ways, bush-tracks, dirt-roads, dead-ends, cul-de-sacs, country lanes and culverts that await the eager but under-prepared traveller. Interventions for children with developmental disorders do not fall into binary categories of "good" and "bad"; however, parents do need to know that some approaches are shameless for their lack of scientific evidence and for their targeting of precious family resources: time, money, and hope. A rough rule of thumb is that the more grandiose the claim, and the greater the abundance of little ™, ®, © and ® symbols you see associated with a product, the more you should sharpen your scepticism. We wish it were not so, but mainstream professionals sometimes stray across the line into employing, promoting, and charging for non-evidence-based approaches. This makes parents' jobs so much harder, and we hope that the principles we have outlined here serve as a useful guide to the complex, unique journey each family travels.

12 Treatment choices in everyday practice

Inevitably, our identities, backgrounds and experiences in SLP/SLT, and the interesting strings we have to our bows, shape our views of professional practice, from the inside out and from the outside in. Between us, we have accumulated, and continue to update and refine, knowledge in diverse areas of academia, clinical linguistics, criminology, education, family therapy, ICT, psychology, public policy, research, teaching, writing, and of course, SLP/SLT. Our workplaces have varied, to include universities; government and private: clinical, education and hospital settings; NGOs, solo and group practices in metropolitan and regional locations, and interdisciplinary, multidisciplinary, and transdisciplinary teams that include family members.

Frequent flyers, between us, we have been honoured with invitations to teach, collaborate, and present continuing professional development (CPD) events in Australia, Brunei, Canada, Denmark, England, Hong Kong, Iceland, Indonesia, Ireland, Jersey, Malaysia, New Zealand, Northern Ireland, Norway, the Philippines, Portugal, Scotland, Singapore, South Africa, Turkey, and the US. We have served as peer-reviewers of articles in some 37 journals[1], collaborated on policy documents, practice guidelines, senate submissions, and position statements, and have been involved, in voluntary capacities, in working with

---

1 ACQuiring Knowledge in Speech, Language and Hearing; Addiction; American Journal of Bioethics; Applied Cognitive Psychology; Advances in Speech Language Pathology; American Journal of Speech Language Pathology; Aphasiology; Australian Family Physician; Australian Journal of Health Promotion; Australian Journal of Learning Difficulties; Australian Journal of Primary Health; Australian Psychologist; Australian Social Work; Asia Pacific Journal of Speech, Language and Hearing; Brain Injury; Canadian Journal of Criminology and Criminal Justice; Canadian Journal of Speech-Language Pathology and Audiology; Child Language Teaching and Therapy; Cleft Palate-Craniofacial Journal; Clinical Linguistics and Phonetics; International Journal of Language and Communication Disorders; Disability, Development and Education; Drugs: Education, Prevention & Policy; Health Education Research; International Journal of Speech, Language, and the Law; International Journal of Speech-Language Pathology; Journal of Applied Research in Intellectual Disabilities; Journal of Clinical Practice in Speech-Language Pathology; Journal of Clinical Speech and Language Studies; Journal of Communication Disorders; Journal of Forensic Psychiatry and Psychology; Journal of Interactional Research in Communication Disorders; Journal of Speech, Language, and Hearing Research; Language Speech and Hearing Services in Schools; Neuropsychological Rehabilitation; Psychology; Crime and Law, and Perspectives on Language Learning and Education.

the APS, ASSBI and LDA, and the SLP/SLT peak bodies, ASHA, IASLT, ISTA, NZSTA, MASH, RCSLT, SASLHA, SHAS and SPA[2], on taskforces and projects.

The upshot is that we strive to be outward-looking and conversant with global affairs, while owning peculiarly SLP/SLT – but not necessarily Australian – worldviews that centre on the importance of providing the best possible services to individuals with communication and swallowing difficulties. This focus is obvious in Chapter 12, where we use SLP/SLT examples in contemplating common dilemmas of everyday practice, and those that come out of left field. We foresee that colleagues in other disciplines, including students, will identify with the information in this chapter, and extrapolate, adapt, and apply it to their own practice situations.

Out of left field

In 2016, a British English teacher, with an MA in English Language Teaching and Linguistics, introduced herself, and asked in an email: "Do you or would you be interested in providing basic screening and speech and language disorder training to English teachers?" The unexpected email raised immediate concerns: territorial, statutory and ethical. Territorial, since all SLPs/SLTs are instilled with their *scope of practice* from day one, as students. Statutory, because, in the UK the RCSLT provides guidelines that support the SLT profession in delivering a high-quality patient and user service, ensuring that SLTs adhere to Health and Care Professions Council (HCPC) legislated standards. Ethical, because SLPs/SLTs everywhere are bound to practise, at all times, to the highest standards of professional competence, following best practice standards, *within their expertise* (Stacey-Knight & Mayo, 2015). So, we are ethically obliged to continually update and extend our knowledge and skills, hold paramount the welfare of those we serve, and sustain quality and safe care of our clients (Chabon et al., 2011).

The writer voiced a wish to "assist this group of learners" with presumed communication difficulties, not necessarily individuals whose speech and language skills had been competently assessed by an SLP/SLT. Inherent in the

---

2 APS: Australian Psychological Society; ASSBI: Australian Society for the Study of Brain Impairment; LDA: Learning Difficulties Australia. ASHA: American Speech-Language-Hearing Association; IASLT: Irish Association of Speech & Language Therapists; ISTA: Indonesian Speech Therapist Association; NZSTA: New Zealand Speech-language Therapists' Association; MASH: Malaysian Association of Speech-Language & Hearing; RCSLT: Royal College of Speech & Language Therapists; SASLHA: South African Speech Language Hearing Association; SHAS: Speech-Language & Hearing Association Singapore; SPA: Speech Pathology Australia.

email was an ethical dilemma[3] for the recipient, and a basic confusion (no matter how benevolent) on the sender's part about the SLP/SLT role, with its requirement for us to ensure that we are "current" in our field:

> "Since the cutbacks in the National Health Service (NHS) in the provision of speech and language therapy to children and adults, [our sector has] been receiving an increased number of learners [who] are children with speech and language disorders or adults who are self-managed. As English teachers, we do not receive any training in speech and language disorders during teacher training, therefore, the majority of English teachers do not have the skills set to assist this group of learners who, theoretically, should be seeking the help of SLTs. I am pondering as to whether a basic training programme covering screening and providing English teachers with basic speech and language tools could be designed and be feasible?"

For us, the idea that a qualified, working professional from another discipline could undertake a short training programme – it is hard to conceive of a teacher with time for a *long* programme – in screening and then "assisting" children with (possibly incorrectly ascertained) speech and language disorders, is disturbing. Questions like this on behalf of a professional group are unusual, but the general public often ask them, revealing hazy concepts of "who should be doing what", and what levels of knowledge and skill are required to underwrite such doing, stimulating us to outline, next, what SLPs/SLTs are, and what we do.

SLP/SLT

There is no difference, other than the name, between a speech-language pathologist (SLP, S-LP) a speech and language therapist (SLT), and a speech pathologist (SP). Certified or full members of the American Speech-Language-Hearing Association (ASHA) which credentials SLPs and audiologists; the Irish Association of Speech & Language Therapists (IASLT), the New Zealand Speech-language Therapists' Association (NZSTA), or the Royal College of Speech &

---

3 The issue was resolved when the points raised in the email were discussed with, and clarified by RCSLT representatives. The story is included here with the permission of both the English teacher and the RCSLT.

Language Therapists (RCSLT) which credentials SLTs; Speech-Language & Audiology Canada—Orthophonie et Audiologie Canada (SAC-OAC) which credentials S-LPs and audiologists; or Speech Pathology Australia (SPA) which credentials SPs, are all uniquely equipped to assess, diagnose, and treat people's *communication* and *swallowing* difficulties across the lifespan. Once qualified, SLPs/S-LPs/SLTs/SPs accept an enduring commitment to career-long professional learning, which is increasingly mandated and regulated by professional bodies.

Mutual Recognition Agreement

Six associations to date: ASHA, IASLT, NZSTA, RCSLT, SAC-OAC and SPA, have signed a mutual recognition agreement (MRA) whereby, with well-defined provisos, members have substantially equivalent credentials. The MRA makes it possible for an SLP/SLT who is a certified or full member of one association to be recognized by, and become a member of, the other five. Whether these practitioners' academic, vocational and clinical educations have spanned four, five, or six years of university study, they all meet the same competency-based occupational standards (C-BOS), with comparable ethical obligations to preserve them. They do so by conforming to their association's Code of Ethics and CPD programme that allows them to maintain membership, retain proficiencies, and extend and upgrade their knowledge and competences, in pursuing "best practice".

Best practice has client care at its heart, and the term denotes professional procedures that are accepted or prescribed as being correct or most effective. Knowing an S-LP/SLP/SLT/SP belongs to one or more MRA associations is no guarantee that they are *currently* up-to-date, but it gives a certain protection to those seeking the services of, or wishing to refer to, legitimate practitioners. That is not to imply that SLPs/SLTs and "speech therapists" recognized by associations in other countries[4] are necessarily "less qualified"; but that it is harder to confidently check credentials.

---

4 SLP/SLT professional organizations that are not MRA signatories include: AKL (Czech Republic), ALF (Denmark), ALO (Luxembourg), AMCAOF (Mexico), APTF (Portugal), ASLAFA (Argentina), ASLP (Malta), CAR-SLP (Cyprus), CISHA (China), DBL (Germany), DIK (Sweden), DKBUD (Turkey), DLOGS (Slovenia), DVL (Switzerland), ELU (Estonia), FLI (Italy), FNO (France), HKAST (Hong Kong), ISHA (India), ISHLA (Israel), ISTA (Indonesia), JAS (Japan), KSLP (Korea), MASH (Malaysia), NLL (Norway), NVLF (Netherlands), PASP (Philippines), PSL (Greece), PZL (Poland), SASLHA (South Africa), SBFA (Brazil), SGPLA (Switzerland), SHAS (Singapore), SLH (Taiwan), SOMEF (Spain), and VVL (Belgium).

Generalists and specialists

Among paediatric SLPs/SLTs is a diminishing proportion of generalists whose clients represent the breadth of childhood communication and swallowing disorders occurring in isolation (e.g., stuttering only), in combination (e.g., stuttering and articulation disorder), or in conjunction with conditions (e.g., cerebral palsy, neurofibromatosis); disorders (e.g., FASD, galactosemia); diseases (e.g., middle ear disease); and syndromes (e.g., Angelman, Fragile-X, Prader-Willi, Velo-Cardio-Facial, or Williams syndromes).

The competencies and scope of SLP/SLT practice have expanded so much that today's clinicians cannot expect to be across current developments in all areas, so most SLPs/SLTs limit their caseloads. For example, some see children with voice and fluency difficulties but not those whose primary needs are for help with language, literacy and speech, and vice versa. Others' caseloads are composed of children with ID ("learning difficulties" in the UK) and/or ASD, and within those populations, children with the gamut of communication, literacy and swallowing issues. Yet others work only with children fitted with hearing aids or cochlear implants; children with craniofacial anomalies; children with dysphagia; or children who have had brain injuries due to accidents, infections, cytotoxic drugs, metabolic disorders, surgery, or tumours. Others see adults *and* children within a total client group, such as AAC users, or individuals who stutter.

The work of some SLPs/SLTs is restricted to particular age bands, notably 0–3 in Early Intervention (EI) and domiciliary settings, or 3 to school-age, or school-aged, or adolescent to young adult in custodial sites. Their modes of service delivery can be "push-in" or "pull-out" in schools; office- or clinic-based; face-to-face in the flesh or via telepractice (teletherapy); or "mobile" – driving, boating or flying between sites. SLPs/SLTs practise in disparate locations: charitable institutions, children's own homes, community health centres, custodial or care facilities, EI centres, hospitals, online, preschools and schools, private practices, social enterprises, university-based clinics, and as volunteers and paid workers in the majority world.

Working in developing communities

Since 1998, CB's www.speech-language-therapy.com has attracted a flow of enquiries and requests for help, often relating to SLP/SLT services in the majority world and in remote places. In the first half of 2016 alone, such email arrived directly from Bali, Bolivia, Cambodia, Ethiopia, Mongolia, Myanmar, Papua New Guinea, Romania, Rwanda, Ukraine and the US.

This one was from the US: "I am recruiting an SLT (I do hope it might be YOU) and an OT who would like to live in Shenzhen for one year to train paraprofessionals on SLT and OT skills for ages 0–8 years old. China has just recognized the need for SLTs. No universities offer it as a major and few courses are offered except via other universities. A CEO of a rehab center for young children wants to offer services, but the therapists would have to speak Chinese, which has many variants. In the interim, the CEO seeks an SLT to train or share basic info to the current teachers/paraprofessionals who have worked with disabled children for years (very experienced and dedicated). Translators are available. If you have a better solution, please share." For the record, CB directed the writer to HKAST, SLP/SLT academics at the University of Hong Kong, the Chinese International Speech-Language and Hearing Association (www.cisha.org.cn) and her own contacts in the PRC. Another 2016 inquiry was from Africa: "We seek a Speech Pathologist to train rehab technician staff to provide the highest quality assessment and therapy services (with a main focus on AAC, ASD and speech) over 6 to 8 weeks in Malawi. We will pay airfares, board and lodgings and meet-greet you in Lilongwe." Like so many of these enquiries, it came with an appeal for a six-figure "suggested sum". CB proffered conservative advice, but as is also usual when an answer is not the one "hoped for", no further correspondence was received.

In our travels, we have seen fully-qualified SLPs/SLTs "make do" with superseded, photocopied (from colour to black and white) and incomplete assessments; tests and intervention materials translated from English to local languages; and culturally inappropriate materials, for instance: the (British) Renfrew Action Picture Test for isiZulu and Xhosa speakers; Brown's Stages (English) "norms" for morphological development applied to Khmer, Tagalog and Vietnamese; and pictorial resources made for the UK and US used with indigenous and non-indigenous Australian, Filipino, Malaysian, New Zealand and South African children. Some fully-qualified SLPs/SLTs also engage, with mixed motives, in "importing" non-evidence-based methods for use by naïve practitioners with vulnerable populations, enjoying Big-Tobacco-style sponsorship.

The TalkTools® Blog (http://blog.talktools.com/2016/slp-and-ot-trip-to-ukraine), for example, records that four Australians, two SLPs and two OTs, volunteered for a week in November 2015 at the Dzherelo Centre in Lviv, Ukraine. The "mission trip" was sponsored by TalkTools®, who also donated (their) merchandise to the centre. The SLPs taught staff how to use TalkTools® exercises and products (see pp. 190–192), "to turn mealtimes into therapy to support the children in developing their oromotor skills. All of the children … required support with the strength and coordination of their jaw. Chewy Tubes with the pre-feeding chewy hierarchy were trialled successfully". Meetings were also held at the Lviv Catholic University, the Polytechnic University and the Military Hospital, where the sponsor's products may have been discussed in an approving light, with no mention of their lack of supporting evidence.

Ethical issues permeate each of these circumstances, in complex, even alien settings where barriers to E³BP far outweigh the facilitators. Doing your best in difficult situations should not equate with knowingly advocating or delivering inferior service, especially when grateful, hospitable, and sometimes adoring recipients believe you offer "the best", and want you back.

Barriers to E³BP

Barriers to E³BP (Dollaghan, 2007) impact most SLPs/SLTs. They include gaps in the evidence base; the expense of purchasing pay-walled research articles; the preference of some clinicians for upholding "tradition" over changing practice (Duchan, 2006, 2010); and little time to read and understand research (Pring, Flood, Dodd, & Joffe, 2012; Roulstone, Wren, Bakopoulou, Goodlad, & Lindsay, 2012; Stephens & Upton, 2013). Poor research literacy makes it hard for some readers to discern which research has methodological merit and clinical relevance for them, and it can contribute to their difficulty understanding the language of, and statistics in, research articles (Kamhi, 2011a; Lof, 2011; Roddam & Skeat, 2010). Confronting such barriers, well-intentioned but time-poor clinicians may access online summaries of research studies, which are sometimes written by seemingly authoritative "experts" with vested (but undeclared) interests in omitting unfavourable studies, "buffing" patchy findings, and over-stating positive reports. These problems may be exacerbated by incomplete knowledge of certain client groups' cultures and languages (e.g., Guiberson & Atkins, 2012; McLeod, Verdon, & Bowen, 2013) in a world of international relocation, migration, refugee dislocation, and philanthropic volunteerism. Barriers can also be imposed by unmanageable workloads, personnel shortages, wait times (Rvachew & Rafaat, 2014), externally enforced constraints to service delivery such as limits to the "therapy hours per client" (Baker, 2012), and "silo" approaches to health, disability and education teams by service providers and individual practitioners. These factors may then contribute to reduced job satisfaction, workforce attrition (McLaughlin, Adamson, Lincoln, Pallant, & Cooper, 2010), and low team morale.

Teams can function ineffectively, impeded by narrow client-eligibility-for-services criteria, rigid policies and attitudes and impermeable professional boundaries, especially where children with ID or ASD are concerned (Cheung, Trembath, Arciuli, & Togher, 2013). This is dispiriting for everyone, particularly clinicians who perceive that the needs and expectations of clients and families are better – if still imperfectly – met, where collaboratively designed and inclusive pathways to care and services exist, via multifaceted eligibility criteria. Overloaded, time-poor clinicians lacking research literacy are probably less likely to read the literature routinely, and many report turning to the Internet for quick, reader-friendly answers (Jansen, Rasekaba, Presnell, & Holland, 2012). When they do, they need good information literacy to pinpoint reliable content and to detect inaccurate, misleading or misguided claims.

Information literacy

The Association of College and Research Libraries (ACRL), a division of the American Library Association (www.ala.org), makes the case for information literacy as the foundation of lifelong learning, across disciplines and learning environments, and at all levels of education.

> *"Information is available through libraries, community resources, special interest organizations, media, and the Internet--and increasingly, information comes to individuals in unfiltered formats, raising questions about its authenticity, validity, and reliability. In addition, information is available through multiple media, including graphical, aural, and textual, and these pose new challenges for individuals in evaluating and understanding it. The uncertain quality and expanding quantity of information pose large challenges for society. The sheer abundance of information will not in itself create a more informed citizenry without a complementary cluster of abilities necessary to use information effectively."*
> ARCL www.ala.org/acrl/standards/
> informationliteracycompetency

The page cited above contains things an information-literate individual is able to do, namely, "to:

1. Determine the extent of information needed

2. Access the needed information effectively and efficiently

3. Evaluate information and its sources critically

4. Incorporate selected information into one's knowledge base

5. Use information effectively to accomplish a specific purpose

6. Understand the economic, legal, and social issues surrounding the use of information, and access and use information ethically and legally"

and this is followed by helpful descriptions of each item listed. Thinking about point 3, we are mindful of professionals and consumers broaching the rich but unpredictable Internet environment to seek information about SLP/SLT – on blogs and websites, in social media, or in Listserv® and other mailing list discussions. The input they need in order to critically *evaluate information* and *evaluate its sources* belongs under the headings: **authority**, **quality**, **usability and accessibility**, and **design**, taking into account the **purpose** and **scope** of the source, and the intended **audience** (which should be stated).

The **authority** of the author(s) should be clear. If a consumer cannot find and understand their credentials, and they do not use scholarly methods that *exclude* overstated claims and puff pieces for products or treatments, it is a signal *not* to take a gamble and to look elsewhere for a reliable source. Reliable informants identify themselves and their locations, and are contactable via a web-based form, email, mail, telephone or in social media. Where relevant, they include appropriate citations from the juried literature to support any claims – indicating how up-to-date it is – present content in a balanced manner, and distinguish fact from opinion. You should not have to provide *your* contact details first in order to connect with an intervention provider.

Assessing **quality**, readers must first check the agenda, purpose and scope of, and intended audience for, the information. Is it for advocacy, sales and marketing, news, policy, propaganda, teaching, or scholarly research purposes? Is it satire disguised as fact? Is it geared to a consumer, student, mass media or professional audience? Is prior knowledge assumed? Is the content accurate, current (that does not necessarily mean recent, as some content stands the test of time; take $E=MC^2$, for example), "checkable", objective, relevant, sufficiently detailed, and pitched to your level of knowledge?

For **usability**, the content must be organized, readable, comprehensive enough, and expressed in language that a motivated consumer can comprehend. Links within the source are useless without **accessibility**. For example, links to pay-walled articles may only be accessible by a privileged few with entrée to the publisher's platform. To accommodate the needs of users with disabilities, the W3C® (www.w3.org) Web Content Accessibility Guidelines should be observed.

Finally, the **design** features of a www-document, including email, may repel or attract. Brief information must be set out appropriately in a way that is easy for the reader to approach, remembering that the once-beloved Comic Sans - especially in blue, and **bold** and *italics*, or horror of horrors, all three <u>underlined</u> – for email, web pages, pdfs and PowerPoint is disdained by many! Lengthy content is better received when shown in a predictable, aesthetically pleasing way, with intuitive navigational aids and an unobtrusive, logical layout that draws readers in.

Disney-grade drawings, graphics and animations are not required, but readable fonts, manageable chunks of text, and colour schemes that aid readability and attentional focus are. The same is true for "printable" and "downloadable" resources that SLPs/SLTs develop and share, or sell, via self-published personal and practice websites and blogs.

The Internet as an evidence source

Researchers in Melbourne, Australia, Jansen et al. (2012) explored the methods that 166 clinical allied health professionals (AHPs) used to access evidence. The most frequently consulted information sources were colleagues in the same profession (84%), search engines such as Google™ (83%), their "clinical experience" (79%), emailed evidence summaries (25%), and web forums (18%). Their respondents cited time and clinical workload as primary obstacles to E^{3}BP, reporting barriers to *implementing* evidence less often than barriers to *finding* it. They concluded that, "Care must be taken to ensure that allied health clinicians have adequate information literacy skills and are aware of accessible, high-quality evidence sources" (p. 154).

Noting Jansen et al. (2012), as well as searching in university electronic databases, we did general web searches. Using both kinds of search allows comparisons between what we find in (mainly pay-walled) electronic journals and reports, with what others find simply by searching the Net, including: Google™, Google Scholar™, Wikipedia®, Open Access journals, the resurfaced Sci-Hub (www.sci-hub.io) nicknamed "Pirate Bay for scientists", or by using #icanhazpdf (plus an email address) in social media. We also stockpiled websites, blogs and Twitter lists, to: (1) help confirm that we have covered the pseudoscientific interventions for children's developmental disorders that are liable to have the greatest impact; and (2) locate the same information that AHP and medical colleagues, families and clients are likely to see on the first page of "returns" in their own web searches.

A fine ideal

Contemplating our "websites and blogs collection" there are three reasons why the Henry Spink Foundation (www.henryspink.org) site stands out. First, the Foundation is based on a fine ideal: "to help families of children with severe disabilities of all kinds", arising from the struggle and resolve of the Spinks to overcome wretched circumstances. Michael and Henrietta Spink have two sons, Henry (b. 1988) and Freddie (b. 1992). Both men are nonverbal and severely disabled, requiring around-the-clock-care since birth (Spink, 2004). The Henry Spink Foundation is a UK independent charity, established by the couple in 1996. Second, it has possibly the largest list of pseudoscientific interventions, many of which the Foundation supports, *anywhere* on the web. Third, it has considerable celebrity endorsement. Its patrons are Darcey Bussell CBE, Felicity Kendal CBE, Timothy Spall OBE, Alastair Stewart OBE, Alan Titchmarsh MBE, and Terry Waite CBE. A web search for Henrietta and Michael Spink reveals ample publicity, reflecting sophisticated media savvy – just what is needed in advocating for severely disabled individuals and the plight of many of their families – and we applaud that.

On www.henryspink.org, they "provide information on conventional and complementary/alternative medicine, therapies and research relating to a very wide range of physical and mental disorders", stating that they "do not make recommendations or favour particular treatments but give you the necessary facts to make choices yourself". The options, with the pros and cons of each intervention, in "fact sheet" form, reflect our worst nightmares around pseudoscience directed at families and children.[5] The "facts" are unattributed (authored anonymously), uncritical, superficial and inaccurate, with much outdated information. To exhibit our concerns, here are five representative excerpts from their reviews of baseless interventions.

---

5 The fact sheet topics include, among others: Acupressure, Acupuncture, Alexander Technique, Aloe Vera, Alternative Treatments For Arthritis, Anthroposophical Medicine, Applied Kinesiology, Aromatherapy, Aston Patterning, Auditory Integration Training, Autogenics, Biofeedback, Brushing Therapy, Candida diet, Chelation Therapy, Chinese Herbalism, Chiropractic, Cranial Osteopathy, Craniosacral Osteopathy, Dance Movement Therapy, Dental Amalgam ("Mercury Poisoning"), Dolphin Therapy, Evening Primrose Oil, Facilitated Communication, the Feingold Food Programme, the Feldenkrais Method, Feuerstein Instrumental Enrichment, Gluten and Casein Allergies, G-therapy, Hellerwork, Herbalism, Higashi School Daily Life Therapy, Homeopathy, Hydrotherapy, Hydrothermal Therapy, Hyperbaric Oxygen Therapy, Hypnotherapy, Intensive Behavioural Therapy (Løvaas Therapy), Irlen Lenses, Ketogenic Diet, Massage Therapy, Meditation, Naturopathy, Neuro-Linguistic Programming, Neurotherapy, Nutritional Therapy, Polarity Therapy, Red Cell Fatty Acid Analysis, Reflexology, Ritalin, Rolfing, Secretin, Shiatsu, Smart Drugs, Sunflower Method, TEACCH, The Son-Rise Programme, The Tomatis Method, Tragerwork, Vega Testing, and Yoga.

Dolphin Therapy, see pages 97–98: "… both sides of the brain enter into synchronization which means there is a far better communication between the left and right sides of the brain, this is an uncommon neurological state, which is typically associated with heightened awareness and increased learning ability."

Chelation Therapy, see pages 276–280: "People who have responded well to chelation therapy often show improvements for some time after the therapy has stopped. As 98% of the chelating agent is passed out of the body within 48 hours, the theory is that prolonged benefits are the result of the body, cleared of toxins, being able to utilise its natural healing forces. Proponents of the therapy believe that many of the vague and unexplained ills experienced by many people could be to do with the toxic environment in which we live, damaging the chemical balance of our systems. They believe that chelation therapy might help to detoxify the body, restoring balance and good health."

Facilitated Communication see pages 154–166: "Opponents to the technique argue that the 'facilitator' can influence or manipulate the users as they attempt to point or type and therefore do the communicating. Recent scientific studies have not been conclusive."

Homeopathy, pages 173–175: "has proved beneficial in the treatment of influenza, asthma, migraine, diarrhoea, fibromyalgia, allergies, digestive system disorders, rheumatism. Generally, it is believed to work well for short term acute illnesses, chronic disorders, immune dysfunction, emotional and mental disorders, skin disorders, or respiratory disorders."

Irlen® Lenses, see pages 240–242: "The lenses may help individuals who suffer from the following disorders providing they have the Irlen® Syndrome: ADD/ADHD, autism, dyslexia, learning difficulties, photosensitive epilepsy."

Readers, attracted by and sympathetic to the undoubted good intentions that put the site there in the first place, and possibly impressed by the Foundation's prominent patrons, need well-honed information literacy to work through it all, objectively. Which brings us back to the interesting topic of cognitive bias. Two of our favourites are blind spot bias: the tendency to see "me" as less biased than "you", or to detect more cognitive biases in others than in oneself; and the Dunning-Kruger effect: the worrying tendency for non-experts to overestimate their ability alongside the tendency for experts to underestimate theirs.

Cognitive bias

A cognitive bias involves wrong reasoning, evaluation, or recall. It occurs when someone clings to beliefs, preferences and preconceptions, despite clearly explained contrary information. At its most extreme, no amount of objective "proof", logic or evidence will sway the person to consider alternative viewpoints. Psychologists study, and incorporate into clinical and education practice, cognitive biases as they relate to reasoning, decision-making, and memory.

Among the common cognitive biases is **confirmation bias**: whereby people tend to look for or interpret information in a way that fortifies their preconceptions and existing beliefs while discrediting information that does not "fit" with what they think. Confirmation bias is evident when supporters of Facilitated Communication (FC) reject evidence that argues against its authenticity. In the case of FC, the disconfirming evidence ranges from confessions by former facilitators (e.g., Boynton, 2012), to damning videos (e.g., Palfreman, 1993) to authoritative research (Schlosser et al., 2014) and expert, peer-reviewed comment (Hemsley & Dann, 2014; Mirenda, 2014a; Travers et al., 2014), to astute journalism (e.g., Auerbach, 2015; Engber, 2015). In attempts to counter this, FC aficionados have volunteered "success stories" (Attfield, 2015; Jasuta, 2015), inauthentic video "evidence" (Finnes, 2015) and, in our direct experience, hounding via social media and menacing telephone calls. Confirmation bias is also apparent when SLPs/SLTs state a provisional diagnosis, of Childhood Apraxia of Speech for example, and proceed to "prove themselves right" rather than weighing all the evidence as a scientist-practitioner should (Finn, Bothe, & Bramlett, 2005; Lof, 2011; Lum, 2002), and perhaps finally identifying a more prevalent, and less severe speech sound disorder.

Self-serving bias is the tendency for people to assess ambiguous information in a way that is beneficial to their interests, and to claim more responsibility for successes than failures (if failures are even acknowledged); and **belief bias** occurs when a person's grasp of the logic of an argument is skewed by their belief in the rightness or wrongness of the conclusion (Gruber et al., 2003). There are many other cognitive biases, including those that are referred to as "effects", such as the Dunning-Kruger effect, above.

The **backfire effect** leads people to react to *disconfirming* evidence by *strengthening* rather than weakening their beliefs. Parents may experience this with their adolescent offspring when they caution against an activity, action, location, purchase or relationship, unintentionally enhancing its appeal. Nyhan,

Reifler, Richey and Freed (2014) found that four public health interventions, devised to alert parents to the risks of communicable diseases and to promote vaccination, had the opposite effect on some parents. The interventions were (1) evidence-based information explaining that MMR vaccination does NOT cause autism; (2) written information about the dangers of the diseases prevented by MMR vaccination; (3) images of children with diseases that would have been prevented by the MMR vaccine; and (4) a dramatic narrative about an infant who almost died of measles. Many participants intensified their misperceptions of vaccines, *amplifying* their resolve to *not* have their children vaccinated, while not one of the four interventions increased parental intent to vaccinate a "future child".

The **bandwagon effect**, or the propensity for "groupthink" or "herd behaviour", sees people acting or believing in certain ways (often impelled more by heart than by head) because others do rather than because there is credible evidence (e.g., using NS-OMT to improve children's speech intelligibility) and the IKEA or not invented here (NIH) effect, or avoidance of criteria, knowledge, products, research or standards developed outside a group (which we have observed in CPD settings, in several countries, where approaches are deemed "too American").

> "Substitute 'damn' every time you're inclined to write 'very'; your editor will delete it and the writing will be just as it should be."
>
> Often attributed to Mark Twain

A very, very intriguing bias is the **authority effect**: the tendency to believe or defer to experts and authors whose words we generally agree with and respect. We like Mark Twain, and quote him to each other, particularly on writing-related matters. We are unsure about the damn quotation above, but we know for certain that he wrote (in *Pudd'nhead Wilson's New Calendar* in *Following the Equator* [Twain, 1897]), "There are those who scoff at the schoolboy, calling him frivolous and shallow. Yet it was the schoolboy who said, 'Faith is believing what you know ain't so.'" So, when we encountered a quotation, ostensibly in the style of Twain, and attributed to him on the Internet, in books, in the 2015 feature film *The Big Short*, and in journal articles, it took a while for us to smell a rat.

> "It ain't what you don't know that gets you into trouble. It's what you know for sure that just ain't so."
>
> Mark Twain never said!

It was easy to establish that the Twain quote was a fake – albeit cited prolifically and sincerely – and to locate a genuine alternative, expressing the same sentiment. It was written by Leo Tolstoy in 1893 and translated into English in 1894, three years before the *Pudd'nhead Wilson* quote.

> "The most difficult subjects can be explained to the most slow-witted man if he has not formed any idea of them already; but the simplest thing cannot be made clear to the most intelligent man if he is firmly persuaded that he knows already, without a shadow of a doubt, what is laid before him."
>
> Tolstoy, 1894, p. 49

Many cognitive biases are related to, if not rooted in, emotional biases and needs, particularly for those clinicians who take people-pleaser behaviour to extremes (forever saying "yes" to avoid a fuss or becoming unpopular), or who allow boundaries between themselves and their clients to blur. Feeling validated and "needed" may be intrinsically rewarding to clinicians, but such ego needs must be kept in check, through participation in wide-ranging CPD, discussion of ideas with peers and mentors, engagement in clinical supervision, and reflection.

What can you say?

It can be daunting for SLPs/SLTs and students to discuss sensitive topics and share concerns about ethics, policies and practices, other than peer-to-peer with close colleagues and privately with dependable confidantes. Most experienced professionals probably unburden themselves *confidentially*, now and again, regarding unprofessional, unethical or unscientific practices in their field. These hushed (or chip-spitting) conversations may be from a fatalistic standpoint that "these things happen" through to a frustrated "but, what can you say?" and a desire not to rock one's own boat or that of others. Sometimes, however, circumstances arise where professionals and students *can* say something, in the here-and-now, or after reflection and advice; particularly when they are asked for an opinion.

These things happen

You, as an SLP/SLT and lifelong learner, may be asked by an employer, senior, or colleague for your "thoughts" or "insights" about a "method" with doubtful credibility, that they have adopted or are considering. Perhaps they are contemplating paying (or even worse, charging parents) for Arrowsmith™, BrainGym®, Brainology®, Cellfield™, Interactive Metronome®, Irlen®, PROMPT©, Reading Recovery™, TalkTools®, Tomatis®, or Verbal Motor Learning (VML) training for you and your colleagues. How do you approach the discussion? What are the risks of speaking out? What are the risks of saying nothing, and thereby giving tacit approval to the non-evidence-based intervention? Do you brandish *Making Sense of Interventions for Children with Developmental Disorders* or Snow (2016) in the boss's face; or better not? Are you experiencing a hint of panic just by thinking about it?

You, as an SLP/SLT student and lifelong learner, may find yourself in a clinic or classroom where assessment and intervention practices, which you are expected to administer under supervision, conflict with what you have learned at university. A common example is the plight of students, whose lecturers counsel against NS-OMT, turning up to clinical placements where treatment rooms bristle with oral motor tools and toys, and supervisors or tutors expect them to run through mouth exercises with children with unclear speech. How do you approach the discussion? How do you feel, thinking about it? What are the risks of "saying something" or the consequences of "saying nothing"? Should you talk to your professional ethics lecturer?

Challenge and risk

McComas (2014, p. 108) contrasts SLPs/SLTs who embrace the opportunity to return to school to do higher degrees with those who "avoid challenges, give up easily, expect success without effort, ignore negative feedback, and are threatened by the successes of others". She portrays practitioners attracted to doctoral education as the people who "seek challenges, persist when they face obstacles, exert effort to reach their goals, use negative feedback to learn, and learn from, and are inspired by, the success of others".

> *"Just as clinicians are encouraged to practice at the top of their licenses, educators can encourage students to practice at the top of their education. By that I mean learners should always be tackling challenging problems and issues, not engaging in work that does not challenge them intellectually. As learners gain more experience in trying to solve challenging problems, two things happen. First, they are learning content as they*

> work. Second, they are learning the process and strategies of
> problem solving, which will make them more skilled in the
> future, enabling them to take on more complex challenges."
>
> McComas, 2014, p. 108

There are parallels between these confronting ideas and the issues around resolving ethical dilemmas. How might we grow as professionals by facing them proactively, applying a casuistry skillset; what are the implications for us, as "learners", if we turn away? For turning away is not "doing nothing"; it is doing something, and as such it has consequences. As problem-solving challenges go, ethical dilemmas are complex and risky. While they are never *easy* to approach, with experience and peer support, and negotiation skills' practice, they become *easier*.

These situations can create cognitive dissonance for the person addressing the dilemma, in the intellectually demanding process of choosing between moral imperatives, where to embrace one will result in contravening another. That is, for an E³BP-committed SLP/SLT, with an ethical dilemma, stating the E³BP case will be uncomfortable, as will saying nothing.

It is central to our professionalism, however, that we do not renege on the E³BP message, or dilute hard-won standards. One mark of a professional is being known as someone who talks the (E³BP) talk, and walks the walk. Sometimes, this means having the courage to change position, in response to a significant shift in the evidence base. Sometimes it means having the courage to hold fast in the face of premature but unfounded excitement about a new treatment.

Casuistry

Ethical frameworks help SLPs/SLTs and students to keep patients, rather than themselves, at the centre of their activities, while *ethical reasoning* is central to clinical reasoning. Casuistry[6], in ethics, is a case-based method of reasoning (Schumann & Alfandre, 2008) that draws on the legal concept of "test cases" or precedents. Casuists use general principles to reason by analogy, comparing clear-cut or resolved cases ("paradigms") with difficult cases, and treating *their* analogous cases similarly. Starting with the moral and practical features of each case, the casuist consults a "taxonomy" or resource file of relevant

---

6 Casuistry /ˈkæʒjuːɪstɹi/ or /ˈkæzjuːɪstɹi/ has another, unflattering definition that equates it to fudging evidence, numbers or facts with the use of clever but unsound reasoning, especially in relation to moral questions, as in sophistry (false arguments intended to deceive).

(to the case) authoritative works or principles, drawn from a Code of Ethics, policy documents and evidence-driven position statements.

Casuistry is valued in many professions, including SLP/SLT (Quail, Sanderson, & Leitão, 2015), as a useful, systematic, flexible way to consider murky ethical dilemmas where how "the rules" are best applied is in doubt. Its forte is its respect for professional (including clinical) experience and E^3BP, its dynamic "growing" of a repertoire of paradigms, and its capacity to advance novice casuists' decision-making skills. It flourishes in workplaces where open dialogue around the ethical, clinical and professional aspects of complex cases is cultivated. It is used to clarify the seriousness and moral significance (for all parties, e.g., client, clinician and employer) of all the elements of the problematic situation, and to determine workable resolutions. Everyone has the opportunity to discuss the *moral* and *practical* pros and cons of identified options.

"Situation ethics" is case-based too, but is different from casuistry. In it, authoritative works and principles are used as guidelines – if at all – without reference to analogous paradigm cases. The situationist understands each case as a unique set of circumstances rather than integral to the wider moral experience. Casuistry varies from deductive, rule-based ethical approaches where a set of rules is considered to be unequivocally applicable in all circumstances. As well, casuistry differs from ethics approaches that rely wholly on good character or virtuous motives, calling for consideration of how to put good character and virtuous motives into practice.

Real-world ethical dilemmas in SLP/SLT

The seven scenarios that follow are anonymized, but real, and here on the assumption that the professionals and consumers concerned were of good character and acted with virtuous motives. There are two examples of workplace practice policies that are incompatible with ethics and E^3BP; two concerning inter-professional relationships, between SLPs/SLTs and OTs, and between SLPs/SLTs and teachers; one epitomizing an intraprofessional disagreement, SLP to SLP; one to do with conflict between an association's policy and a member's principles; and finally, a conflict between all three aspects of the evidence arm of the E^3BP triangle, where a client's beliefs, preferences, community and culture are at variance with the evidence base and the clinical judgement and expertise of a competent practitioner.

Scenario 1

As an experienced clinician, you have secured your dream job in a private practice. You learn belatedly that screening assessments, not thorough evaluations, are the norm and that you are expected to provide intervention with minimal data on clients' strengths, difficulties and treatment needs. You know that doing a detailed assessment is time-consuming, considering it as time well spent, as it streamlines the process of establishing goals and delivering the best possible, explicitly principled, individualized intervention. You feel your professional autonomy and ethics will be compromised if you accede, and that this is not such a fabulous job after all.

Scenario 2

Your cash-strapped government-funded agency adopts a "magic six weeks" policy, where children are seen for intervention in six-week blocks. Management justifies the decision through a disingenuous nod to "equal rights", citing risible "evidence" from a flawed study. Your view is that, under this policy, E^{3}BP will be impossible, with parents (who trust and rely on the skills and professionalism of the agency's personnel) hoodwinked into accepting that limited bursts of intervention constitute best practice, and that their children will not be short-changed.

Scenario 3

Members of your youthful E^{3}BP-focused SLP/SLT department decry using NS-OMT to achieve speech and language goals. The senior OTs in your newly-established transdisciplinary team, however, use them with gusto to accomplish sensory integration goals with children and adolescents with ID who are nonverbal and/or on the autism spectrum. Having discussed the ethics and practicalities of the situation (Kenny, Lincoln, & Balandin, 2010; Mårtensson, Fors, Wallin, Zander, & Nilsson, 2016), and looked at the casuistry paradigms you amassed in your student days, you and your SLP/SLT team are concerned that the now tenuous team dynamics will be irreparably damaged if the OTs' practices are questioned – besides, who will speak first?

Scenario 4

The teachers in a school you visit enthuse over a university-based CPD training on "brain based learning", and want to fill you in on the right-brain, left-brain, whole-brain "secrets" they have learned from a charismatic education professor about how to influence children's brain chemistry – to "train the brain" when children have literacy difficulties. Furthermore, they are already using some of the techniques, and would like you to absorb them into your sessions with the children you see who have various combinations of speech, language and literacy difficulties. You have worked hard to earn friendly alliances with the teachers, and know that when it comes to classroom practice they prefer to trust their gut instincts, the advice of fellow teachers, and personal experience, and resent "outside" (NIH or IKEA effect) research being "quoted at them".

Scenario 5

An SLP/SLT colleague mentions over coffee that he has recommended to a bilingual family that they speak English, and not Spanish to their preschooler, Tomás, who has unclear speech and late language milestones in both his languages. You understand from Goldstein (2015) that solid research evidence speaks against this advice. In the wise words of Kohnert (2008, p. 105): "A disorder in bilinguals is not caused by bilingualism or cured by monolingualism".

Scenario 6

Your professional association's periodic news magazine advertises events that attract CEUs or CPD points[7]. You see one such advertisement in the current issue. It falls within an area of practice with a client group that interests you greatly, as the topic of your PhD research. Your excellent grasp of the relevant literature, and the presenter's unfortunate reputation, tell you the particular "angle" the workshop will focus on is spurious, is not research-based, and that the information and products on offer will be suspect. While you do not intend to attend, you see this as the last straw, for only recently the same magazine has run effusive articles on non-evidence-based dolphin therapy, executive functioning interventions, Social Thinking®, and swimming-pool-based treatment for children with apraxia, ASD, cerebral palsy and Ds. Do you complain in writing, telephone the Action Center, post something (potentially defamatory) in a discussion list, freak out on Facebook, tantrum in Twitter, or hold your (reluctant) peace?

---

7 Of the Mutual Recognition Agreement (MRA) signatories, ASHA issues Continuing Education Units (CEUs), IASLT, NZSTA, RCSLT, and SPA have CPD Points, and SAC-OAC has Continuing Education Equivalents (CEEs). SASHLA also has CPD Points.

Scenario 7

With 10 months of consistent therapy attendance and conscientious home follow-up, Robert-Louis, a 7-year-old with ASD, progresses well with his pragmatic language skills. Nevertheless, his mother, Windsong, has been slow to warm to you, appearing wary. Finally, she confides that Robert-Louis has been having chelation and Samonas™ Sound Therapy for years. She believes that with the good results she is seeing, speech therapy will soon be unwarranted – though they will continue with their long-time homeopath and chiropractor, and a new-found Irlen® specialist, who says Scotopic Sensitivity (or Visual Stress) explains the boy's poor eye-contact. Indeed, the Irlen® practitioner says that an SLP/SLT is not the ideal professional to work on "eye-related issues". Then Windsong asks, "Are *you* OK with us finishing up next week?"

Motivations

1. It is well known among her colleagues that the private practice employer in Scenario 1 claims that she is so experienced as an SLP/SLT that she can diagnose this-that-or-the-other disorder "at 50 paces" ("ASD at 50 paces", "CAS at 50 paces", "Dyslexia at 50 paces"; you get the picture). Evidently, she is so skilled in speed-spotting CAS at a distance of 38.1 metres, that she identifies it three times as frequently as the population incidence suggests! She lets "her people" know that, in all sincerity, she only employs experienced clinicians because she expects them to have similar diagnostic acumen, to "be able to get children into the therapy they need without a lot of mucking about with time-wasting assessments".

2. The "magic six weeks" policy in Scenario 2 is based in equality rather than equity principles, and a "needs must" mentality, where management reasons that it is "fairer" for all to receive some therapy than for fewer to receive enough. There are no clinical outcome measures in place that clinicians can apply to counter that logic. Instead, they find "creative" (deceptive) ways to manipulate the record-keeping system so that some children – especially those with severe difficulties and good prognostic indicators – are seen for intervention with the same intensity, but for longer. Their parents are complicit, and sworn to secrecy.

3. In Scenario 3, the senior OTs are adamant that their implementation of NS-OMT is evidence based. They hold that it fits with their traditional

conceptualization of sensory integration dysfunction, citing Ayres (1972) even though, eight years later, an academic Educational Psychologist reviewed such programmes and concluded, "Current evidence shows that there are no accepted standards for identifying children in need of sensory integration therapy; assessment procedures associated with the therapy have low reliability and validity; and the therapeutic procedures used have not been shown to improve sensory integrative processing skills or academic skills like reading" (Bochner, 1980; and see Lang et al., 2012 for a more recent systematic review, with similar conclusions). When the OTs are timidly pressed by the inexperienced and "junior" SLPs/SLTs for recent evidence, the mood sours. The SLPs/SLTs retreat but, as they have recently read Alvesson and Spicer (2016), are guilt-ridden: are they trading their professional values and ethics for a quiet life?

4. The teachers in Scenario 4 are aglow with enthusiasm, recalling the entertaining CPD event away from classroom pressures, dismissing or forgetting the learning theory they covered as students in psychology lectures. Unencumbered by backgrounds in human neurology or linguistics, they are enthralled by the mysterious process of unlocking "brain based learning" for literacy. They are struck too, by how "lovely and approachable" the professor is, despite her distinguished reputation, important-sounding qualifications and the dizzying commercial success of her brain plasticity books and video self-training packages. It emerges, however, that while the professor – with all her pretty flow charts, infographics, anatomy drawings and emotive anecdotes – is eminent, her academic background is in education leadership and business management, and not in cognitive science, literacy, neurology (neuroanatomy, neurophysiology, neuropsychology, or neuroscience) or psychology. It is not that the teachers are especially gullible, but rather that their low information and research literacy in relevant disciplines leaves them prey to misinformation, and the authority effect has worked a treat.

5. Tomás's SLP in Scenario 5 quotes a CPD event he attended in 1999 to justify his erroneous "monolingualism as a cure for multilingualism woes" stance. He believed it then; he believes it now; and he believes that there is no reason to change.

6. We do not doubt the motives of the Association's news magazine's products and services advertising team in accepting ads for non-evidence-

based continuing education opportunities that yield CEUs or CPD or Pro-D points. Why would they *not* accept them from approved CE/CPD/Pro-D providers? We do wonder, however, about the quality of the checks and balances, or lack of, that allow presenters of non-evidence-based training – including those that directly or indirectly flog their wares to participants and ultimately their clients – to pass muster with some Continuing Education Boards and CPD Coordinators and committees.

7. Windsong and the E^3BP-intent therapist in Scenario 7 are chalk and cheese in some respects, but united in the sense that each wants the best for Robert-Louis. Windsong, now in her mid-40s, grew up in a hippie commune in northern New South Wales and, like her family, prefers CAM, healers, and the tranquil counsel of a Swami in a hinterland riverbank Ashram. She vigorously opposes orthodox medicine, including antibiotics and vaccines, is sensitive to disapproval (disclosing that she occasionally volunteers that she does not know the identity of Robert-Louis' father, to quietly test for a reaction so as to know who she is dealing with), and deflects information that conflicts with her harmonious world view with a blissful smile.

Responding

There are four-way correspondences between Scenario 1's inadequate assessment protocols, Scenario 2's arbitrary intervention dosages, an RCSLT web poll, and conversations with and between discouraged SLTs across the UK. One poll question was, "Do you have to carry out therapy that you know is not evidence based?" Of the 178 respondents, 113 (63.5%) said yes (reported as 65% in the June, 2016 *Bulletin*, p. 6), according with results of formal surveys of SLT clinical practice (e.g., Pring et al., 2012; Joffe, 2015), and spurring further discussion. Local service provision is described as being inequitable and non-evidence-based, disproportionately driven by budget and caseload throughput demands, with a variety of protocols and strategies in place calculated to ration services. Protocols in schools (including maintained special schools for pupils with severe learning difficulties, and other maintained special schools), specialist centres, and local authorities, contracted by NHS Clinical Commissioners can include: long wait times, absence of early identification and EI, limited opportunities for workforce development (discipline-specific training or CPD), no therapy for children before 4 or after 11 years of age, exclusively consultation-based

SLT management with no direct therapy provided to any child at any age, and (those magic) 6-week therapy blocks with long intervals between them.

In preparing to confront Scenarios 1 and 2, and analogous ones, practitioners using a casuistry approach can acquaint themselves with, and include in their taxonomies, the rousing words of the (superseded in 2015[8]) *No Child Left Behind Act* (NCLB, 2001). In NCLB, the term "scientifically based research", used over 100 times in the Act, was comprehensively defined as research "that:

- employs systematic, empirical methods that draw on observations or experimentation;

- involves rigorous data analyses that are adequate to test the stated hypotheses and justify the conclusions drawn;

- relies on measurements or observational methods that provide reliable and valid data across evaluators and observers, across multiple measurements and observations, and across studies by the same or different investigators;

- is evaluated using experimental or quasi-experimental designs in which individuals, entities, programs, or activities are assigned to different conditions and with appropriate controls to evaluate the effects of the conditions of interest, with a preference for random-assignment experiments, or other designs to the extent that those designs contain within-condition or across-condition controls;

- ensures experimental studies are presented in sufficient detail and with clarity to allow for replication or, at a minimum, offer the opportunity to build systematically on their findings;

- has been accepted by a peer-reviewed journal or approved by a panel of independent experts through a comparably rigorous, objective scientific review."

---

8 NCLB's successor: *Every Student Succeeds Act* (ESSA, 2015) was signed into law by President Barack Obama in December 2015, rescinding several of the most unpopular provisions of NCLB.

"I need to follow this path"

If you can say, "I need to follow *this* path because the law dictates it, and to do otherwise would be illegal, unethical and against my principles", you take a strong position. Depending where you practise, it may not be possible to quote government legislation ("the law") such as *ESSA*, but we *all* can use our Codes of Ethics, within a casuistry framework, to explain and defend an ethical standpoint and facilitate open discussion. If you are nervous with this approach, if confronting and discussing issues with policymakers and managers is new for you, or you feel "junior" in the situation, prepare, discuss, rehearse and role-play beforehand. Gather the support and consider the advice of like-minded peers and mentors. You may not be able to take them to meetings, but you will feel buoyed up by their encouragement, less alone, and better informed.

Make an appointment with the relevant person (or people), specifically to talk about the issue rather than it being an agenda item on a longer list. Have your facts and the vital points you must make written down and ready, and plan to be the calmest, steadiest, least belligerent, and most determined person in the room. Offer to send a progress summary of the encounter, and suggest yourself as host for a subsequent meeting or forum where the issue can be surveyed and debated thoughtfully, by those affected, from various angles. Never be shrill, use your professionalism as a shield and not a hidey-hole, and remember, Rome wasn't built in a day.

Professional relationships and evidence

Our examples of interprofessional and intraprofessional dilemmas were between SLPs/SPTs (Scenario 1), SLPs/SLTs and OTs (Scenario 3), and SLPs/SLTs and teachers (Scenario 4). It might be the most direct route into the topic, but citing *ethics* up front, in an Ethics of Care approach, may also be the surest way to deprive an important, adult conversation of oxygen. Differences over practice are probably best tackled via the evidence (E^3BP) route, starting from the honest standpoint that *you* don't know it all.

In a sincere and respectful effort to expand your knowledge, and avoiding an adversarial, combative or denigrating air, ask the other professional, "where are you coming from?", "what can you tell me about this?" and (politely) "where is your evidence?" If they provide evidence, read it carefully, putting preconceptions aside. By asking for, and examining evidence supporting *their* position you create an opening for them to request evidence for *yours*.

If they ask for your evidence, take your time (that's code for "Don't shoot from the lip") and give them one, preferably brief, clearly written, reference to the highest possible level of evidence in support of your view: handing them a copy of the article. This approach frees both parties to discover "news of a difference" (Bateson, 1972), potentially facilitating constructive discussion. You might find that you don't have it entirely right, and that you have added to your knowledge-base, and vice versa. You may persuade, or be persuaded, or meet someone half-way.

Professional associations' policies, principles and practice

Was there *ever* a profession that did not moan about its professional association on the one hand, and defend to the Nth degree on the other? Probably not. In the case of SLP/SLT, we *are* our professional associations: our respective associations represent us, are comprised of us, and are represented by us. We share a primary goal: that of providing high-quality, ethical care to clients and their families. Our associations want to be proud of us and the way we uphold values, principles and ethics, and we want to be proud of them, across those same domains. So, when an association – ASHA, IASLT, NZSTA, RCSLT, SAC-OAC, SPA, etc. – slips up, there is an inescapable reaction from at least some of its members, and sometimes from non-members.

Professional associations are not infallible, beyond criticism, or remote from the day-to-day work we do. As part of their remit they constantly canvas "ordinary" members' views, urge participation in association activities (advisory panels, boards, editorial and ethics committees, conferences, meetings, policy development, position papers, publicity campaigns (e.g., Better Hearing and Speech Month: May in the US; Speech & Hearing Month: May in Canada; Speech Pathology Week: August in Australia; SLT Awareness Week in NZ: September), publications, social media, interest groups, and more, seek member feedback and act on it. They also appoint expert volunteers from the profession, and paid qualified staff, to respond to ethical breaches.

If you are concerned that an action, advertisement, CPD, CEU or Pro-D activity, or information disseminated by a speaker your association supports conflicts significantly with evidence or ethics, your responsibility to the association and to yourself *is* to say something, professionally, in confidence to the right person, through proper channels. Often, an effective starting point is to telephone or email the association, state the nature of the concern, and ask how they suggest you might proceed. While you are at it, consider what you can contribute to your professional association, over and above your annual dues and constructive feedback – you may be just the proactive person they need.

Client–professional relationships

> "I see science literacy as kind of a vaccine against charlatans who would try to exploit your ignorance."
> Neil deGrasse Tyson, 2009

Clinicians can take certain steps *early* in the setup of the therapeutic contract that are calculated to *proactively* ward off conflict when clients' beliefs and preferences clash with the currently-available evidence base, and clinical judgement. One step is to introduce, without pontification, the topic of "science". Let it be known, from the outset, that you are a "scientist-practitioner". A simple strategy, in the context of describing your treatment approach to a parent, AHP colleague or teacher, is to say things like, "I want _____'s intervention to be based in the best science" and, when discussing your intervention, to comment along the lines of, "There is good science behind this technique" and "This may look like pure fun and games; but strong scientific research says, 'do it'". This establishes a foundation for answering queries about pseudoscience. If asked, "What's your view on XYZ intervention?" possible lead-ins might be, "Well, you know how I feel about science – have you looked at it from that angle, or would you like me to check it out?" or, "Last time I read about it there did not seem to be science in its favour – but I will find out if things have changed, and let you know one way or the other".

While the words "science", "research" and "scientific research" may strike a chord with clients, harping on about "EBP", "E^{3}BP", and "levels of evidence", and ear bashing them about THE PEER-REVIEWED LITERATURE, may be counterproductive. People are, quite rightly, put off by grandiose statements of commitment to E^{3}BP, and condescending clinicians who take the moral high ground, becoming preachy on the topic. We must never present, or think of ourselves as "superior" because of our duty to E^{3}BP, since by authentically embracing it we take on concurrent commitments to intellectual humility, curiosity and leadership. Clinicians who are dedicated to E^{3}BP are flexible thinkers and lifelong learners who value scholarship, change their minds and their practice over time in response to new empirical evidence, theoretical shifts and societal changes. By contrast, SLPs/SLTs who do not commit to and pursue E³BP will lean towards maintaining an invariant course, irrespective of how the world around them is changing.

When it comes to questions of evidence, clients, especially those with good Baloney Radar, can make it easy for us, as in the exchange below, shared in a tweet by an SLP colleague!

> *Patient: Acupuncture for dry mouth – any good?*
>
> *SLP: Well...*
>
> *Patient: ...or is it bullshit?*
>
> *SLP: Yeah, it's bullshit.*
>
> *Patient: OK, good to know.*
>
> THAT WAS IT

Windsong took forever to trust her son's therapist, but when she felt ready to divulge the CAM interventions Robert-Louis was receiving, her question, "Are *you* OK with us finishing up next week?" left an opening for the therapist to put the case for continuing his SLP/SLT intervention, that objective assessment indicated would result in more progress. Simultaneously, appreciating that Windsong had known and valued the homeopath and chiropractor for years, and that the Irlen® specialist was white-anting the SLP/SLT role in a way that "spoke" to her, was a warning to resist dismissing them as quacks (not in so many words), or even mildly challenging their contributions. Why feed the backfire effect? Maintaining Windsong's trust (and face) is the only way to leave the way clear for Robert-Louis to have further access to SLP/SLT.

In discussing options and choices with clients, in a narrative ethics approach, it is vital to listen carefully and respectfully and to determine what is going on. After all, they are talking to you, which means that at some level they are interested in, or even need your response. Don't second-guess their narrative, or make assumptions about why they are sharing their opinions and concerns – though you could ask, "Why now?" to take the conversation forward productively. When families detect disapproval, antagonism or your disappointment that they favour a non-evidence-based approach they, justifiably, go into protective mode and are uncomfortable saying what is on their minds, inducing, in game theory terms, a lose-lose situation. Acknowledge the person's courage in speaking up, recognize their genuine intent, remember that everyone does their best, and all parents seek the best for their children. Try to establish this as a *mutual* goal.

Why pounce on Windsong, deflating her confidence or leading her to a point where she feels she is betraying her community's beliefs and practices?

What if you let that rest, and listen well to what she thinks? Might her resistance to your stance on the hazardous and potentially life-threatening practice of chelation dissolve, or at least lessen? Because, you will *have* to say something, in keeping with your shared purpose of doing the best for Robert-Louis, keeping him safe. This will be a delicate conversation where you suppress any urge to manipulate or coerce, knowing that it is not your role to compete with parents, or to win an ideological debate.

Sometimes, in our professional and private lives, we must stand up and be counted. That will mean expressing an informed view in a way that is forthright, unambiguous, courteous, and unapologetic. "That is not advisable because of the risks" is forthright, unambiguous, courteous (in the right tone, with the right face), and unapologetic; "That's not such a great idea" and "I wouldn't do that in your shoes", "I'm not too sure about that", and "Well, I don't know...", are not. It is not helpful if clinicians prevaricate, dither, sit on the fence, and respond vaguely when asked about dangerous pseudoscientific interventions (e.g., chelation, chiropractic subluxation for infants, toddlers and children, and risky diets), high-risk non-interventions (e.g., withholding vaccination; and homeopathic vaccines), interventions that jeopardize health (e.g., the GF, CF and GFCF diets), and scientifically discredited interventions (e.g., FC).

In some less dangerous situations (than chelation, subluxation, non-vaccination, and risky diets) – remembering that you might not be able to accurately define all of the dangers – find out what the family feels their child gains from participation in a non-E^3BP approach. If their answers are unconvincing, and the intervention appears to be so much hocus pocus or a money-making racket, there is one way to go. That is, for you to explain that, based on current knowledge, the approach will at the very least create a significant *opportunity cost*: consuming valuable time in which the child could engage in approaches more likely to yield long-term gains. In this connection, Travers (2016) discusses, helpfully, opportunity costs of non-evidence-based interventions in special education contexts.

All of these, and more, entail opportunity cost: Arrowsmith™, Auditory Integration Training (Berard Method, Johansen Individualized Auditory Stimulation, Samonas™ Sound Therapy, The Listening Program®, Therapeutic Listening™, and Tomatis®), Behavioural Optometry, BrainGym®, Cellfield™, Etalon, Fast ForWord®, GemIIni™ Discrete Video Modelling, HEGL/Heguru™, Interactive Metronome®, Irlen®, Kinesiotaping, Learning Breakthrough™, Myofascial Release, MNRI®, the McGuire Program, NS-OMT, PROMPT©, Reading Recovery™, Shichida™, the Son-Rise Program®, Solisten®, TalkTools®, Therapeutic Speech Massage, and Verbal Motor Learning (VML).

Resources

An SLP/SLT casuist's "taxonomy" or resource file starts with authoritative works or principles drawn from their professional association's Code of Ethics, policy documents and evidence-based position statements that guide and remind them of workplace responsibilities. Professional associations develop and distribute additional resources, employ staff who will help members and the public when ethical issues arise (including facilitating conciliation at a "non-official" level), and offer training. For example, the RCSLT provides, on its website, an interactive Evidence-Based Clinical Decision-Making Tool, and Communicating Quality Live. SPA offers open access to the 2015 Ethics supplement (http://speechpathologyaustralia.cld.bz/JCPSLP-Vol-17-Supplement-1-2015-lores#24) to the *Journal of Clinical Practice in Speech-Language Pathology*. SPA also has on its website an excellent self-guided-learning Ethics Education Package, and templates for considering ethical dilemmas using a Principles-Based Reasoning Decision Making Protocol, a Casuistry Approach, an Ethics of Care Approach, and a Narrative Approach. ASHA has Evidence-Based Practice resources (www.asha.org/Research/EBP) that include Evidence maps, as well as Ethics Resources (www.asha.org/Practice/ethics/default) associated with its Code of Ethics, updated in March 2016.

Rules of engagement

Ethical thinking and critical thinking are pivotal in SLP/SLT professional and clinical practice, underpinning E^3BP. In all discussions with families and colleagues, know that there are two main categories of non-evidence-based practice. First, interventions for which the science arguing conclusively *against* them is "in"; and second, interventions that have been inadequately studied, so that anecdotal, testimonial accounts, and perhaps a handful of methodologically weak published studies are all that are currently available. In the second category, however, there should be a theoretically sound, biologically-plausible explanation for *why* an approach *might* work, and a reasoned explanation of *how* it is supposed to work: the therapeutic mechanism associated with the intervention (Clark, 2003).

> "Our knowledge of language development and impairment should put us in a strong position when we write for audiences with receptive language difficulties, or for others who come

> *from a wide range of educational backgrounds. We are used to modifying our spoken language and many of us are experienced in giving verbal explanations or presentations to clients and carers."*
> Rosemarie Hayhow, in Dobinson and Wren, 2013, p. 207

In addressing ethical dilemmas, whether verbally or in writing, argue your position logically, in language that consumers and professionals can comprehend, ensuring that you have a close understanding of the science involved. Know that real-life ethical dilemmas are rarely textbook cases in which a "right" way must be discerned from a "wrong" way. Sometimes resolving an ethical dilemma requires identification of the least-worst course of action, because all of the options entail risks of some form. Avoid inflicting *ad hominem* attacks, and deflect them if they come your way (there is a skill in that, and it can be learned), playing the argument and not the person or the profession, and keeping the client's welfare to the forefront – always.

Epilogue

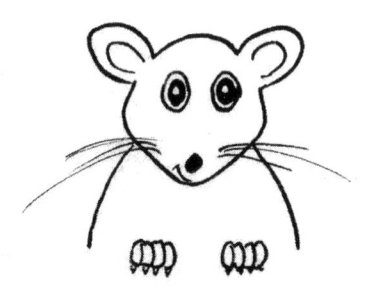

STIRRING THE POSSUM
"To liven things up, create a disturbance, raise issues that others wish left dormant"
G.A. Wilkes, A Dictionary of Australian Colloquialisms

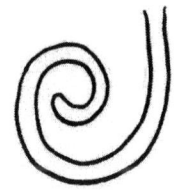

Helen Rippon

As a joint venture, *Making Sense of Interventions for Children's Developmental Disorders* represents two years of camaraderie, backgrounding, and steady collaborative writing. It involved heavy lifting at times, defying the sheer magnitude of the task, and contending with the dreary particulars of unconvincing but widely-adopted theories and methodologies, which we cover in about half of this book. Dissecting the pseudoscientific interventions, and their tangible and potential impacts on clients, colleagues, and the body of knowledge was truly disheartening. By contrast, the overall experience of co-authorship was thoroughly enjoyable, especially when exploring, discussing and writing about the wealth of practicable, theoretically sound, evidence-based, and promising treatments that occupy the other half, countering the disappointing dross.

We became adept at lifting each other's spirits through the trying patches – when our preference would have been to read about interesting research, and new or confirming evidence, in the field of intervention for children's developmental disorders – with the solid support of our families, friends and colleagues. There has also been a stream of encouragement from a globally scattered and delightful Twitter-following of academic, education and health professionals. There are naysayers and voluble CAM promoters among them, but the collegial stalwarts recommend readings; offer opinions, ideas, information, and links; reply, argue, like, re-tweet, and make us laugh; boldly stirring the possum, and urging us on via the book's *ongoing* Twitter handle, @TxChoices.

@TxChoices

Tx or T_x is medical shorthand for "treatment". We intended "treatment *choices*" to signpost that parents, clinicians, and educators must *choose* from various options, including watchful waiting, when considering clinical and educational interventions for children with the disorders we have discussed: ASD, cerebral palsy, communication disorders, dysphagia, emotional difficulties, ID, literacy difficulties, sensory impairments, specific learning disability, and more. Of course, T_x for *treatment* is different from TX for *Texas* – which the scope of our project occasionally felt bigger than – or T-X for *The-Terminatrix*[1], the shapeshifting personification of the fate that we fantasize will befall opportunity-time-and-money-sucking, hope-wasting, fad interventions: termination.

Where are they now?

Generally, fads persist, or go away and re-emerge as variations of themselves, but the idea of their ceasing is not entirely fantasy. Some, like Nullifire fire-resistant-paint inventor Wynford Dore's Dyslexia Dyspraxia Attention Treatment (DDAT), redubbed The Dore Program, *did* terminate. The Dore Achievement Centres empire, across Australia, NZ, the UK and US, bloomed around futile physical exercises purported to cure a fictional disorder called CDD (cerebellar developmental delay), supposedly stimulating the cerebellum and accelerating its development. The Dore Program enterprise proved less fireproof than its namesake's paint, and was bankrupted in 2009, with Professors Dorothy Bishop (Bishop, 2007; and see www.slideshare.net/deevybishop/the-dore-programme-evaluation), Max Coltheart, Maggie Snowling (see

---

[1] The-Terminatrix (T-X) is a gynoid (of female appearance) antagonist in *Terminator 3: Rise of the Machines*. The T-X is designed to not only terminate humans but also rogue Terminators reprogrammed by the Resistance, as "anti-terminator terminators".

www.abc.net.au/4corners/content/2007/s1997916.htm) and other scientists (e.g., Stephenson & Wheldall, 2006) effectively wielding the flamethrowers. This termination occurred only after incalculable hours, opportunities and funds were wasted by parents lured to a "revolutionary drug-free dyslexia remedy...hailed a wonder cure by experts". We won't say that he was *sent* to Coventry; just that Mr Dore's education-related activities seem now to be limited to being owner-director of Brigade Clothing Ltd, a Coventry-based schoolwear manufacturing company. Alas, the Dore Program's legacy lingers; for example, www.doreusa.com delivers it to over 60 US schools, with new owners, DOREctors and Partnership AmbassaDOREs (so called), and Learning Breakthrough™ (www.learningbreakthrough.com) the "core therapy" used by Dore is still coining it in.

Other pseudoscience profiteers who have emerged from the flames, to operate shamelessly in fields where they were once roundly condemned and brought to book, include the de-registered, discredited, and currently US-based Andrew Wakefield whose lethal anti-vaccination crusade continues unabated. The fitfully updated website www.gillianmckeith.com scarcely hints that Gillian McKeith enterprises remain operational, but her Facebook page and 42,000-follower Instagram account suggest that she has a profitable business around nutrition advice (which she is still unqualified to dispense), book sales, TV series (in Portugal at the time of writing) and the joys of detox, colonic irrigation, Goji Berries, Raw Shelled Hemp Seeds, and Gold of Pleasure Oil. Reports of FC's demise were premature, and Facilitated Communication continues to flourish in its own name and more latterly the Rapid Prompting Method, Soma® RPM, and Supported Typing, and to fool and harm the unwary.

Keep up the good work

As systematic Sagittarians and Arians (see page 99 for unbelievable proof), issuing report cards, we would stack the reputable interventions neatly, and rate them according to their levels of evidence (Dollaghan, 2007), writing in their comments sections, "keep up the good work". In the process, we would ask an important, and carefully framed question about each clinical or educational intervention, namely: "What is the level of evidence (if any) for XYZ?" rather than, "Is XYZ an evidence-based practice?".

Could try harder

In the next pile would be approaches that have a degree of face validity and show some promise, but that are not yet supported by sufficient quality evidence, and await initial, or further and more searching, *independent* evaluation. In their comments we would pen, "could try harder".

Could try harder

Animal Assisted Intervention	PODD
Autism Seminars for Families	PECS™
Brainology® (Growth Mind-set)	PRISM
Camphill	Positive Behaviour Support
Circle Time	RIP IT UP Reading©
Controlled Crying	SCERTS®
DIR®, DIRFloortime®	Schufried CogniPlus and NeuroMite training
Early Bird, Early Bird Plus	Social Stories™
LAMP	Social Thinking®
LEAP	SOS Feeding Solutions
Lindamood-Bell®	Speech Buddies™
Low FODMAP Diet for ASD	STAR Feeding Therapy
MindsetMaker™ (Growth Mind-set)	Talking Mats
Multisensory Approach (to CAS)	TEACCH®
Neurofeedback	The Hanen Programs® More than Words
Non-speech Oral Movements (NSOM)	Triple-P Positive Parenting
Orton-Gillingham / Multi-Sensory Structured Language Program	Tuning into Kids
PROMPT©	Video Modelling

No convincing evidence

Finally, there would be the possibly irredeemable "no research support" heap, destined for the shredder, of our first-170-or-so approaches whose developers appear to make no effort to produce real scientific evidence, because they are doing nicely, thank you very much, without it; or they have no capacity to produce it; or they cling doggedly to highly a contested line that their "evidence" and testimonials are sufficient "proof" and robust evidence to the contrary can be conveniently dismissed or ignored.

Is a "fad" a craze, passing phase, practice or interest followed for a time with exaggerated zeal? If it is, some pseudoscientific theories and treatments transcend fad status by their very persistence in the face of critical scientific scrutiny, and sometimes, bad press. Sadly, some of them have a firm foothold in mainstream clinical practice and education. Here they are.

Epilogue

No convincing evidence

ACNlatitudes	Dynamic Baby Gymnastics
Acupressure	Dyslexie
Acupuncture	Epsom Salts Baths
Affinity Therapy; Disney Therapy	Etalon: Anna Deeter
Alkaline diet	Facilitated Communication
Anthroposophic Medicine	FAILSAFE eating
Anthroposophic Therapeutic Speech	Fast ForWord™
Apraxia Speaks Speech Diet	Feingold Food Program
Aromatherapy	Feuerstein Instrumental Enrichment
Arrowsmith Program™	ForBrain® Bone Conduction Headset
Aston Patterning	GAPS Nutritional Protocol
Auditory Integration Treatments	GemIIni™
Baby Sign Language	GF (gluten free) diet for ASD
Balance 360 Clean Eating Nutrition	GFCF diet for ASD
Balanced Literacy	Glenn Doman™ Method
Beckman Oral Motor	Gut and Physiology Diet
Behavioural Optometry	Gut and Psychology Diet
Berard AIT Method	HEGL/Heguru™
Bioindividual Nutrition®	Hellerwork® Structural Integration
Bleach Therapy	Higashi School Daily Life
Body Ecology Diet (BED); Kefir	Hippotherapy
Body Work	Holding Therapy
Boot Camp	Homeopathic Vaccination
Brain Balance®	Homeopathy
BrainGym®	HOP Baby
Brainwork	Horseboy Method
Brainy Baby®	Hyperbaric Oxygen Therapy (HBOT)
Brainy Child	iLs Integrated Listening Systems
Brushing and Icing	Interactive Metronome®
Candida (Cleanse) Diet	Intrinsic Touch Therapy
CEASE Therapy	Irlen® Lenses
Cellfield™	Johansen Individualized Auditory Stimulation
CF (Casein free) Diet for ASD	Jones Geniuses Accelerated Education
Chelation	Juice Plus+®
Chirophonetics	Kill Your Lisp
Chiropractic	Kill Your Stutter
Concept Mapping (CO-OP)	Kinesio Taping for Oral Motor Issues
Cogmed Working Memory Training	Kinesiology
Craniosacral Therapy/Craniosacral Osteopathy	KipOnline
Crispiani Method	Learning Breakthrough™
Cry it Out	Learning Styles Theory
Davis Dyslexia Program	LearningRx
Defeat Autism Now Diet	Left-brain-right-brain Dominance Theory
Discrete Video Modelling	Løvaas Method
Dolphin Therapy	Lupron Therapy
Dore Program	Magnetic Pulse Therapy

Continued...

Interventions for Children with Developmental Disorders

Marte Meo	Sensory Rooms
Master Mineral Solution	Shichida™
McGuire Program	Smacking
MDT Method: Elad Vashdi	Son-Rise Program®
Mercury Learning Systems	Sound Therapy
Miracle Mineral Solution (MMS)	Specific Carbohydrate Diet
MNRI®	Speech Diet
Multi-cueing (aka Searchlights)	Spiritual Nutrition
Multiple Intelligences	Stem Cell Therapy (for ASD)
Multisensory Listening Therapy for ASD	Sunflower Method
Myofascial Release	Supported Typing
Naturopathy	Switch On Reading
Neurolinguistic Programming™	TalkTools® - for SSD
NS-OMT for SSD	Testosterone Regulation
NOW!® Programs	The Children of the Rainbow
NutriiVeda	The Children's Reflexology Programme
Opioid Excess Theory	The Listening Program®
Oral Placement Therapy for SSD	The Three-Cuing System
Osteopathy	Therapeutic Listening™
Play Project	Therapeutic Speech Massage
Polarity Therapy	Therapeutic Touch Therapy
Primary Movement®	Third Brain
Psychodynamic Intervention for ASD	Tomatis®, Solisten®
Psychological Astrology	Trager (Tragerwork)
Psychoneurology	Transcranial Magnetic Stimulation
Pulsed Magnetic Field Therapy	Type to Communicate
Rainbow Diet	Vega Testing (Vega Machine)
Rapid Prompting Method (RPM)	VML Method: Elad Vashdi
RDI™	Vocal Science™
RDIconnect™	WeeHands™
Reading Recovery™	Weighted vests
ReadingWise	Whole Brain Learning
Reflexology	Whole Brain/Brain Based Teaching
Responsive Teaching	Whole Language
Rolfing	Wilson reading System®
Samonas™ Sound Therapy	Wrapping Therapy (Packing Therapy)
Searchlights (aka Multi-cueing)	Xlens
Secretin Injections (for ASD)	Yeast Free Diet
Sensory Diet	Your Baby Can Learn
Sensory Integration Therapy	ZEBR. Reframing Autism

Although the "no research support" list is long, we could easily double it without straying from unscientific interventions that large numbers of clinicians, teachers and parents will try – in a spirit of trust and hope – and even endorse. We trust you will not try any of them: not a one, as they are devoid of scientific support, and as such will fail your sons and daughters, clients, students, you, and anyone who emulates you.

Go on, convince us

As proponents of scientific research (see pages 5–6), scientist-practitioners, and authors we value scholarship, change our minds in response to robust new empirical evidence, and are happy to consider reasoned theoretical shifts. If you feel that "your" intervention for children with developmental disorders – one you administer as a health professional or educator, one you have embraced as helpful for your child or for the children in your classroom or home-school room, or one you promote and benefit from financially – has been put on the "no convincing evidence" list unfairly or in error, please write. When you do, provide no testimonials; and don't tell us that seeing is believing, that it "works for you", or that you "don't know why it works, but it does". Simply send relevant, independent peer-reviewed supporting publications from at least one high-quality (not a Beall's List predatory one; see pages 293–294) journal.

One article in one reputable journal could well see you achieve a place on the "could try harder list". Replication of your findings, reported in journals of good standing, could keep you there, or might earn our, and the scientific community's "keep up the good work" seal! Whether you send equivocal, modest, or good-quality evidence, we will gladly review it and amend any future editions of this book accordingly, mention your positive efforts on our website (CB) and blog (PS), and acknowledge your contribution in social media. We can't say fairer than that.

Gold

As we have outlined, there are many principled but not necessarily glamorous interventions, supported by diverse grades of research evidence, for parents and professionals to choose from when we join forces to address children's treatment needs. We have also stressed that ethical, properly credentialed, currently up-to-date, mainstream health and education practitioners are uniquely qualified to responsibly guide parents through the sometimes difficult selection process. Such professionals can critically appraise the science behind interventions, identifying and avoiding pseudoscientific false promises.

At the same time, parents, whether well-versed or naïve in matters of science, are entitled to interrogate we professionals' preferences, negotiate with us, and guide us towards reflecting upon and reviewing our clinical and teaching practices and perspectives. Trusting in each other's capacities, and holding to the principle that the best hope for children's progress lies in "the science" and good communication between parties, we can choose optimal approaches and modify treatment plans rationally without jumping onto some faddy bandwagon in response to each child's needs and progress. Equally, when we collaborate and hear each other, we are in a strong position to resist aggressive marketing and to say "no" to interventions that lack scientific support. Mainstream education has an opportunity here to show leadership in eschewing charismatic salesfolk and their shiny, new, untested neurofandangles, in favour of the hard yards of painstakingly engaging with scientifically validated approaches.

We hope that *Making Sense of Interventions for Children's Developmental Disorders* will prove to be a good little guide in this endeavour, and that you will find your intervention gold.

References

Aburahma, S.K., Khader, Y.S., Alzoubi, K., & Sawalha, N. (2010). Complementary and alternative medicine use in a pediatric neurology clinic. *Complementary Therapies in Clinical Practice, 16(3)*, 117–120.

Adams, D., Dagenais, S., Clifford, T., Baydala, L., King, W.J., Hervas-Malo, M. Moher, D., & Vohra, S. (2013). Complementary and Alternative Medicine use by pediatric specialty outpatients. *Pediatrics, 131(2)*, 225–232.

Afkari, S. (2007). Measuring frequency of spontaneous swallowing. *Australasian Journal of Physical and Engineering Sciences in Medicine, 30(4)*, 313–317.

Aisen, M.L., Kerkovich, D., Mast, J., Mulroy, S., Wren, T.A., Kay, R.M., & Rethlefsen, S.A. (2011). Cerebral palsy: Clinical care and neurological rehabilitation. *The Lancet Neurology, 10(9)*, 844–852.

Altunc, U., Pittler, M.H., & Ernst, E. (2007). Homeopathy for childhood and adolescence ailments: Systematic review of randomized clinical trials. *Mayo Clinic Proceedings, 82(1)*, 69–75.

Alvesson, M. & Spicer, A. (2016). (Un) Conditional surrender? Why do professionals willingly comply with managerialism? *Journal of Organizational Change Management, 29(1)*, 29–45.

American Academy of Pediatrics (2009). *AAP Policy: Vision Problems Do Not Cause Dyslexia*. Retrieved 6 January 2016 from www.healthychildren.org/English/news/Pages/AAP-Policy-Vision-Problems-Do-Not-Cause-Dyslexia.aspx

American Academy of Pediatrics (2011, 2012). *Policy Statement: Sensory Integration Therapies for Children with Developmental and Behavioral Disorders*. Retrieved 13 May 2016 from http://pediatrics.aappublications.org/content/129/6/1186

American Psychiatric Association. (2013). *Diagnostic and Statistical Manual of Mental Disorders* (5th ed.) (DSM-5®). Washington, D.C.: Author.

Aras, M.H., Göregen, M., Güngörmüş, M., & Akgül, H.M. (2010). Comparison of diode laser and Er:YAG lasers in the treatment of ankyloglossia. *Photomedicine and Laser Surgery, 28(2)*, 173–177.

Araújo, D.D.F. & Almondes, K.M.D. (2014). Sleep and cognitive performance in children and pre-adolescents: A review. *Biological Rhythm Research, 45(2)*, 193–207.

ASHA (1995). *Facilitated Communication* [Position Statement]. Retrieved 22 January 2016 from www.asha.org/policy

American Academy of Pediatrics, Attention Deficit Sub-Committee (2011). ADHD: Practice guideline for the diagnosis, evaluation, and treatment of attention-deficit/hyperactivity disorder in children and adolescents. *Pediatrics, 28(5)*.

ASHA (2004). Auditory integration training [Technical Report]. Available from http://www.asha.org/policy

ASHA (2007a). *Childhood Apraxia of Speech* [Technical Report]. Retrieved 26 December, 2015 from www.asha.org/docs/html/TR2007-00278.html

ASHA (2007b). *Childhood Apraxia of Speech* [Position Statement]. Retrieved 26 December 2015 from www.asha.org/policy

Arns, M., Heinrich, H., & Strehl, U. (2014). Evaluation of neurofeedback in ADHD: The long and winding road. *Biological Psychology, 95*, 108–115.

Arrowsmith-Young, B. (2013). *The Woman Who Changed Her Brain: How I Left My Learning Disability Behind and Other Stories of Cognitive Transformation.* New York: Free Press.

Attfield, R. (2015). Typing to communicate—Overcoming stigma. *International Communication Project.* Retrieved 2 April 2016 from www.internationalcommunicationproject.com/profile/typing-to-communicate-overcoming-stigma/

Auerbach, D. (2015). Facilitated Communication is a cult that won't die. www.slate.com/articles/health_and_science/medical_examiner/2015/11/facilitated_communication_pseudoscience_harms_people_with_disabilities.html

Augustine, M.B., Swift, K.M., Harris, S.R., Anderson, E.J., & Hand, R.K. (2016). Integrative medicine: Education, perceived knowledge, attitudes, and practice among Academy of Nutrition and Dietetics Members. *Journal of the Academy of Nutrition and Dietetics, 116(2)*, 319–329.

Australian Association for Infant Mental Health (2013). *Controlled Crying. Position Paper No. 1.* Retrieved 9 May 2016 from https://aaimhi.sslsvc.com/key-issues/position-statements-and-guidelines/AAIMHI-Position-paper-1-Controlled-crying.pdf

Australian Childhood Foundation (2010). *Making Space for Learning.* Ringwood: Australian Childhood Foundation. www.childhood.org.au

Australian Health Practitioner Regulation Agency (2014). *Guidelines for Advertising Regulated Health Services.* Retrieved 19 July 2016 from www.ahpra.gov.au/documents/default.aspx?record=WD14%2F13127&dbid=AP&chksum=vHkDZCBUPtLJ%2Fx1D8bR85A%3D%3D.

Australian Institute of Health and Welfare: Chrisopoulos, S., Harford, J.E. & Ellershaw, A. (2016). *Oral Health and Dental Care in Australia: Key Facts and Figures 2015.* Cat. no. DEN 229. Canberra: AIHW.

Ayres, A.J. (1972). *Sensory Integration and Learning Disorders.* Los Angeles, CA: Western Psychological Services.

Ayres, A.J. & Robbins, J. (2005). *Sensory Integration and the Child: Understanding Hidden Sensory Challenges.* Torrance, CA: Western Psychological Services.

BDA: The Association of UK Dietitians (2014). Dietitian, Nutritionist, Nutritional Therapist or Diet Expert? A comprehensive guide to roles and functions. Retrieved 26 January 2016 from www.bda.uk.com/about/about_bda/dietitians

BMJ (2016, May). *BMJ Confidential.* Simon Singh: Challenging pseudoscience. *353: i2776.*

Baddeley, A.D. & Hitch, G. (1974). Working memory. *Psychology of Learning and Motivation, (8)*, 47–89.

Bailey, J.S. & Burch, M. (2016). *Ethics for Behavior Analysts*, 3rd edition. New York, NY: Routledge.

Bailey, R.L., Parette, H.P., Stoner, J.B., Angell, M.E., & Carroll, K. (2006). Family members' perceptions of augmentative and alternative communication device use. *Language, Speech, and Hearing Services in Schools, 37(1)*, 50–60.

Baker, E. (2012). Optimal intervention intensity in speech-language pathology. *International Journal of Speech-Language Pathology, 14(5)*, 478–485.

Baldwin, S. (2011). Myth busting: How reading is taught in a Waldorf school. Retrieved 8 January 2016, from www.blog.bellalunatoys.com/2011/waldorf-reading.html

Barbaro, J. & Dissanayake, C. (2009). Autism spectrum disorders in infancy and toddlerhood: A review of the evidence on early signs, early identification tools, and early diagnosis. *Journal of Developmental & Behavioral Pediatrics, 30(5)*, 447–459.

Barkley, R.A. (2014). Sluggish cognitive tempo (concentration deficit disorder?): Current status, future directions, and a plea to change the name. *Journal of Abnormal Child Psychology, 42(1)*, 117–125.

Barkley, R.A. (2015). Concentration deficit disorder (sluggish cognitive tempo). In *Attention Deficit Hyperactivity Disorder: A Handbook for Diagnosis and Treatment* (pp. 267–313). New York: Guilford Press.

Barnett, W.S. (2011). Effectiveness of early educational intervention. *Science, 333(6045)*, 975–978.

Bartick, M. & Smith, L.J. (2014). Speaking out on safe sleep: Evidence-based infant sleep recommendations. *Breastfeeding Medicine, 9(9)*, 417–422.

Barton, E.E., Reichow, B., Schnitz, A., Smith, I.C., & Sherlock, D. (2015). A systematic review of sensory-based treatments for children with disabilities. *Research in Developmental Disabilities, 37*, 64–80.

Bateson, G. (1972). *Steps to an Ecology of Mind*. Chicago, IL: Chicago University Press.

Baydala, L. & Wikman, E. (2001). The efficacy of neurofeedback in the management of children with attention deficit/hyperactivity disorder. *Paediatrics & Child Health, 6(7)*, 451.

Beauchamp, R.A., Willis, T.M., Betz, T.G., Villanacci, J., Leiker, R.D., Rozin, L., Brown, M.J., Homa, D.M., Dignam, T.A., & Morta, T. (2006). Deaths associated with hypocalcemia from chelation therapy – Texas, Pennsylvania, and Oregon, 2003–2005. *Journal of the American Medical Association, 295*, 2131–2133.

Becker, S.P. (2013). Topical review: Sluggish cognitive tempo: Research findings and relevance for pediatric psychology. *Journal of Pediatric Psychology, 38(10)*, 1051–1057.

Beebe, D.W. (2011). Cognitive, behavioral, and functional consequences of inadequate sleep in children and adolescents. *Pediatric Clinics of North America, 58(3)*, 649–665.

Bell, V., Bishop, D.V., & Przybylski, A.K. (2015). Editorial: The debate over digital technology and young people. Needs less shock and more substance. *BMJ, 351*, h3064.

Benson, J.D., Parke, C.S., Gannon, C., & Muñoz, D. (2013). A retrospective analysis of the sequential oral sensory feeding approach in children with feeding difficulties. *Journal of Occupational Therapy, Schools, & Early Intervention, 6(4),* 289–300.

Beukelman, D.R. & Mirenda, P. (2005). *Augmentative and Alternative Communication: Supporting Children and Adults with Complex Communication Needs.* Baltimore, Paul H. Brookes.

Bellini, S. & Akullian, J. (2007). A meta-analysis of video modeling and video self-modeling interventions for children and adolescents with autism spectrum disorders. *Exceptional Children, 73(3),* 264–287.

Benedetti, F., Mayberg, H S., Wager, T.D., Stohler, C.S., & Zubieta, J.K. (2005). Neurobiological mechanisms of the placebo effect. *The Journal of Neuroscience, 25(45),* 10390-10402.

Bennett-Levy, J., Richards, D.A., Farrand, P., Christensen, H., Griffiths, K.M., Kavanagh, D.J., ... & Proudfoot, J. (2010). Low intensity CBT interventions: A revolution in mental health care. *Low Intensity CBT Interventions, 13,* 3–18.

Bergin, T. (2013). *The Evidence Enigma: Correctional Boot Camps and other Failures in Evidence-based Policymaking.* Surrey: Ashgate Publishing.

Biesiekierski, J.R., Peters, S.L., Newnham, E.D., Rosella, O., Muir, J.G., & Gibson, P.R. (2013). No effects of gluten in patients with self-reported non-celiac gluten sensitivity after dietary reduction of fermentable, poorly absorbed, short-chain carbohydrates. *Gastroenterology, 145(2),* 320–328.

Biesta, G. (2007). Why "what works" won't work: Evidence-based practice and the democratic deficit in educational research. *Educational Theory, 57(1),* 1–22.

Biklen, D. (1990). Communication unbound. Autism and praxis. *Harvard Education Review, 60(3),* 291–314.

Biklen, D.P. (1993). *Communication Unbound: How Facilitated Communication is Challenging Traditional Views of Autism and Ability/Disability.* New York, NY: Teachers College Press.

Biklen, D. & Burke, J. (2006). Presuming competence. *Equity & Excellence in Education, 39(2),* 166–175.

Bishop, D.V.M. (2007). Curing dyslexia and attention-deficit hyperactivity disorder by training motor co-ordination: Miracle or myth? *Journal of Paediatrics and Child Health, 43(10),* 653–655.

Bishop, D.V.M. (2012, January 23). BishopBlog: Psychoanalytic treatment for autism: Interviews with French analysts [Web log post]. Retrieved January 23, 2016 from www.deevybee.blogspot.co.uk/2012/01/psychoanalytic-treatment-for-autism.html

Bishop, D.V.M (2013). Research review: Emanuel Miller Memorial Lecture 2012 – Neuroscientific studies of intervention for language impairment in children: Interpretive and methodological problems. *Journal of Child Psychology & Psychiatry, 54(3),* 247–259.

Bishop, D.V.M. (2014). Ten questions about terminology for children with unexplained language problems, *International Journal of Language & Communication Disorders, 49(4),* 381–415.

Bishop, D.V.M., Snowling, M.J., Thompson, P.A., & Greenhalgh, T., & CATALISE consortium (2016). CATALISE: A multinational and multidisciplinary Delphi consensus study identifying language impairments in children. *PLoS ONE, 11(7)*, e0158753. DOI:10.1371/journal.pone.0158753

Bishop, D.V.M, Whitehouse, A., Watt, H., & Line, E. (2008). Autism and diagnostic substitution: Evidence from a study of adults with a history of developmental language disorder. *Developmental Medicine & Child Neurology, 50(5)*, 341–345.

Bitter, J.R. (2013). *Theory and Practice of Family Therapy and Counseling, 2nd edition*. Belmont, CA: Brooks Cole: Cengage Learning.

Bitter, J.R. (2015). Counselling children and their families experiencing SSD: systemic interventions for speech-language professionals. In C. Bowen, *Children's Speech Sound Disorders, 2nd edition* (pp. 127–132). Oxford: Wiley-Blackwell.

Blischack, D.M. & Cheek, M. (2001). A lot of work keeping everything controlled: A class research project. *American Journal of Speech-Language Pathology, 10(1)*, 10–16.

Blakemore, S.J. & Choudhury, S. (2006). Development of the adolescent brain: Implications for executive function and social cognition. *Journal of Child Psychology and Psychiatry, 47(3–4)*, 296–312.

Blunden, S.L., Thompson, K.R., & Dawson, D. (2011). Behavioural sleep treatments and night time crying in infants: Challenging the status quo. *Sleep Medicine Reviews, 15(5)*, 327–334.

Blyton, E. (1951). Famous Five 10: *Five on a Hike Together*. London UK: Hodder Children's Books.

Bochner, S. (1980). Sensory integration therapy and learning disabilities: A critique. *Australian Occupational Therapy Journal, 27(3)*, 125–137.

Bowen, C. (1998). *Speech-language-therapy dot com*. Retrieved 8 January 2016 from www.speech-language-therapy.com

Bowen, C. (2015). *Children's Speech Sound Disorders, 2nd edition*. Oxford: Wiley-Blackwell.

Boynton, J. (2012). Facilitated Communication—what harm it can do: Confessions of a former facilitator. *Evidence-based Communication Assessment and Intervention, 6(1)*, 3–13.

Bradford, D. & Wan, W-Y. (2015). *Reading Recovery: A Sector-Wide Analysis*. Sydney: Centre for Education Statistics and Evaluation.

Bradshaw, J. (2013). The use of augmentative and alternative communication apps for the iPad, iPod and iPhone: An overview of recent developments. *Tizard Learning Disability Review, 18(1)*, 31–37.

Bradshaw, J., Steiner, A.M., Gengoux, G., & Koegel, L.K. (2015). Feasibility and effectiveness of very early intervention for infants at-risk for autism spectrum disorder: A systematic review. *Journal of Autism and Developmental Disorders, 45(3)*, 778–794.

Brady, N.C., Fleming, K., Thiemann-Bourque, K., Olswang, L., Dowden, P., Saunders, M.D., & Marquis, J. (2012). Development of the Communication Complexity Scale. *American Journal of Speech-Language Pathology, 21(1)*, 16–28.

Brainex Corporation (2015a). *About the Arrowsmith Program*. Retrieved 6 January 2016 from www.arrowsmithschool.org/arrowsmithprogram/

Brainex Corporation (2015b). Arrowsmith Program Research Summary Document, Toronto, ON: Author. Retrieved 6 January 2016 from www.arrowsmithschool.org/arrowsmithprogram-background/pdf/Research%20Summary.pdf

Brakes, P. & Williamson, C. (2007). Dolphin assisted therapy: Can you put your faith in DAT? *Whale and Dolphin Conservation Society, 21*.

Brignell, A., Song, H., Zhu, J., Suo, C., Lu, D., & Morgan, A.T. (2016). Communication intervention for autism spectrum disorders in minimally verbal children. *Cochrane Database of Systematic Reviews* 2016, Issue 8. Art. No.: CD012324. DOI: 10.1002/14651858.CD012324

Brinkmann, S., Reilly, S., & Meara, J.G. (2004). Management of tongue-tie in children: A survey of paediatric surgeons in Australia. *Journal of Paediatric Child Health, 40(11)*, 600–605.

Brunner, M., Hemsley, B., Palmer, S., Dann, S., & Togher, L. (2015). Review of the literature on the use of social media by people with traumatic brain injury (TBI). *Disability and Rehabilitation, 37(17)*, 1511–1521.

Buckingham, J., Wheldall, K., & Beaman-Wheldall, R. (2013). Why Jaydon can't read. The triumph of ideology over evidence in teaching reading. *Policy*, 29(3), 21–32.

Buie, T. (2013). The relationship of autism and gluten. *Clinical Therapeutics, 35(5)*, 578–583.

Burnett, N. & Thorsborne, M. (2015). *Restorative Practice and Special Needs*. London, UK: Jessica Kingsley.

Buyck, I. & Wiersema, J.R. (2014). Resting electroencephalogram in attention deficit hyperactivity disorder: Developmental course and diagnostic value. *Psychiatry Research, 216(3)*, 391–397.

Buryk, M., Bloom, D., & Shope, T. (2011). Efficacy of neonatal release of ankyloglossia: A randomized trial. *Pediatrics, 128(2)*, 280–288.

Campbell-McBride, N. (2010). *Gut and Psychology Syndrome. Natural Treatment of Autism, ADD, ADHD, Dyslexia, Dyspraxia, Depression and Schizophrenia, 2nd edition*. White River Junction, VT: Medinform Publishing.

Cannon, G. & Leitzmann, C. (2016). *New Nutrition Science*. Oxford: Wiley-Blackwell.

Carey, B., O'Brian, S., Lowe, R., & Onslow, M. (2014). Webcam delivery of the Camperdown Program for adolescents who stutter: A Phase II trial. *Language, Speech, and Services in Schools, 45(4)*, 314–324.

Carr, D. & Felce, J. (2007). The effects of PECS™ teaching to phase III on the communicative interactions between children with autism and their teachers. *Journal of Autism and Developmental Disorders, 37*, 724–737.

Cefai, C., Ferrario, E., Cavioni, V., Carter, A., & Grech, T. (2014). Circle time for social and emotional learning in primary school. *Pastoral Care in Education, 32(2)*, 116–130.

Cellfield Pty Ltd. (2015). Frequently asked questions, Southport, QLD, Author. Retrieved 6 January 2016 from www.cellfield.com/faqs.php

Chabon, S., Morris, J., & Lemoncello, R. (2011). Ethical deliberation: A foundation for evidence-based practice. *Seminars in Speech and Language, 32(4),* 298–308.

Chacko, A., Feirsen, N., Bedard, A.C., Marks, D., Uderman, J.Z., & Chimiklis, A. (2013). Cogmed working memory training for youth with ADHD: A closer examination of efficacy utilizing evidence-based criteria. *Journal of Clinical Child & Adolescent Psychology, 42(6),* 769–783.

Chan, J. & Nankervis, K. (2014). Stolen voices: Facilitated communication is an abuse of human rights. *Evidence-Based Communication Assessment and Intervention, 8(3),* 151–156.

Chapman, J.W., Tunmer, W.E., & Prochnow, J.E. (2001). Does success in the Reading Recovery program depend on developing proficiency in phonological processing skills? A longitudinal study in a whole language instructional context, *Scientific Studies in Reading, 5,* 141–17.

Cheung, G., Trembath, D., Arciuli, J., & Togher L. (2013). The impact of workplace factors on evidence-based speech-language pathology practice for children with autism spectrum disorders. *International Journal of Speech-Language Pathology, 15(4),* 396–406.

Christon, L.M., Mackintosh, V.H., & Myers, B.J. (2013). Use of complementary and alternative medicine (CAM) treatments by parents of children with autism spectrum disorders. *Research in Autism Spectrum Disorders, 7(3),* 466–474.

Corbett, B.A., Key, A.P., Qualls, L., Fecteau, S., Newsom, C., Coke, C., & Yoder, P. (2016). Improvement in social competence using a randomized trial of a theatre intervention for children with autism spectrum disorder. *Journal of Autism and Developmental Disorders, 46(2),* 658–672.

Cross, M. (2011). *Children with Social, Emotional, and Behavioural Difficulties and Communication Problems: There is Always a Reason, 2nd edition.* London: Jessica Kingsley.

Cichero, J.A.Y. (2016), Introducing solid foods using baby-led weaning vs. spoon-feeding: A focus on oral development, nutrient intake and quality of research to bring balance to the debate. *Nutrition Bulletin, 41(1),* 72–77.

Cırık, V. & Efe, E. (2015). The use of complementary and alternative medicine by children. *Journal of Family Medicine & Community Health, 2(2),* 1031–1035.

Clark, H.M. (2003). Neuromuscular treatments for speech and swallowing: A tutorial. *American Journal of Speech-Language Pathology, 12(4),* 400–415.

Clarke, G., Debar, L., Lynch, F., Powell, J., Gale, J., O'Connor, E., ... & Hertert, S. (2005). A randomized effectiveness trial of brief cognitive-behavioral therapy for depressed adolescents receiving antidepressant medication. *Journal of the American Academy of Child & Adolescent Psychiatry, 44(9),* 888–898.

Clay, M.M. (1993). *Reading Recovery: A Guidebook for Teachers in Training.* Portsmouth, NH: Heinemann.

Cogo-Moreira, H., Andriolo, R.B., Yazigi, L., Ploubidis, G.B., Brandão de Ávila, C.R., & Mari, J.J. (2012). Music education for improving reading skills in children and adolescents with dyslexia. *Cochrane Database of Systematic Reviews* Issue 8. Art. No.: CD009133.

Cohen, N.J. (2001). *Language Impairment and Psychopathology in Infants, Children, and Adolescents.* Thousand Oaks, CA: Sage Publications.

Commissioner for Children and Young People (2007). *Creating Calmer Classrooms.* Melbourne: Child Safety Commissioner. www.ccyp.vic.gov.au

Communication Matters (2013). Shining a light on Augmentative and Alternative Communication. Retrieved 10 July 2016 from www.communicationmatters.org.uk/shining-a-light-on-aac

Cortese, S., Ferrin, M., Brandeis, D., Buitelaar, J., Daley, D., Dittmann, R. W., ... & Zuddas, A. (2015). Cognitive training for attention-deficit/hyperactivity disorder: Meta-analysis of clinical and neuropsychological outcomes from randomized controlled trials. *Journal of the American Academy of Child & Adolescent Psychiatry, 54(3),* 164–174.

Cortese, S., Ferrin, M., Brandeis, D., Holtmann, M., Aggensteiner, P., Daley, D., ... & Sonuga-Barke, E. J. (2016). Neurofeedback for attention-deficit/hyperactivity disorder: Meta-Analysis of clinical and neuropsychological outcomes from randomized controlled trials. *Journal of the American Academy of Child & Adolescent Psychiatry, 55(6),* 444–455.

Cook, H. (2015). Tighter management of restraints used in schools. The Age. Retrieved July 11 2016 from www.theage.com.au/victoria/tighter-management-of-restraints-used-in-schools-20150903-gjemo1.html

Coyne, J.C. & Kwakkenbos, L. (2013). Triple P-Positive Parenting programs: The folly of basing social policy on underpowered flawed studies. *BMC Medicine, 11(1),* 1.

Cress, C.J. & Marvin, C.A. (2003) Common questions about AAC services in early intervention. *Augmentative and Alternative Communication, 19(4),* 254–272.

Crispiani, P. & Palmieri, E. (2015). Improving the fluidity of whole word reading with a dynamic coordinated movement approach. *Asia Pacific Journal of Developmental Differences, 2(2),* 158–183.

Crooke, P.J. & Olswang, L.B. (2015). Practice-based research: Another pathway for closing the research–practice gap. *Journal of Speech, Language, and Hearing Research, 58(6),* S1871–S1882.

Crossley, R. & Remington-Gurney, J. (1992). Getting the words out: Facilitated communication training. *Topics in Language Disorders, 12(4),* 29–45.

Davis, T.N., O'Reilly, M., Kang, S., Rispoli, M., Sigafoos, J., Lancioni, G., Copeland, D., Attai, S., & Mulloy, A. (2013). Chelation treatment for autism spectrum disorders: A systematic review. *Research in Autism Spectrum Disorders, 7(1),* 49–55.

Dawson, G., Rogers, S., Munson, J., Smith, M., Winter, J., Greenson, J., Donaldson A., & Varley J. (2010). Randomized, controlled trial of an intervention for toddlers with autism: The Early Start Denver Model. *Pediatrics, 125(1),* e17–23.

De Been, I. & Beijer, M. (2014). The influence of office type on satisfaction and perceived productivity support. *Journal of Facilities Management, 12(2),* 142–157.

de Jager, T. & du Toit, P. (2009). Beginner teacher professional development: An action research and Whole Brain learning approach to peer mentoring. Retrieved June 18, 2016 from www.academia.edu

de Sonneville-Koedoot, C., Stolk, E., Rietveld, T., & Franken, M-C. (2015) Direct versus indirect treatment for preschool children who stutter: The RESTART randomized trial. PLoS ONE *10(7)*, e0133758. DOI:10.1371/journal.pone.013375

de Wit, E., Visser-Bochane, M.I., Steenbergen, B., van Dijk, P., van der Schans, C.P., & Luinge, M.R. (2016). Characteristics of auditory processing disorders: A systematic review. *Journal of Speech, Language, and Hearing Research, 59(2)*, 384–413.

Dekker-Lee, S., Howard-Jones, N.C., & Jolles, P. (2012). Neuromyths in education: Prevalence and predictors of misconceptions among teachers. *Frontiers in Psychology, 18*, http://dx.doi.org/10.3389/fpsyg.2012.00429

Delaney, A.L. (2015). Special considerations for the pediatric population relating to a swallow screen versus clinical swallow or instrumental evaluation, *SIG 13 Perspectives on Swallowing and Swallowing Disorders (Dysphagia), 24(1)*, 155–161.

Des Roches Rosa, S., Myers, J.B., Ditz, L., Willingham, E., & Greenburg, C. (2011). *Thinking Person's Guide to Autism*. Redwood City, CA: Deadwood City Publishing.

Dekker-Lee, S., Howard-Jones, N.C. & Jolles, P. (2012). Neuromyths in education: Prevalence and predictors of misconceptions among teachers. *Frontiers in Psychology, 18*, http://dx.doi.org/10.3389/fpsyg.2012.00429

Delano, M.E. (2007). Video modeling interventions for individuals with autism. *Remedial & Special Education, 28(1)*, 33–42.

DeLoache, J.S., Chiong, C., Sherman, K., Islam, K., Vanderborght, M., Troseth, G.L., & O'Doherty, K. (2010). Do babies learn from baby media? *Psychological Science, 21(11)*, 1570–1574.

De Rubeis, S., He, X., Goldberg, A.P., Poultney, C.S., Samocha, K., Cicek, A.E., Kou, Y. et al. (2014). Synaptic, transcriptional, and chromatin genes disrupted in autism. *Nature, 515 (7526)*, 209–215.

DeStefano, F., Price, C.S., & Weintraub, E. S. (2013). Increasing exposure to antibody-stimulating proteins and polysaccharides in vaccines is not associated with risk of autism. *Journal of Pediatrics, 163(2)*, 561–567.

Dionne, M. & Martini, R. (2011). Floor time play with a child with autism: A single-subject study. *Canadian Journal of Occupational Therapy, 48(3)*, 196–203.

Dicke, T., Elling, J., Schmeck, A., & Leutner, D. (2015). Reducing reality shock: The effects of classroom management skills training on beginning teachers. *Teaching and Teacher Education, 48*, 1–12.

Dockrell, J.E., Ricketts, J., Charman, T., & Lindsay, G. (2014). Exploring writing products in students with language impairments and autism spectrum disorders. *Learning and Instruction, 32*, 81–90.

Dollaghan, C.A. (2007). *The Handbook for Evidence-based Practice in Communication Disorders*. Baltimore, MD: Paul H. Brookes.

Donohoe, C., Topping, K., & Hannah, E. (2012). The impact of an online intervention (Brainology) on the mindset and resiliency of secondary school pupils: A preliminary mixed methods study. *Educational Psychology, 32(5)*, 641–655.

Donvan, J. & Zucker, C. (2016a). *In a Different Key: The Story of Autism.* New York, NY: Penguin Random House.

Donvan, J. & Zucker, C. (2016b). The early history of autism in America. *Smithsonian Magazine,* Retrieved August 5 2016 from http://www.smithsonianmag.com/science-nature/early-history-autism-america-180957684/

Douglas, P.S. & Hill, P.S. (2013). Behavioral sleep interventions in the first six months of life do not improve outcomes for mothers or infants: A systematic review. *Journal of Developmental & Behavioral Pediatrics, 34(7),* 497–507.

Duchan, J F. (2006). How conceptual frameworks influence clinical practice: Evidence from the writings of John Thelwall, a 19th-century speech therapist. *International Journal of Language & Communication Disorders, 41,* 735–744.

Duchan, J.F. (2010). The early years of language, speech, and hearing services in U.S. Schools. *Language, Speech, and Hearing Services in Schools, 41(2),* 152–160.

Duncombe, M.E., Havighurst, S.S., Kehoe, C.E., Holland, K.A., Frankling, E.J., & Stargatt, R. (2014). Comparing an emotion- and a behavior-focused parenting program as part of a multsystemic intervention for child conduct problems. *Journal of Clinical Child & Adolescent Psychology, 45(3),* 1–15.

Durkin, K. & Barber, B. (2002). Not so doomed: Computer game play and positive adolescent development. *Journal of Applied Developmental Psychology, 23(4),* 373–392.

Durkin, K., Boyle, J., Hunter, S., & Conti-Ramsden, G. (2013). Video games for children and adolescents with special educational needs. *Journal of Psychology, 221(2),* 79–89.

Dweck, C.S. (2007). The secret to raising smart kids. *Scientific American Mind, 18(6),* 36–43.

Dye, B.A., Thornton-Evans, G., Li, X., & Iafolla, T.J. (2015). *Dental caries and sealant prevalence in children and adolescents in the United States, 2011–2012. NCHS Data Brief, no 191.* Hyattsville, MD: National Center for Health Statistics.

Dye, B.A., Xianfen, L., & Beltrán-Aguilar, E.D. (2012). *Selected Oral Health Indicators in the United States 2005–2008. NCHS Data Brief, no. 96.* Hyattsville, MD: National Center for Health Statistics, Centers for Disease Control and Prevention.

ESSA (2015). Every Student Succeeds Act of 2015, Pub. L. No. 114-95 § 114 Stat. 1177 (2015–2016).

Edwards, D.K. & Marlise Martin, S. (2011). Protecting children as feeding skills develop. *SIG 13 Perspectives on Swallowing and Swallowing Disorders (Dysphagia), 20(3),* 88–193.

Efron, D., Jarman, F., & Barker, M. (1997). Methylphenidate versus dexamphetamine in children with attention deficit hyperactivity disorder: A double-blind, crossover trial. *Pediatrics, 100(6),* e6–e6.

Einfeld, S.L. & Tonge, B.J. (1996). Population prevalence of psychopathology in children and adolescents with intellectual disability: II Epidemiological findings. *Journal of Intellectual Disability Research, 40,* 99–109.

Eisenberger, N.I. (2012). The pain of social disconnection: Examining the shared neural underpinnings of physical and social pain. *Nature Reviews Neuroscience, 13(6),* 421–434.

Elder, J.H. (2008). The gluten-free, casein-free diet in autism: An overview with clinical implications. *Nutrition in Clinical Practice, 23(6),* 583–588.

Elliott, J.G. & Grigorenko, E.L. (2014). *The Dyslexia Debate.* New York, NY: Cambridge University Press.

Engber, D. (2015). The strange case of Anna Stubblefield. *The New York Times Magazine.* Retrieved 3 April 2016 from http://www.nytimes.com/2015/10/25/magazine/the-strange-case-of-anna-stubblefield.html?_r=0

Ernst, E. (1999). Prevalence of complementary/alternative medicine for children: A systematic review. *European Journal of Pediatrics, 158(1),* 7–11.

Ernst, E. (2015). *A Scientist in Wonderland: A Memoir of Searching for Truth and Finding Trouble.* Upton Pyne: Imprint Academic.

Eschler, C., Klein, J., & Overby, M. (2010, November). Ankyloglossia: Current beliefs and practice patterns of speech-language pathologists. Poster presentation. American Speech-Language-Hearing Association Convention, Philadelphia, PA.

Evans, S., Meekings, S., Nuttall, H.E., Jasmin, K.M., Boebinger, D., Adank, P., & Scott, S.K. (2014). Does musical enrichment enhance the neural coding of syllables? Neuroscientific interventions and the importance of behavioral data. *Frontiers in Human Neuroscience, 8,* Article 964, 1–4.

Fardet, A. & Rock, E. (2014). Toward a new philosophy of preventive nutrition: From a reductionist to a holistic paradigm to improve nutritional recommendations. *Advances in Nutrition, 5,* 430–446.

Fabiano, G.A., Pelham, W.E., Coles, E.K., Gnagy, E.M., Chronis-Tuscano, A., & O'Connor, B.C. (2009). A meta-analysis of behavioral treatments for attention-deficit/hyperactivity disorder. *Clinical Psychology Review, 29(2),* 129–140.

Farrell, M.L. & Sherman, G.F. (2011). Multisensory structured language education. In J. Birsh (Ed.), *Multisensory Teaching of Basic Language Skills, 3rd edition* (pp. 25–43). Baltimore: Paul H. Brookes.

Federal Trade Commission (2016). Lumosity to pay $2 million to settle FTC deceptive advertising charges for its "brain training" program. Retrieved July 1, 2016 from www.ftc.gov/news-events/press-releases/2016/01/lumosity-pay-2-million-settle-ftc-deceptive-advertising-charges

Feinstein, A. (2010). *History of Autism: Conversations with the Pioneers.* London, UK: Wiley-Blackwell.

Ferguson, C.J. & Donnellan, M.B. (2014). Is the association between children's baby video viewing and poor language development robust? A reanalysis of Zimmerman, Christakis, and Meltzoff (2007). *Developmental Psychology, 50(1),* 129–137.

Fernandez-Duque, D., Evans, J., Christian, C., & Hodges, S.D. (2015). Superfluous neuroscience information makes explanations of psychological phenomena more appealing. *Journal of Cognitive Neuroscience, 27(5),* 926–944.

Fey, M.E., Kamhi, A.G., & Richard, G.J. (2012). Letter to the Editor. Auditory training for children with auditory processing disorder and language impairment: A response to Bellis, Chermak, Weihing and Musiek. *Language, Speech and Hearing Services in Schools, 43(3)*, 387–392.

Fields-Meyer, T. (2011). *Following Ezra: What One Father Learned About Gumby, Otters, Autism, and Love from his Extraordinary Son*. New York, NY: New American Library.

Finn, P., Bothe, A., & Bramlett, R. (2005). Science and pseudoscience in communication disorders: Criteria and applications. *American Journal of Speech-Language Pathology, 14(3)*, 172–186.

Finnes, S. (2015). Speaking through a Letterboard. *International Communication Project*. Retrieved 2 April 2016 from www.internationalcommunicationproject.com/profile/755/

Flora, S.J.S. & Pachauri, V. (2010). Chelation in metal intoxication. *International Journal of Environmental Research and Public Health, 7(7)*, 2745–2788.

Foorman, B.R., Francis, D.J., Fletcher, J.M., Schatschneider, C., & Mehta, P. (1998). The role of instruction in learning to read: Preventing reading failure in at-risk children. *Journal of Educational Psychology, 90*, 1–15.

Fox, M. (n.d.). Like mud, not fireworks. *The Place of Passion in the Development of Literacy*, Retrieved April 7, 2015 from http://memfox.com/for-teachers/for-teachers-like-mud-not-fireworks/#more-1551

Foxx, R.M. & Mulick, J.A. (2016). *Controversial Therapies for Autism and Intellectual Disabilities: Fad, Fashion, and Science in Professional Practice, 2nd edition*. New York, NY: Routledge.

Fraker, C. & Walbert, L. (2011). Treatment of selective eating and dysphagia using pre-chaining and food chaining© Therapy Programs, *SIG 13 Perspectives on Swallowing and Swallowing Disorders (Dysphagia), 20(3)*, 75–81.

François, C., Grau-Sánchez, J., Duarte, E., & Rodriguez-Fornells, A. (2015). Musical training as an alternative and effective method for neuro-education and neuro-rehabilitation. *Frontiers in Psychology, 6, Article 475*, 1–15.

Freeman, J., Simonsen, B., Briere, D.E., & MacSuga-Gage, A.S. (2014). Pre-service teacher training in classroom management. A review of state accreditation policy and teacher preparation programs. *Teacher Education and Special Education: The Journal of the Teacher Education Division of the Council for Exceptional Children, 37(2)*, 106–120.

Fulton, E., Eapen, V., Črnčec, R., Walter, A., & Rogers, S. (2014). Reducing maladaptive behaviors in preschool-aged children with autism spectrum disorder using the Early Start Denver Model. *Frontiers in Pediatrics, 2:40*. DOI: 10.3389/fped.2014.00040 http://journal.frontiersin.org/article/10.3389/fped.2014.00040/full

Gajos, J.M. & Beaver, K.M. (2016). The effect of omega-3 fatty acids on aggression: A meta-analysis. *Neuroscience & Biobehavioral Reviews, 69(Oct)*, 147–158.

Galuschka, K., Ise, E., Krick, K., & Schulte-Körne, G. (2014). Effectiveness of treatment approaches for children and adolescents with reading disabilities: A meta-analysis of randomized controlled trials. *PLOS One*. DOI: 10.1371/journal.pone.0089900

Gambrill, E. (2012). *Propaganda and the Helping Professions*. New York, NY: Oxford University Press.

Gardner, H. (2003). Multiple Intelligences after Twenty Years. Invited Address, American Educational Research Association, 21 April 2003. Retrieved 8 February 2016 from http://ocw.metu.edu.tr/pluginfile.php/9274/mod_resource/content/1/Gardner_multiple_intelligent.pdf

Gardner, H. (2011). *Frames of Mind: The Theory of Multiple Intelligences, 3rd edition*. New York, NY: Basic Books.

Gathercole, S.E. & Alloway, T.P. (2008). *Working Memory and Learning: A Practical Guide for Teachers*. London: Sage.

Gathercole, S.E., Dunning, D.L., & Holmes, J. (2012). Cogmed training: Let's be realistic about intervention research. *Journal of Applied Research in Memory and Cognition*, 1(3), 201–203.

Gensini, G.F., Conti, A.A., & Conti A. (2005). Past and present of "what will please the lord": An updated history of the concept of placebo. *Minerva Medica*, 96(2), 121–124.

Gerber, S., Brice, A., Capone, N., Fujiki, M., & Timler, G. (2012). Language use in social interactions of school-age children with language impairments: An evidence-based systematic review of treatment. *Language, Speech and Hearing Services in the Schools*, 43(2), 235–249.

Geretsegger, M., Elefant, C., Mössler, K.A., & Gold, C. (2014). Music therapy for people with autism spectrum disorder. *Cochrane Database of Systematic Reviews*, 6.

Gershoff, E.T. & Bitensky, S.H. (2007). The case against corporal punishment of children: Converging evidence from social science research and international human rights law and implications for US public policy. *Psychology, Public Policy, and Law*, 13(4), 231.

Gevensleben, H., Rothenberger, A., Moll, G.H., & Heinrich, H. (2012). Neurofeedback in children with ADHD: Validation and challenges. *Expert Review of Neurotherapeutics*, 12(4), 447–460.

Goldacre, B. (2007). Advertising: What's wrong with Gillian McKeith. *The Guardian*. Retrieved 24 January 2016 from www.theguardian.com/media/2007/feb/12/advertising.food

Goldacre, B. (2008). *Bad Science*. London: Fourth Estate.

Goldstein, B. (2015). Providing clinical services to multilingual children with SSD. In C. Bowen, *Children's speech sound disorders 2nd edition* (pp. 148–153). Oxford: Wiley-Blackwell.

Gordon, R.L., Fehd, H.M., & McCandliss, B.D. (2015). Does music training enhance literacy skills? A meta-analysis. *Frontiers in Psychology*, 6, Article 177, 1–16.

Gorski, D. (2015). Prince of pseudoscience. Retrieved April 7, 2015 from http://www.slate.com/articles/health_and_science/medical_examiner/2015/03/prince_charles_visits_washington_d_c_and_kentucky_homeopathy_and_anti_gm.html

Gough, P.B. & Hillinger, M.L. (1980). Learning to read: An unnatural act. *Bulletin of the Orton Society*, 30, 179–196.

Gow, R.V., Hibbel, J.R., & Parletta, N. (2015). Current evidence and future directions for research with omega-3 fatty acids and attention deficit hyperactivity disorder. *Current Opinion in Clinical Nutrition and Metabolic Care, 18(2)*, 133–138.

Gray, C. & Garand, J. (1993). Social stories: Improving responses of students with autism with accurate social information. *Focus on Autistic Behavior, 8*, 1–10.

Graziano, P.A., Calkins, S.D., & Keane, S.P. (2011). Sustained attention development during the toddlerhood to preschool period: Associations with toddlers' emotion regulation strategies and maternal behaviour. *Infant and Child Development, 20(6)*, 389–408.

Green, B.C., Johnson, K.A., & Bretherton, L. (2014). Pragmatic language difficulties in children with hyperactivity and attention problems: An integrated review. *International Journal of Language and Communication Disorders, 49(1)*, 15–29.

Greenfield, S. (2015). *Mind Change: How Digital Technologies are Leaving their Mark on our Brains.* New York: Random House.

Grosche, M. & Volpe, R.J. (2013). Response-to-intervention (RTI) as a model to facilitate inclusion for students with learning and behaviour problems. *European Journal of Special Needs Education, 28(3)*, 254–269.

Gruber, F.A., Lowery, S.D., Seung, H-K, & Deal, R. (2003). Approaches to speech/language intervention and the true believer. *Journal of Medical Speech-Language Pathology, 11(2)*, 95–104.

Gujral, N., Freeman, H.J., & Thomson, A.B.R. (2012). Celiac disease: Prevalence, diagnosis, pathogenesis and treatment, *World Journal of Gastroenterology, 18(42)*, 6036–6059.

Gunter, C.D. & Koenig, M.A. (2016). Fads and controversial treatments in speech-language. pathology. In R.M. Foxx and J.A. Mulick (Eds), *Controversial Therapies for Autism and Intellectual Disabilities: Fad, Fashion, and Science in Professional Practice, 2nd edition.* New York, NY: Routledge.

Guiberson, M. & Atkins, J. (2012). Speech-language pathologists' preparation, practices, and perspectives on serving culturally and linguistically diverse children. *Communication Disorders Quarterly, 33(3)*, 169–180.

Hagopian, L.P., Fisher, W.W., Sullivan, M.T., Acquisto, J., & LeBlanc, L.A. (1998). Effectiveness of functional communication training with and without extinction and punishment: A summary of 21 inpatient cases. *Journal of Applied Behavior Analysis, 3*, 211–235.

Hattie, J. (2008). *Visible Learning: A Synthesis of over 800 Meta-Analyses Relating to Achievement.* Abingdon: Routledge.

Hattie, J. (2014). *Self-Concept.* Hove: Psychology Press.

Hale, L. & Guan, S. (2015). Screen time and sleep among school-aged children and adolescents: A systematic literature review. *Sleep Medicine Reviews, 21*, 50–58.

Havighurst, S.S., Wilson, K.R., Harley, A.E., Kehoe, C., Efron, D., & Prior, M.R. (2013). "Tuning into Kids": Reducing young children's behavior problems using an emotion coaching parenting program. *Child Psychiatry & Human Development, 44(2)*, 247–264.

Hawe, P. & Potvin, L. (2009). What is population health intervention research? *Canadian Journal of Public Health, 100(1)*, 8–14.

Hawking, S. (2013). *My Brief History*. New York, NY: Bantam Books.

Hayes, H. & Snow, P. (2013). Oral language competence and restorative justice processes: Refining preparation and the measurement of conference outcomes. *Trends & Issues in Crime and Criminal Justice, 463*, 1–7.

Hayhow, R. (2013). Sharing your findings. in C. Dobinson & Y. Wren (Eds), *Creating Practice-Based Evidence: A Guide for SLTs*. Guildford, UK: J&R Press.

Hempenstall, K. (2012). Response to intervention: Accountability in action. *Australian Journal of Learning Difficulties, 17(2)*, 101–131.

Hemphill, S.A., Toumbourou, J.W., Herrenkohl, T.I., McMorris, B.J., & Catalano, R.F. (2006). The effect of school suspensions and arrests on subsequent adolescent antisocial behavior in Australia and the United States. *Journal of Adolescent Health, 39(5)*, 736–744.

Hemsley, B. (2012). Ethical issues in augmentative and alternative communication. *Journal of Clinical Practice in Speech-Language Pathology, 14(2)*, 88–92.

Hemsley, B. & Dann, S. (2014). Social media and social marketing in relation to facilitated communication: Harnessing the affordances of social media for knowledge translation, *Evidence-Based Communication Assessment and Intervention, 8(4)*, 187–206.

Hennessy, K. & Hennessy, K. (2013). *Anything but Silent: Our Family's Journey through Childhood Apraxia of Speech*. Tarentum, PA: Word Association Publishers.

Hill, L. (2015, February 24). Can psychological astrology help to understand a child with communication difficulties? [Web log post]. Retrieved January 26, 2016 from www.smarttalkersblog.com/2015/02/how-can-psychological-astrology-help-to.html

Hiscock, H., Bayer, J.K., Hampton, A., Ukoumunne, O.C., & Wake, M. (2008). Long-term mother and child mental health effects of a population-based infant sleep intervention: Cluster-randomized, controlled trial. *Pediatrics, 122(3)*, e621–e627.

Hoover, W.A. & Gough, P.B. (1990). The simple view of reading. *Reading and Writing, 2(2)*, 127–160.

Hodge, M. (2010). Intervention for developmental dysarthria. In A.L. Williams, S. McLeod, & R.J. McCauley (Eds), *Interventions for Speech Sound Disorders in Children* (pp. 557–578). Baltimore, MD: Paul H. Brookes.

Hofmann, S.G. (2011). *An Introduction to Modern CBT: Psychological Solutions to Mental Health Problems*. Chichester: John Wiley & Sons.

Hogan, M., Westcott, C., & Griffiths, M. (2005). Randomized, controlled trial of division of tongue-tie in infants with feeding problems. *Journal of Paediatrics and Child Health, 41(5–6)*, 246–250.

Holtmann, M., Sonuga-Barke, E., Cortese. S., & Brandeis, D. (2014). Neurofeedback for ADHD: A review of current evidence. *Child and Adolescent Psychiatric Clinics of North America, 23(4)*, 789–806.

Homer, M. & Carbajal, P. (2015). Swallowing and feeding services in the schools: From therapy to the dinner table. *SIG 13 Perspectives on Swallowing and Swallowing Disorders (Dysphagia), 24(4)*, 155–161.

Hornickel, J. & Kraus, N. (2013). Unstable representation of sound: A biological marker of dyslexia. *The Journal of Neuroscience, 33(8)*, 3500–3504.

Horner, S., Simonelli, A.M., Schmidt, H., Cichowski, K., Hancko, M., Zhang, G., & Ross, E.S. (2014). Setting the stage for successful oral feeding: The impact of implementing the SOFFI feeding program with medically fragile NICU infants. *Journal of Perinatal and Neonatal Nursing, 28(1)*, 59–68.

Houghton, K., Schuchard, J., Lewis, C., & Thompson, C. (2013). Promoting child-initiated social-communication in children with autism: Son-Rise Program intervention effects. *Journal of Communication Disorders, 46(5–6)*, 495–506.

Housego, E. & Burns, C. (1994). Are you sitting too comfortably? A critical look at 'circle time' in primary classrooms. *English in Education, 28(2)*, 23–30.

Howard-Jones, P.A. (2014). Neuroscience and education: Myths and messages. *Nature Reviews Neuroscience, 15*, 817–824.

Hulme, C. & Melby-Lervåg, M. (2012). Current evidence does not support the claims made for CogMed working memory training. *Journal of Applied Research in Memory and Cognition, 1(3)*, 197–200.

Hysing, M., Pallesen, S., Stormark, K.M., Jakobsen, R., Lundervold, A.J., & Sivertsen, B. (2015). Sleep and use of electronic devices in adolescence: Results from a large population-based study. *BMJ open, 5(1)*, e006748.

Hutchins, S.D. (2016). Communing with dolphins. *The ASHA Leader, 21(1)*, 22–23.

Iacono, T., West, D. Bloomberg, K., & Johnson, H. (2009). Reliability and validity of the revised Triple C: Checklist of Communicative Competencies for adults with severe and multiple disabilities. *Journal of Intellectual Disability Research, 53(1)*, 44–53.

Institute for Multisensory Language Education (n.d.). *Orton Gillingham Approach*. Retrieved 6 January 2016 from www.multisensoryeducation.net.au/?mact=News,cntnt01,detail,0&cntnt01articleid=27&cntnt01returnid=163

International Communication Project. Retrieved 11 July 2016 from www.internationalcommunicationproject.com

International Dyslexia Association (n.d.). *Multisensory Structured Language Teaching*. Retrieved 12 March 2016 from https://eida.org/multisensory-structured-language-teaching/

International Society for Augmentative and Alternative Communication (2014). *Position Statement on Facilitated Communication*. Retrieved 23 January 2016 from http://valid.org.au/documents/isaac_fc_position_statement.pdf

Isaacson, R. (2009). *The Horse Boy: A Father's Quest to Heal His Son*. New York, NY: Little, Brown and Company.

Jansen, L., Rasekaba, T., Presnell, S., & Holland, A.E. (2012). Finding evidence to support practice in allied health: Peers, experience and the internet. *Journal of Allied Health, 41(4)*, 154–161.

Janssen, M., Toussaint, H.M., van Mechelen, W., & Verhagen, E.A. (2014). Effects of acute bouts of physical activity on children's attention: A systematic review of the literature. *Springerplus, 3(1)*, 1.

Jasuta, S. (2015). Helping others speak through Facilitated Communication. *International Communication Project*. Retrieved 2 April 2016 from www.internationalcommunicationproject.com/profile/763/

Jegatheesan, B., Beetz, A., Ormerod, E., Johnson, R., Fine, A., Yamazaki, K., Dudzik, C., Garcia, R.M., & Choi, G. (2014). International Association of Animal-Human Interactions Organizations (IAHAIO) White Paper: Definitions for Animal Assisted Intervention and Animal Assisted Activity and Guidelines for Wellness of Animals Involved. Columbia, MO: IAHAIO.

Jennings, P. (2004). *The Reading Bug...and How You Can Help Your Child to Catch It*. London: Penguin Books.

Jerger, J. & Musiek, F. (2000). Report of the consensus conference on the diagnosis of auditory processing. *Journal of the American Academy of Audiology, 11(9)*, 467–474.

Joffe, V. (2015). Common practice in speech sound disorders in UK. In C. Bowen, *Children's Speech Sound Disorders, 2nd edition* (pp. 244–246). Oxford: Wiley-Blackwell.

Jones, L., Bellis, M.A., Wood, S., Hughes, K., McCoy, E., Eckley, L., ... & Officer, A. (2012). Prevalence and risk of violence against children with disabilities: A systematic review and meta-analysis of observational studies. *The Lancet, 380*(9845), 899–907.

Justus, T.C. & Ivry, R.B. (2001). The cognitive neuropsychology of the cerebellum. *International Review of Psychiatry, 13(4)*, 276–282.

Kamhi, A. (2004). A meme's eye view of speech-language pathology. *Language, Speech, and Hearing Services in Schools, 35(2)*, 105–111.

Kamhi, A.G. (2011a). Balancing certainty and uncertainty in clinical practice. *Language, Speech, and Hearing Services in Schools, 42(1)*, 59–64.

Kamhi, A.G. (2011b). What speech-language pathologists need to know about auditory processing disorder. *Language, Speech, and Hearing Services in Schools, 42(3)*, 265–272.

Karkhaneh, K., Clark, B. Ospina, M.B., Seida, J.C., Smith, V., & Hartling, L. (2010). Social Stories™ to improve social skills in children with autism spectrum disorder: A systematic review. *Autism, 14(6)*, 641–662.

Keats, L.F. (n.d.). Can your child's diet boost her intelligence? Retrieved on 26 January 2016 from www.woolworthsbabyandtoddlerclub.com.au/toddler/toddlers-health-and-nutrition/can-your-childs-diet-boost-his-intelligence/

Kemp-Koo, D. (2013). A case study of the Learning Disabilities Association of Saskatchewan (LDAS) Arrowsmith Program. Doctor of Philosophy thesis, University of Saskatchewan, Saskatoon.

Kenny, B., Lincoln, M., & Balandin, S. (2010). Experienced speech-language pathologists' responses to ethical dilemmas: An integrated approach to ethical reasoning. *American Journal of Speech-Language Pathology, 19(3)*, 121–134.

Kenrick, K. & Day, A.S. (2014). Coeliac disease: Where are we in 2014? *Australian Family Physician, 43(10)*, 674–678.

Kent, R.D. (2015). Nonspeech oral movements and oral motor disorders: A narrative review *American Journal of Speech-Language Pathology, 24(4)*, 763–789.

Kiefer, M., Schuler, S., Mayer, C., Trumpp, N. M., Hille, K., & Sachse, S. (2015). Handwriting or typewriting? The influence of pen-or keyboard-based writing training on reading and writing performance in preschool children. *Advances in Cognitive Psychology, 11(4)*, 136.

Klingberg, T., Forssberg, H., & Westerberg, H. (2002). Training of working memory in children with ADHD. *Journal of Clinical and Experimental Neuropsychology, 24(6)*, 781–791.

Kohnert, K. (2008). *Language Disorders in Bilingual Children and Adults.* San Diego, CA: Plural Publishing.

Krafnick, A.J., Flowers, D.L., Napoliello, E.M., & Eden, G.F. (2011). Gray matter volume changes following reading intervention in dyslexic children. *Neuroimage, 57(3)*, 733–741.

Kraus, N., Slater, J., Thompson, E.C., Hornickel, J., Strait, D.L., Nicol, T., & White-Schwoch, T. (2014a). Music enrichment programs improve the neural encoding of speech in at-risk children. *The Journal of Neuroscience, 34(36)*, 11913–11918.

Kraus, N., Slater, J., Thompson, E.C., Hornickel, J., Strait, D.L., Nicol, T., & White-Schwoch, T. (2014b). Auditory learning through active engagement with sound: Biological impact of community music lessons in at-risk children. *Frontiers in Neuroscience, 8, Article 351*, 1–12.

Kolb, D. (1985). *Learning Style Inventory.* Boston, MA: McBer.

Kuhn, T.S. (1977). *The Essential Tension: Selected Studies in Scientific Tradition and Change.* Chicago, IL: University of Chicago Press.

Kurtz, P. F., Boelter, E.W., Jarmolowicz, D.P., Chin, M.D., & Hagopian, L.P. (2011). Analysis of functional communication training as an empirically supported treatment for problem behavior displayed by individuals with intellectual disabilities. *Research in Developmental Disabilities, 32*, 2935–2942.

Labat, H., Ecalle, J., Baldy, R., & Magnan, A. (2014). How can low-skilled 5-year-old children benefit from multisensory training on the acquisition of the alphabetic principle? *Learning and Individual Differences, 29*, 106–113.

Lang, R., O'Reilly, M., Healy, O., Rispoli, M., Lydon, H., Streusand, W., Davis, T., Kang, S., Sigafoos, J., Lancioni, G., Didden, R., & Giesbers, S. (2012). Sensory integration therapy for autism spectrum disorders: A systematic review. *Research in Autism Spectrum Disorders, 6(3)*, 1004–1018.

Leach, T. & Lewis, E. (2013). Children's experiences during circle-time: A call for research-informed debate. *Pastoral Care in Education, 31(1)*, 43–52.

Leaf, J.B., Kassardjian, A., Oppenheim-Leaf, M.L., Cihon, J.H., Taubman, R., Leaf, R., & McEachin, J. (2016). Social Thinking®: Science, psuedoscience, or antiscience? *Behavior Analysis in Practice, 9(2)*, 152–157.

Lear, C.S.C., Flanagan, J.B., & Moorrees, C.F.A. (1965). The frequency of deglutition in man. *Archives of Oral Biology, 10(1)*, 83–99.

Lee, A.S-Y., & Gibbon, F.E. (2015). Non-speech oral motor treatment for developmental speech sound disorders in children. *Cochrane Database of Systematic Reviews 2015, Issue 3*. Art. No.: CD009383. DOI: 10.1002/14651858.CD009383.pub2

Leekam, S. (2013). Diagnostic interview for social and communication disorders. In *Encyclopedia of Autism Spectrum Disorders* (pp. 926–931). New York: Springer.

Leitão, S., Scarinci, N., & Koenig, C. (2015). Ethical reflections: Readability of speech pathology reports. *Journal of Clinical Practice in Speech-Language Pathology, 17(Supp. 1)*, 30–32.

Levin, S. (2015). *Unlocked: A Family Emerging from the Shadows of Autism*. New York, NY: Skyhorse Publishing.

Levy, S.E. & Hyman, S.L. (2015). Complementary and alternative medicine treatments for children with autism spectrum disorders. *Child and Adolescent Psychiatric Clinics of North America, 24(1)*, 117–143.

Lewin, T. (2009, Oct 23). No Einstein in your crib? Get a refund, *New York Times*, retrieved from www.nytimes.com/2009/10/24/education/24baby.html?_r=0 on December 11, 2015.

Liao, S.T., Hwang, Y.S., Chen, Y.J., Lee, P., Chen, S.J., & Lin, L.Y. (2014). Home-based DIR/Floortime intervention program for preschool children with autism spectrum disorders: Preliminary findings. *Physical & Occupational Therapy in Pediatrics, 34(4)*, 356–367.

Liberman, I.Y. (1971). Basic research in speech and the lateralisation of language: Some implications for reading disability. *Bulletin of the Orton Society, 21*, 71–87.

Liesemer, K., Bratton, S.L., Zebrack, C.M., Brockmeyer, D., & Statler, K.D. (2011). Early post-traumatic seizures in moderate to severe pediatric traumatic brain injury: Rates, risk factors, and clinical features. *Journal of Neurotrauma, 28(5)*, 755–762.

Lilienfeld, S.O., Lynn, S.J. & Lohr, J.M. (2015). Science and pseudoscience in clinical psychology. Initial thoughts, reflections, and considerations. In S.O. Lilienfeld, S.J. Lynn, and J.M. Lohr (Eds), *Science and Pseudoscience in Clinical Psychology*, 2nd edition (pp. 1–16). New York: Guilford Press.

Lilienfeld, S.O., Marshall, J., Todd, J.T., & Shane, H.C. (2014). The persistence of fad interventions in the face of negative scientific evidence: Facilitated communication for autism as a case example. *Evidence-Based Communication Assessment and Intervention, 8(2)*, 62–101.

Listen and Learn Centre (2014). *Interactive Metronome in Australia*, Retrieved 8 January 2016 from http://listenandlearn.com.au/interactive-metronome/

Lof, G.L. (2011). Science-based practice and the speech-language pathologist. *International Journal of Speech-Language Pathology, 13(3)*, 189–196.

Logan, K J. (2014). *Fluency Disorders*. San Diego, CA: Plural Publishing.

Loher, S. & Roebers, C.M. (2013). Executive functions and their differential contribution to sustained attention in 5–8-year-old children. *Journal of Educational and Developmental Psychology, 3(1)*, 51.

Longcamp, M., Zerbato-Poudou, M.T., & Velay, J. L. (2005). The influence of writing practice on letter recognition in preschool children: A comparison between handwriting and typing. *Acta Psychologica, 119(1)*, 67–79.

Lord, C., Risi, S., Lambrecht, L., Cook Jr, E.H., Leventhal, B.L., DiLavore, P.C., ... & Rutter, M. (2000). The Autism Diagnostic Observation Schedule—Generic: A standard measure of social and communication deficits associated with the spectrum of autism. *Journal of Autism and Developmental Disorders, 30(3)*, 205–223.

Lord, C., Rutter, M., & Le Couteur, A. (1994). Autism Diagnostic Interview-Revised: A revised version of a diagnostic interview for caregivers of individuals with possible pervasive developmental disorders. *Journal of Autism and Developmental Disorders, 24(5)*, 659–685.

Lorenz, K. (1990). Cereals and schizophrenia. In Y. Pomeranz (Ed.) *Advances in Cereal Science and Technology*. St. Paul MN: American Association of Chemists.

Lown, J. (2002). Circle Time: The perceptions of teachers and pupils. *Educational Psychology in Practice, 18(2)*, 93–102.

Lum, C. (2002). *Scientific Thinking in Speech and Language Therapy*. Mahwah, NJ: Lawrence Erlbaum Associates.

Lyon, G.R. (n.d.). Converging evidence: Reading research–What it takes to read. Retrieved 13 March 2016 from www.childrenofthecode.org/interviews/lyon.htm#Instructionalcasualties

Macdonald, A. (2011). *Solution-Focused Therapy: Theory, Research & Practice*. London, UK: Sage Publications Ltd.

Mankad, D., Dupuis, A., Smile, S., Roberts, W., Brian, J., Lui, T., Genore, L., Zaghloul, D., Iaboni, A.... (2015). A randomized, placebo controlled trial of omega-3 fatty acids in the treatment of young children with autism. *Molecular Autism*, Retrieved 15 August 2016 from https://molecularautism.biomedcentral.com/articles/10.1186/s13229-015-0010-7

Mariën, P., Ackermann, H., Adamaszek, M., Barwood, C.H., Beaton, A., Desmond, J., ... & Leggio, M. (2014). Consensus paper. Language and the cerebellum: An ongoing enigma. *The Cerebellum, 13(3)*, 386–410.

Mårtensson, P., Fors, U., Wallin, S., Zander, U., & Nilsson, G.H. (2016). Evaluating research: A multidisciplinary approach to assessing research practice and quality. *Research Policy, 45(3)*, 593–603.

Marinus, E., Mostard, M., Segers, E., Schubert, T.M., Madelaine, A., & Wheldall, K. (2016). A special font for people with dyslexia: Does it work and, if so, why? *Dyslexia*. Early online 19 May 2016. DOI: 10.1002/dys.1527

Marzano, R.J., Marzano, J.S., & Pickering, D.J. (2003). *Classroom Management That Works. Research-Based Strategies for Every Teacher*. Alexandria, VA: Association for Supervision and Curriculum Development (ASCD).

Masand, P.S. & Gupta, S. (2002). Long-term side effects of newer-generation antidepressants: SSRIS, venlafaxine, nefazodone, bupropion, and mirtazapine. *Annals of Clinical Psychiatry, 14(3)*, 175–182.

Matson, J.L., Adams, H.L., Williams, L.W., & Reiske, R.D. (2013). Why are there so many unsubstantiated treatments in autism? *Research in Autism Spectrum Disorders, 7(3)*, 466–474.

Maul, C.A., Findley, B.R., & Nicolson Adams, A. (2015). *Behavioral Principles in Communicative Disorders: Applications to Assessment and Treatment.* San Diego, CA: Plural Publishing.

McArthur, G.M. (2009). Auditory processing disorders: Can they be treated? *Current Opinion in Neurology, 22,* 137–143.

McCabe, D.P. & Castel, A.D. (2008). Seeing is believing: The effect of brain imaging on judgments of scientific reasoning. *Cognition, 107,* 343–352.

McCauley, R.J., Strand, E., Lof, G.L., Schooling, T., & Frymark, T. (2009). Evidence-based systematic review: Effects of nonspeech oral motor exercises on speech, *American Journal of Speech-Language Pathology, 18(4),* 343–360.

McComas, K.L. (2014). *Dig Your in Heels and Fight! How Women Become Researchers in Communication Sciences and Disorders.* Guildford, UK: J&R Press.

McGraw, P. (n.d.). Increasing your child's intellectual performance. Retrieved 26 January 2016 from hwww.drphil.com/articles/article/189

McGuire, D. (2015). *Beyond Stuttering: The McGuire Programme for Getting Good at the Sport of Speaking.* London: Souvenir Press.

McKean, C., Mensah, F.K., Eadie, P., Bavin, E.L., Bretherton, L., Cini, C., & Reilly S. (2015). Levers for language growth: Characteristics and predictors of language trajectories between 4 and 7 years. PLoS One, *10(8),* e0134251. DOI:10.1371/journal.pone.0134251

McLaughlin, E.G., Adamson, B.J., Lincoln, M.A., Pallant. J.F., & Cooper, C.L. (2010). Turnover and intent to leave among speech pathologists. *Australian Health Review, 34(2),* 227–233.

McLeod, S., Verdon, S., & Bowen, C. (2013). International aspirations for speech-language pathologists' practice with multilingual children with speech sound disorders: Development of a position paper. *Journal of Communication Disorders, 46,* 375–387.

Medwell, J. & Wray, D. (2007). Handwriting: What do we know and what do we need to know? *Literacy, 41(1),* 10–15.

Mercado-Deane, M.G., Burton, E.M., Harlow, S.A., Glover, A.S., Deane, D.A., Guill, M.F., & Hudson, V. (2001). Swallowing dysfunction in infants less than 1 year of age. *Pediatric Radiology, 31(6),* 423–428.

Merzenich, M.M., Jenkins, W.M., Johnston, P., Schreiner, C., Miller, S.L., & Tallal, P. (1996). Temporal processing deficits of language-learning impaired children ameliorated by training. *Science, 271,* 77–81.

Messner, A.H. & Lalakea, M.L. (2000). Ankyloglossia: Controversies in management. *International Journal of Pediatric Otorhinolaryngology, 54(2–3),* 123–31.

Millard, S.K., Nicholas A., & Cook F.M. (2008). Is parent-child interaction therapy effective in reducing stuttering? *Journal of Speech, Language and Hearing Research, 51(3),* 636–650.

Miller, C. (n.d.). How anxiety leads to disruptive behavior. *Child Mind Institute.* Retrieved 22 February 2016 from www.childmind.org/en/posts/articles/2013-3-26-anxiety-and-disruptive-behavior

Mills, K.L. (2014). Effects of Internet use on the adolescent brain: Despite popular claims, experimental evidence remains scarce. *Trends in Cognitive Sciences, 18(8),* 385-387.

Mindell, J., Kuhn, B., Lewin, D.S., Meltzer, L.J., & Sadeh, A. (2006). Behavioral treatment of bedtime problems and night wakings in infants and young children. *Sleep, 29(10),* 1263.

Mindell, J.A., Telofski, L.S., Wiegand, B., & Kurtz, E. S. (2009). A nightly bedtime routine: Impact on sleep in young children and maternal mood. *Sleep, 32(5),* 599-606.

Mirenda, P. (1997). Supporting individuals with challenging behavior through functional communication training and AAC: Research review. *Augmentative & Alternative Communication, 13(4),* 207-207.

Mirenda, P. (2014a). Comments and a personal reflection on the persistence of facilitated communication. *Evidence-Based Communication Assessment and Intervention, 8(2),* 1-9.

Mirenda, P. (2014b). Revisiting the mosaic of supports required for including people with severe intellectual or developmental disabilities in their communities. *Augmentative and Alternative Communication, 30(1),* 19-27.

Moats L. C. (2000). *Whole Language Lives On. The Illusion of "Balanced" Reading Instruction.* Washington, DC: Thomas Fordham Foundation.

Moats, L.C. (2009). Teaching spelling to students with language and learning difficulties. In G.A. Troia (Ed.). *Instruction and Assessment for Struggling Writers. Evidence-Based Practices* (pp. 269-289). New York, NY: Guilford Press.

Moats, L.C. (2010). *Speech to Print. Language Essentials for Teachers, 2nd edition.* Baltimore: Paul H. Brookes Publishing.

Montee, B.B., Miltenberger, R.G., & Wittrock, D. (1995). An experimental analysis of Facilitated Communication. *Journal of Applied Behavior Analysis, 28,* 189-200.

Moore, T. (2013). Teamwork in early childhood intervention services: Recommended practices. National Disability Insurance Scheme (NDIS). Retrieved 11 July 2016 from www.ndis.gov.au.

Morlock, L., Reynolds, J., Fisher, S., & Comer, R. J. (2015). Video modeling and word identification in adolescents with Autism Spectrum Disorder. *Child Language Teaching and Therapy, 31(1),* 101-111.

Morris, C.R. & Agin, M.C. (2009). Syndrome of allergy, apraxia, and malabsorption: Characterization of a neurodevelopmental phenotype that responds to omega 3 and vitamin E supplementation. *Alternative Therapies in Health and Medicine, 15(3),* 34-43.

Moynihan, R. & Henry, D. (2006). The fight against disease mongering: Generating knowledge for action. *PLOS Medicine, 3(4),* 0425-0428.

Mulloy, A., Lang, R., O'Reilly, M., Sigafoos, J., Lancioni, G., & Rispoli, M. (2012). Gluten-free and casein-free diets in the treatment of autism spectrum disorders: A systematic review. *Research in Autism Spectrum Disorders, 4(3),* 328-339.

Murphy, C.F. & Schochat, E. (2013). Effects of different types of auditory temporal training on language skills: A systematic review. *Clinics, 68(10),* 1364-1370.

Murphy, J. & Cameron, L. (2008). The effectiveness of Talking Mats® with people with intellectual disability. *British Journal of Learning Disabilities, 36(4),* 232-241.

MUSEC: Macquarie University Special Education Centre (2015, June). *MUSEC Briefings,* Retrieved 29 May 2016 from www.musec.mq.edu.au/community_outreach/musec_briefings/

Myklebust, H. (1954). *Auditory Disorders in Children.* New York, NY: Grune & Stratton.

NCLB (2001). No Child Left Behind Act of 2001, Pub. L. No. 107-110, § 115, Stat. 1425 (2002).

Naidu, S., Wilkinson, J.M., & Simpson, M.D. (2005). Attitudes of Australian pharmacists toward complementary and alternative medicines. *Annals of Pharmacotherapy, 39(9),* 1456-1461.

National Autism Center (2015). *Findings and Conclusions: National Standards Project, Phase 2.* Randolph, MA: Author.

National Health and Medical Research Council (2015). *Evidence on the Effectiveness of Homeopathy for Treating Health Conditions.* Canberra: NHMRC. Retrieved 11 July 2016 from www.nhmrc.gov.au/guidelines-publications/cam02

National Prescribing Service (2000). *What is Polypharmacy?* Retrieved 19 March 2016 fromwww.nps.org.au/__data/assets/pdf_file/0003/15780/news13_polypharmacy_1200.pdf

National Reading Panel (2000). *Teaching Children to Read: An Evidence-Based Assessment of the Scientific Research Literature on Reading and its Implications for Reading Instruction.* www.nichd.nih.gov/publications/pubs/nrp/documents/report.pdf

National Research Council (2001). *Educating Children with Autism.* Committee on Educational Interventions for Children with Autism. Catherine Lord and James P. McGee, (Eds). Division of Behavioral and Social Sciences and Education. Washington, DC: National Academy Press.

New South Wales Department of Education and Training (2016). *Reading Recovery: A Research-Based Early Intervention Program.* Retrieved 7 July 2016 from www.curriculumsupport.education.nsw.gov.au/earlyyears/reading_recovery/research.htm

Nicholson, T. (2011). The Orton-Gillingham approach: What is it? Is it research-based? *LDA Bulletin, July,* 9-11.

Norbury, C.F. (2014). Practitioner Review: Social (pragmatic) communication disorder conceptualization, evidence and clinical implications. *Journal of Child Psychology and Psychiatry, 55,* 204-216.

Norris, J.A. & Damico, J.S. (1990*). Whole language in theory and practice: Implications for language intervention. Language, Speech & Hearing Services in Schools, 21(4),* 212-220.

Norwood, K.W., Slayton, R.L., Liptak, G.S., & Murphy, N.A. (2013). Oral health care for children with developmental disabilities, *Pediatrics, 131(3),* 614-619.

Nyhan, B., Reifler, J., Richey, S., & Freed, G. L. (2014). Effective Messages in Vaccine Promotion: A Randomized Trial. Pediatrics, 133(4), 1-8. Oberman, L.M., Enticott, P.G., Casanova, M.F., Rotenberg, A., Pascual-Leone, A., & McCracken, J.T. (2015). Transcranial magnetic stimulation (TMS) therapy for autism: An international consensus conference held in conjunction with the international meeting for autism research on May 13th and 14th, 2014. *Frontiers in Human Neuroscience, 8(1034)*, 1–3.

O'Brian, S., Iverach, L., Jones, M., Onslow, M., Packman, A., & Menzies, R. (2013). Effectiveness of the Lidcombe Program for early stuttering in Australian community clinics. *International Journal of Speech-Language Pathology, 15(6)*, 593–603.

O'Callahan, C., Macary, S., & Clemente, S. (2013). The effects of office-based frenotomy for anterior and posterior ankyloglossia on breastfeeding. *International Journal of Pediatric Otorhinolaryngology, 77(5)*, 827–832.

Odom, S.L., Boyd, B., Hall, L., & Hume, K. (2010). Evaluation of comprehensive treatment models for individuals with Autism Spectrum Disorders. *Journal of Autism and Developmental Disorders, 40*, 425–436.

O'Haire, M.E. (2010). Companion animals and human health: Benefits, challenges, and the road ahead. *Journal of Veterinary Behavior: Clinical Applications and Research, 5(5)*, 226–234.

O'Haire, M.E. (2013). Animal-assisted intervention for autism spectrum disorder: A systematic literature review. *Journal of Autism and Developmental Disorders, 43(7)*, 1606–1622.

Olswang, L.B. (1998). Treatment efficacy research. In C.M. Frattali (Ed.), *Measuring Outcomes in Speech-Language Pathology* (pp. 134–150). New York, NY: Thieme.

O'Neill, S.C. & Stephenson, J. (2014). Evidence-based classroom and behaviour management content in Australian pre-service primary teachers' coursework: Wherefore art thou? *Australian Journal of Teacher Education (Online), 39(4)*, 1.

Oxenham, S. (2016). Thousands of fMRI brain studies in doubt due to software flaws. *New Scientist*. https://www.newscientist.com/article/2097734-thousands-of-fmri-brain-studies-in-doubt-due-to-software-flaws/ Accessed 14 August 2016.

Paas, F., Van Gog, T., & Sweller, J. (2010). Cognitive load theory: New conceptualizations, specifications, and integrated research perspectives. *Educational Psychology Review, 22(2)*, 115–121.

Paivio, A. (1986). *Mental Representations: A Dual Coding Approach*. New York: Oxford University Press.

Pajareya, K. & Nopmaneejumruslers, K. (2011). A pilot randomized controlled trial of DIR/Floortime™ parent training intervention for pre-school children with autistic spectrum disorders. *Autism, 15(2)*, 1–15.

Pajareya, K. & Nopmaneejumruslers, K. (2012). A one-year prospective follow-up study of a DIR/Floortime parent training intervention for preschool children with autistic spectrum disorders. *Journal of the Medical Association of Thailand, 95(9)*, 1184–1193.

Palfreman, J. (1993, Oct 19). Frontline: Prisoners of Silence. WGBH Educational Foundation. Retrieved 2 April 2016 from www.pbs.org/wgbh/pages/frontline/programs/transcripts/1202.html

Pashler, H., McDaniel, M., Rohrer, D., & Bjork, R. (2008). Learning styles concepts and evidence. *Psychological Science in the Public Interest, 9(3)*, 105–119.

Patel, A.D. (2011). Why would musical training benefit the neural encoding of speech? The OPERA hypothesis. The relationship between music and language. *Frontiers in Psychology*, 2, Article 142, 1–14.

Patino, E. (2014). *Sensory Integration Therapy: What It Is and How It Works*. Retrieved 13 May 2016 from https://www.understood.org/en/learning-attention-issues/treatments-approaches/alternative-therapies/sensory-integration-therapy-what-it-is-and-how-it-works

Paul, P. (2006, Jan 8). Want a brainier baby? Time. Retrieved 11 December 2015 from ilabs.washington.edu/news/TIME_BrainierBaby_Jan_06.pdf

Paull, J. (2011). The secrets of Koberwitz: The diffusion of Rudolf Steiner's Agriculture Course and the founding of biodynamic agriculture, *Journal of Social Research & Policy*, 2(1), 19–29.

Paunesku, D., Walton, G.M., Romero, C., Smith, E.N., Yeager, D.S., & Dweck, C.S. (2015). Mind-set interventions are a scalable treatment for academic underachievement. *Psychological Science*. DOI: 0956797615571017

Pennington, L., Parker, N.K., Kelly, H., & Miller, N. (2016). Speech therapy for children with dysarthria acquired before three years of age. *Cochrane Database of Systematic Reviews*, 2016, Issue 7. Art. No.: CD006937. DOI: 10.1002/14651858.CD006937.pub3

Petrenko, C.L. (2013). A review of intervention programs to prevent and treat behavioral problems in young children with developmental disabilities. *Journal of Developmental and Physical Disabilities*, 25(6), 651–679.

Pfeiffer, B.A., Koenig, K., Kinnealey, M., Sheppard, M., & Henderson L. (2011). Effectiveness of sensory integration interventions in children with autism spectrum disorders: A pilot study. *American Journal of Occupational Therapy*, 65(1), 72–85.

Pistorius, M. (2013). *Ghost Boy: The Miraculous Escape of a Misdiagnosed Boy Trapped Inside His Own Body*. Nashville, TN: Thomas Nelson.

Poil, S.S., Bollmann, S., Ghisleni, C., O'Gorman, R.L., Klaver, P., Ball, J., ... & Michels, L. (2014). Age dependent electroencephalographic changes in attention-deficit/hyperactivity disorder (ADHD). *Clinical Neurophysiology*, 125(8), 1626–1638.

Polanczyk, G.V., Willcutt, E.G., Salum, G.A., Kieling, C., & Rohde, L.A. (2014). ADHD prevalence estimates across three decades: An updated systematic review and meta-regression analysis. *International Journal of Epidemiology*, 43(2), 434–442.

Ponsford, J., Bayley, M., Wiseman-Hakes, C., Togher, L., Velikonja, D., McIntyre, A.,... Tate, R. (2014). INCOG recommendations for management of cognition following traumatic brain injury, Part II: Attention and information processing speed. *Journal of Head Trauma Rehabilitation*, 29(4), 321–337.

Porter, G. & Cafiero, J. (2009). Pragmatic organization dynamic display (PODD) communication books: A promising practice for individuals with autism spectrum disorders. *Perspectives on Augmentative and Alternative Communication*, 18, 121–129.

Posadzki, P., Alotaibi A., & Ernst E. (2012). Adverse effects of homeopathy: A systematic review of published case reports and case series. *International Journal of Clinical Practice*, 66(12), 1178–1188.

Posner, J.B., Saper, C.B., Schiff, N. & Plum, J.B. (2007). *Plum and Posner's Diagnosis of Stupor and Coma*. New York: Contemporary Neurology.

Price, A.M., Wake, M., Ukoumunne, O.C., & Hiscock, H. (2012). Five-year follow-up of harms and benefits of behavioral infant sleep intervention: Randomized trial. *Pediatrics*, *130(4)*, 643–651.

Prideaux, L., Marsh, K.A., & Caplygin, D. (2005). Efficacy of the Cellfield intervention for reading difficulties: An integrated computer-based approach targeting deficits associated with dyslexia. *Australian Journal of Learning Disabilities*, *10(2)*, 51–62.

Pring, T., Flood, E., Dodd, B., & Joffe, V. (2012). The working practices and clinical experiences of paediatric speech and language therapists: A national UK survey. *International Journal of Language and Communication Disorders*, *47(6)*, 696–708.

Prior, M. & Cummins, R. (1992). Questions about Facilitated Communication and autism. *Journal of Autism and Developmental Disorders*, *22(3)*, 331–337.

Prior, M., Roberts, J.M.A., Rodger, S., Williams, K., & Sutherland, R. (2011). A review of the research to identify the most effective models of practice in early intervention of children with autism spectrum disorders. Australian Government Department of Families, Housing, Community Services and Indigenous Affairs (FaCSIA), Australia.

Prizant, B.M. & Fields-Meyer, T. (2015). *Uniquely Human: A Different Way of Seeing Autism*. New York, NY: Simon & Schuster.

Prizant, B.M. & Rubin, E. (1999). Contemporary issues in interventions for autism spectrum disorders: A commentary. *Journal of the Association for Persons with Severe Handicaps*, *24(3)*, 199–208.

Prizant, B., Wetherby, A.M., Rubin, E., Laurent, A.C., & Rydell, P. (2006). *The SCERTS Model: A Comprehensive Educational Approach for Children with Autism Spectrum Disorders*. Baltimore, MD: Paul H. Brookes.

Punja, S., Shamseer, L., Hartling, L., Urichuk, L., Vandermeer, B., Nikles, J. & Vohra S. (2016). Amphetamines for attention deficit hyperactivity disorder (ADHD) in children and adolescents. *Cochrane Database of Systematic Reviews*, Issue 2.Art. No.: CD009996. DOI: 10.1002/14651858.CD009996.pub2.

Quail, M., Sanderson, B., & Leitão, S. (2015). Ethical reasoning in clinical education: Achieving the balance. *Journal of Clinical Practice in Speech-Language Pathology*, *17(Supp. 1)*, 70–74.

Queensland Government (2015). *Final Report for the Evaluation of Queensland's Youth Boot Camps*. https://publications.qld.gov.au/dataset/final-report-for-the-evaluation-of-queenslands-youth-boot camps/resource/a654be83-cd7f-43b3-b6cd-cdf2c9c8b48d

Quincy, J. (MDCCLXXXVII [1787]). Lexicon physico-medicum; or, a new medicinal dictionary. Explaining the difficult terms used in the several branches of the profession, And in such Parts of Natural Philosophy, As are introductory thereto. With an Account of The things signified by such terms. The tenth edition, with new improvements from the latest authors. London, UK: T. Longman in Paternoster Row.

RCSLT (2011). *Developmental Verbal Dyspraxia* [Policy Statement]. Retrieved 11 July 2016 from www.rcslt.org

Randi, J. (2002) Homeopathy: The Test, BBC Horizon Programme Transcript, retrieved 2 November 2016 from www.bbc.co.uk/science/horizon/2002/homeopathyrandi.shtml

Rapley, G. (2011). Baby-led weaning: Transitioning to solid foods at the baby's own pace. *Community Practitioner, 84(6)*, 20–23.

Rasberry, C.N., Lee, S.M., Robin, L., Laris, B.A., Russell, L.A., Coyle, K.K., & Nihiser, A.J. (2011). The association between school-based physical activity, including physical education, and academic performance: A systematic review of the literature. *Preventive Medicine, 52*, S10–S20.

Ray, C. (2016). Inbox: Use of dolphins. *The ASHA Leader, 21(4)*, 5. Retrieved 19 June 2016 from http://leader.pubs.asha.org/article.aspx?articleid=2506037

Rayner, C., Denholm, C., & Sigafoos, J. (2009). Video-based intervention for individuals with autism: Key questions that remain unanswered. *Research in Autism Spectrum Disorders, 3(2)*, 291–303.

Reichow, B. (2012). Overview of meta-analyses on early intensive behavioral intervention for young children with autism spectrum disorders. *Journal of Autism and Developmental Disorders, 42(4)*, 512–520.

Reiner, C. & Willingham, D. (2010). The myth of learning styles. *Change, Sept–Oct*, 33–35.

Rice, M.L. (2014). Advocating for SLI. *International Journal of Language & Communication Disorders, 49(4)*, 402–405.

Richard, G.J. (2011). The role of the Speech-Language Pathologist in identifying and treating children with auditory processing disorder. *Language, Speech, and Hearing Services in Schools, 42(3)*, 297–302.

Richdale, A., Francis, A., Gavidia-Payne, S., & Cotton, S. (2000). Stress, behaviour, and sleep problems in children with an intellectual disability. *Journal of Intellectual and Developmental Disability, 25(2)*, 147–161.

Richdale, A.L. & Schreck, K.A. (2009). Sleep problems in autism spectrum disorders: Prevalence, nature, and possible biopsychosocial aetiologies. *Sleep Medicine Reviews, 13(6)*, 403–411.

Ritchie, K.D. & Goeke, J.L. (2006). Orton-Gillingham and Orton-Gillingham-based reading instruction: A review of the literature. *The Journal of Special Education, 40(3)*, 171–183.

Ritter, M.R., Colson, K.A., & Park, J. (2013). Reading intervention using interactive metronome in children with language and reading impairment: A preliminary investigation. *Communication Disorders Quarterly, 34(2)*, 106–119.

Roberts, G., Quach, J., Spencer-Smith, M., Anderson, P.J., Gathercole, S., Gold, L., ... & Wake, M. (2016). Academic outcomes 2 years after working memory training for children with low working memory: A randomized clinical trial. *JAMA Pediatrics, 170(5)*, e154568–e154568.

Roberts J.M.A. & Prior, M. (2006). A review of the research to identify the most effective models of practice in early intervention services for children with Autism Spectrum Disorders (ASD). Australian Government Department of Health and Ageing (DoHA).

Roberts, J.M.A. & Williams, K. (2016). Autism spectrum disorder: Evidence-based/evidence-informed good practice for supports provided to preschool children, their families and carers. Retrieved 29 July 2016 from https://myplace.ndis.gov.au/ndisstorefront/index.html

Roddam, H. & Skeat, J. (2010). *Embedding Evidence-Based Practice in Speech and Language Therapy: International Examples.* Oxford: Wiley-Blackwell.

Rogers, S.J. & Dawson, G. (2010). *Early Start Denver Model for Young Children with Autism: Promoting Language, Learning, and Engagement.* New York: The Guilford Press.

Rogers, S.J., Estes, A., Lord, C., Vismara, L., Winter, J., Fitzpatrick, A.... (2012). Effects of a brief Early Start Denver Model (ESDM)–based parent intervention on toddlers at risk for autism spectrum disorders: A randomized controlled trial. *Journal of the American Academy of Child & Adolescent Psychiatry, 51(10),* 1052–1065.

Romski, M., Sevcik, R.A., Barton-Hulsey, A., & Whitmore, A.S. (2015). Early intervention and AAC: What a difference 30 years makes. *Augmentative and Alternative Communication, 31(3),* 181–202.

Roethlisberger, F.J. & Dickson, W. (1939). *Management and the Worker.* Cambridge, MA: Harvard University Press.

Ross, E. & Fuhrman, L. (2015). Supporting oral feeding skills through bottle selection, *SIG 13 Perspectives on Swallowing and Swallowing Disorders (Dysphagia), 24(2),* 50–57.

Ross, S.W., Romer, N., & Horner, R.H. (2013). Teacher well-being and the implementation of schoolwide positive behavior interventions and supports. *Journal of Positive Behavior Interventions, 14(2),* 118–128.

Rose, J. (2006). *Independent Review of the Teaching of Early Reading.* UK: Department for Education and Skills.

Rosenthal, R. & Jacobson, L. (1968). *Pygmalion in the Classroom: Teacher Expectation and Pupils' Intellectual Development.* London: Holt, Rinehart & Winston.

Roulstone, S., Wren, Y., Bakopoulou, I., Goodlad, S., Lindsay, G. (2012). *Exploring Interventions for Children and Young People with Speech, Language and Communication Needs: A Study of Practice.* London: Department for Education.

Rowe, K. (2005). *Australia's National Inquiry into the Teaching of Literacy.* Melbourne: ACER.

Royal Australasian College of Physicians (2008). *A Consensus Approach for the Paediatrician's Role in the Diagnosis and Assessment of Autism Spectrum Disorders in Australia.* Retrieved 4 June 2016 from www.racp.edu.au/docs/default-source/advocacy-library/pa-pol-a-consensus-approach-for-the-paediatricians-role-in-the-diagnosis-and-assessment-of-autism.pdf

Rueda, M.R., Posner, M.I., & Rothbart, M.K. (2005). The development of executive attention: Contributions to the emergence of self-regulation. *Developmental Neuropsychology, 28(2),* 573–594.

Rupela, V., Velleman, S.L., & Andrianopoulos, M.V. (2016). Motor speech skills in children with Down syndrome: A descriptive study. *International Journal of Speech-Language Pathology, 18(5),* 483–492

Russell, L.M. (2014). Closing the dental divide. *Medical Journal of Australia, 201(11)*, 641–642.

Rvachew, S. (2015). *Autism is a Neurodevelopmental Disorder.* Retrieved 6 January 2015 from www.developmentalphonologicaldisorders.wordpress.com/2015/02/01

Rvachew, S. & Brosseau-Lapré, F. (2012). *Developmental Phonological Disorders: Foundations of Clinical Practice.* San Diego, CA: Plural Publishing.

Rvachew, S. & Brosseau-Lapré, F. (2018). *Developmental Phonological Disorders: Foundations of Clinical Practice, 2nd edition.* San Diego, CA: Plural Publishing.

Rvachew, S. & Rafaat, S. (2014). Report on benchmark wait times for pediatric speech sound disorders. *Canadian Journal of Speech-Language Pathology and Audiology, 38*, 82–96.

Sadleir, L.G., Paterson, S., Smith, K.R., Redshaw, N., Ranta, A., Kalnins, R., ... & Scheffer, I.E. (2015). Myoclonic occipital photosensitive epilepsy with dystonia (MOPED): A familial epilepsy syndrome. *Epilepsy Research, 114*, 98–105.

Sadoski, M. & Paivio, A. (2004). A dual coding theoretical model of reading. In R.B. Ruddell and N.J. Unrau (Eds), *Theoretical Models and Processes of Reading, 5th edition* (pp. 1329–1362). Newark, DE: International Reading Association.

Sagan, C. (1996). *Does Truth Matter? Science, Pseudoscience, and Civilization.* Skeptical Inquirer, 20(2) March/April. Retrieved 9 August 2016 from www.csicop.org/si/show/does_truth_matter_science_pseudoscience_and_civilization

Sallows, G.O. & Graupner, T.D. (2005). Intensive behavioral treatment for children with autism: Four-year outcome and predictors. *American Journal on Mental Retardation, 110(6), 417–438.*

Saloviita, T. (2016). Does linguistic analysis confirm the validity of facilitated communication? *Focus on Autism and Other Developmental Disabilities.* Published online, 2 May 2016, DOI: 10.1177/1088357616646075 1–9

Sandbank, M. & Yoder, P. (2016). The association between parental mean length of utterance and language outcomes in children with disabilities: A correlational meta-analysis. *American Journal of Speech-Language Pathology, 25(2)*, 240–251.

Sanders, M.R., Mazzucchelli, T.G., & Studman, L.J. (2004). Stepping Stones Triple P: The theoretical basis and development of an evidence-based positive parenting program for families with a child who has a disability. *Journal of Intellectual and Developmental Disability, 29(3)*, 265–283.

Sanders, M.R., Turner, K.M.T., & Markie-Dadds, C. (2002). The development and dissemination of the Triple P-Positive Parenting Program: A multilevel evidence-based system of parenting and family support. *Prevention Science, 3*, 173–198.

Santangelo, T. & Graham, S. (2015). A comprehensive meta-analysis of handwriting instruction. *Educational Psychology Review, 28(2)*, 1–41.

Satir, V. (1972). *Peoplemaking.* Palo Alto, CA: Science and Behavior Books.

Scarborough, H.S. & Brady, S.A. (2002). Toward a common terminology for talking about speech and reading: A glossary of the 'phon' words and some related terms. *Journal of Literacy Research, 34*, 299–334.

Schlosser, R.W., Balandin, S., Hemsley, B., Iacono, T., Probst, P., & von Tetzchner, S. (2014). Facilitated Communication and authorship: A systematic review. *Augmentative and Alternative Communication, 30(4)*, 359–368.

Schmidt, R. A., & Lee, T. D. (2011). *Motor Control and Learning: A Behavioural Emphasis*, 5th edition. Champaign, IL: Human Kinetics.

Schumann, J.H. & Alfandre, D. (2008). Clinical ethical decision making: The four topics approach. *Seminars in Medical Practice, 11*, 36–42.

Schreibman, L. (2005). *The Science and Fiction of Autism*. Cambridge: Harvard University Press.

Schwarz, A. (2014). Idea of new attention disorder spurs research, and debate. *The New York Times*, April 11. Accessed 17 July 2016 from http://mobile.nytimes.com/2014/04/12/health/idea-of-new-attention-disorder-spurs-research-and-debate.html

Serry, T., Rose, M., & Liamputtong, P. (2014). Reading Recovery teachers discuss Reading Recovery: A qualitative investigation. *Australian Journal of Learning Difficulties, 19(1)*, 61–73.

Sherry, M. (2016). Facilitated communication, Anna Stubblefield and disability studies. *Disability & Society. 31(7)*, 974–982.

Shinaver III, C.S., Entwistle, P.C., & Söderqvist, S. (2014). Cogmed WM training: Reviewing the reviews. *Applied Neuropsychology: Child, 3(3)*, 163–172.

Shire, S.Y. & Jones, N. (2015). Communication partners supporting children with complex communication needs who use AAC: A systematic review. *Communication Disorders Quarterly, 37*, 3–15.

Shriberg, L.D., Potter, N.L., & Strand, E.A. (2011). Prevalence and phenotype of childhood apraxia of speech in youth with galactosemia. *Journal of Speech, Language, and Hearing Research, 54(2)*, 487–519.

Shukla-Mehta, S., Miller, T., & Callahan, K.J. (2010). Evaluating the effectiveness of video instruction on social and communication skills training for children with autism spectrum disorders: A review of the literature. *Focus on Autism and Other Developmental Disabilities, 25(1)*, 23–36.

Sibley, M.H., Kuriyan, A.B., Evans, S.W., Waxmonsky, J.G., & Smith, B.H. (2014). Pharmacological and psychosocial treatments for adolescents with ADHD: An updated systematic review of the literature. *Clinical Psychology Review, 34(3)*, 218–232.

Silberman, S. (2015). *NeuroTribes: The Legacy of Autism and the Future of Neurodiversity*. Crows Nest, NSW: Allen & Unwin.

Singer, J. (2016). *NeuroDiversity: The Birth of an Idea*. Judy Singer: Sydney NSW, Amazon Digital Services.

Sinha, Y., Silove, N., Wheeler, D., & Williams, K. (2006). Auditory integration training and other sound therapies for autism spectrum disorders: A systematic review. *Archives of Disease in Childhood, 91(12)*, 1018–1022.

Singh, A., Uijtdewilligen, L., Twisk, J.W., Van Mechelen, W., & Chinapaw, M.J. (2012). Physical activity and performance at school: A systematic review of the literature including a methodological quality assessment. *Archives of Pediatrics & Adolescent Medicine, 166(1)*, 49–55.

Singh, S. & Ernst, E. (2008). *Trick or Treatment? Alternative Medicine on Trial*. Ealing, UK: Bantam Press.

Skinder-Meredith, A.E. (2015). Speech characteristics rating form. In C. Bowen, *Children's Speech Sound Disorders, 2nd edition* (pp. 312–318). Oxford: Wiley-Blackwell.

Sloan, S. & Ponsford, J. (2013). Managing cognitive problems following TBI. In J. Ponsford, S. Sloan, & P. Snow (eds), *Traumatic Brain Injury: Rehabilitation for Everyday Adaptive Living, 2nd edition* (pp. 99–132). London: Psychology Press.

Sonuga-Barke, E. J., Brandeis, D., Cortese, S., Daley, D., Ferrin, M., Holtmann, M., ... & Dittmann, R. W. (2013). Nonpharmacological interventions for ADHD: systematic review and meta-analyses of randomized controlled trials of dietary and psychological treatments. *American Journal of Psychiatry, 170*, 275–289.

Snow, P.C. (2009). Child maltreatment, mental health and oral language competence: Inviting Speech Language Pathology to the prevention table. *International Journal of Speech Language Pathology, 11(12)*, 95–103.

Snow, P.C. (2013). *The Snow Report*. Retrieved 27 January 2016 from www.pamelasnow.blogspot.com

Snow, P. C. (2014). Why not everyone is enthusiastic about the Arrowsmith Program. *The Snow Report*. Retrieved 5 January 2016 from www.pamelasnow.blogspot.com

Snow, P.C. (2016). Elizabeth Usher Memorial Lecture: Language is literacy is language— Positioning speech-language pathology in education policy, practice, paradigms and polemics. *International Journal of Speech-Language Pathology, 18(3)*, 216–228.

Snow, P.C. & Douglas, J. (2017) Psychosocial aspects of pragmatic language difficulties. In L. Cummings (Ed.) *Research in Clinical Pragmatics* (pp. 617-649), Cham, Switzerland: Springer-Verlag.

Snow, P.C. & Powell, M.B. (2011). Youth (in)justice: Oral language competence in early life and risk for engagement in antisocial behaviour in adolescence. *Trends & Issues in Crime and Criminal Justice, 435*, 1–6.

Snow, P.C., Powell, M.B. & Sanger, D.D. (2012). Oral language competence, young speakers and the law. *Language, Speech & Hearing Services in Schools, 43(4)*, 496–506.

Snow, P.C., Woodward, M., Mathis, M., & Powell, M.B. (2015). Language functioning, mental health and alexithymia in incarcerated young offenders. *International Journal of Speech-Language Pathology, 18(1)*, 20–31.

Söderqvist, S. & Nutley, S. (nd). Cogmed *Working Memory Training Claims & Evidence –Extended Version V.4*. Pearson. Retrieved 30 June 2016 from www.cogmed.com.au/userfiles/CogmedClaimsEvidenceV4.pdf

Sofronoff, K., Jahnel, D., & Sanders, M. (2011). Stepping Stones Triple P seminars for parents of a child with a disability: A randomized controlled trial. *Research in Developmental Disabilities, 32(6)*, 2253–2262.

Solomon, A. (2012). *Far from the Tree: Parents, Children, and the Search for Identity*. New York, NY: Scribner, US edition.

Solomon, A. (2013). *Far from the Tree: A Dozen Kinds of Love*. New York, NY: Scribner, UK edition.

Spaulding, L S., Mostert, M.P., & Beam, A.P. (2010). Is Brain Gym® an effective educational intervention? *Exceptionality, 18(1)*, 18–30.

Speech Pathology Association of Australia (2015). *Clinical Practice — Guides, Information Sheets and Frequently Asked Questions (FAQs): Advertising*. Melbourne: Author.

Speech Pathology Association of Australia (2009). *Position Paper: Evidence Based Speech Pathology Practice for Individuals with Autism Spectrum Disorder*. Melbourne: Author.

Speech Pathology Australia (2012). *Augmentative and Alternative Communication Clinical Guideline*. Melbourne: Author.

Spencer-Smith, M. & Klingberg, T. (2015). Benefits of a working memory training program for inattention in daily life: A systematic review and meta-analysis. *PloS one, 10(3)*, e0119522.

Spink, H. (2004). *Henrietta's Dream: A Mother's Search for a Better Life for Henry and Freddie*. London: Hodder & Stoughton.

Stacey-Knight, C.L. & Mayo, R. (2015). Comparing the codes of ethics of the six signatory associations of the Mutual Recognition Agreement. *International Journal of Speech-Language Pathology, 17(4)*, 421–430.

Stephenson, J. (2016). We need to know more about providing effective support for communication partners of children who use augmentative and alternative communication. *Evidence-Based Communication Assessment and Intervention, 10(1)*, 1–6.

Stephenson, J. & Wheldall, K. (2008). Miracles take a little longer: Science, commercialisation, cures and the Dore program. *Australasian Journal of Special Education, 32(1)*, 67–82.

Stockard, J. (2010). Promoting reading achievement and countering the "fourth-grade slump": The impact of Direct Instruction on reading achievement in fifth grade. *Journal of Education for Students Placed at Risk, 15(3)*, 218–240.

Storebø, O.J., Ramstad, E., Krogh, H.B., Nilausen, T.D., Skoog, M., Holmskovm M., Rosendal, S,, Groth, C., Magnusson, F.L., Moreira-Maia, C.R., Gillies, D., Buch Rasmussen, K., Gauci, D., Zwi, M., Kirubakaran, R., Forsbøl, B., Simonsen, E. & Gluud, C. (2015). Methylphenidate for children and adolescents with attention deficit hyperactivity disorder (ADHD). *Cochrane Database of Systematic Reviews*, Issue 11. Art. No.: CD009885. DOI: 10.1002/14651858.CD009885.pub2.

Strain, P.S. & Bovey II, E.H. (2011). Randomized, controlled trial of the LEAP model of early intervention for young children with autism spectrum disorders. *Topics in Early Childhood Special Education, 31(3)*, 133–154.

References

Strong, G.K., Torgerson, C.J., Torgerson, D., & Hulme, C. (2011). A systematic meta-analytic review of evidence for the effectiveness of the 'Fast ForWord' language intervention program. *Journal of Child Psychology & Psychiatry, 52(3)*, 224–235.

Steehler, M.W., Steehler, M.K., & Harley, E.H. (2012). A retrospective review of frenotomy in neonates and infants with feeding difficulties. *International Journal of Pediatric Otorhinolaryngology, 76(9)*, 1236–1240.

Stephens, D. & Upton, D. (2012). Speech and language therapists' understanding and adoption of evidence-based practice. *International Journal of Therapy and Rehabilitation, 19(6)*, 328–334.

Stephenson, J. & Wheldall, K. (2006). Macquarie University Special Education Centre. *MUSEC Briefings, 11*. Retrieved 29 June 2016 from www.musec.mq.edu.au/community_outreach/musec_briefings/

Strong, G.K., Torgerson, C.J., Torgerson, D., & Hulme, C. (2011). A systematic meta-analytic review of evidence for the effectiveness of the 'Fast ForWord' language intervention program. *Journal of Child Psychology & Psychiatry, 52(3)*, 224–235.

Suskind, R. (2014). *Life, Animated: A Story of Sidekicks, Heroes and Autism*. Glendale, CA: Kingswell.

Sutton, M. (Ed.) (2015). *The Real Experts: Readings for Parents of Autistic Children*. Fort Worth, TX: Autonomous Press.

Sydney Morning Herald (2010). *Persistence and Passion Speak Loudest*. Retrieved 22 January 2016 from www.smh.com.au/comment/obituaries/persistence-and-passion-speak-loudest-20101031-178v0.html

Szatmari, P., Georgiades, S., Duku, E., Bennett, T.A., Bryson, S., Fombonne, E., Mirenda, P., Roberts, W., Smith, I.M., Vaillancourt, T. et al. (2015). Developmental trajectories of symptom Severity and adaptive functioning in an inception cohort of preschool children with Autism Spectrum Disorder. *JAMA Psychiatry, 72(3)*, 276–283.

Tallal, P., Miller, S.L., Bedi, G., Byma, G., Wang, X., Nagarajan, S.S., Jenkins, W.M., & Merzenich, M.M. (1996). Language comprehension in language-learning impaired children improved with acoustically modified speech. *Science, 271*, 81–84.

Taylor, J. (2010). Psychotherapy for people with learning disabilities: Creating possibilities and opportunities. A review of the literature. *Journal of Learning Disabilities and Offending Behaviour, 1(3)*, 15–25.

Taylor, L.E., Swerdfeger, A.L., & Eslick, G.D. (2014). Vaccines are not associated with autism: An evidence-based meta-analysis of case-control and cohort studies. *Vaccine, 32(29)*, 3623–3629.

Thapar, A., Cooper, M., Eyre, O., & Langley, K. (2013). Practitioner review: What have we learnt about the causes of ADHD? *Journal of Child Psychology and Psychiatry, 54(1)*, 3–16.

Thoyre, S.M., Pados, B.F., Park, J., Estrem, H., Hodges, E.A., McComish, C., Van Riper, M., & Murdoch, K. (2014). Development and content validation of the Pediatric Eating Assessment Tool (Pedi-EAT). *American Journal of Speech-Language Pathology, 23(1)*, 46–59.

Tierney, A. & Kraus, N. (2013). Music training for the development of reading skills. Applying brain plasticity to advance and recover human ability. *Progress in Brain Research, 207*, 209–241.

Todd, A.J., Carroll, M.T., Robinson, A. & Mitchell, E.K.L. (2015). Adverse events due to chiropractic and other manual therapies for infants and children: A review of the literature. *Journal of Manipulative and Physiological Therapeutics, 38(9),* 699–712. Retrieved 31 December 2016 from http://dx.doi.org/10.1016/j.jmpt.2014.09.008

Todd, J.T. (2016). Old horses in new stables: Rapid Prompting, Facilitated Communication, science, ethics, and the history of magic. in R. Foxx & J.A. Mulick (Eds), *Controversial Therapies for Autism and Intellectual Disabilities: Fad, Fashion, and Science in Professional Practice,* 2nd edition (pp. 372–409). New York, NY: Routledge.

Tolstoy, L. (1894). *The Kingdom of God is Within You.* New York, NY: The Cassell Publishing Co.

Toner, D., Giordano, T., & Handler, S.D. (2014). Office frenotomy for neonates: Resolving dysphagia, parental satisfaction and cost-effectiveness. *ORL Head and Neck Nursing, 32(2),* 6–7.

Tostanoski, A., Lang, R., Raulston, T., Carnett, A., & Davis, T. (2013). Voices from the past: Comparing the rapid prompting method and facilitated communication. *Developmental Neurorehabilitation, 17(4),* 219–223.

Travers, J.C. (2016). Evaluating claims to avoid pseudoscientific and unproven practices in special education. *Intervention in School and Clinic,* Published early online 18 August 2016. DOI: 10.1177/1053451216659466

Travers, J.C., Ayres, K., Simpson, R.L., & Crutchfield, S. (2016). Fad, pseudoscientific, and controversial interventions. In R. Lang, T. Hancock, & N. Singh (Eds), *Early Intervention for Young Children with Autism Spectrum Disorders* (pp. 257–293). New York, NY: Springer.

Travers, J.C., Tincani, M., & Lang, R. (2014). Facilitated communication denies people with disabilities their voice. *Research and Practice for Persons with Severe Disabilities, 39(3),* 195–202.

Tunmer, W.E., Chapman, J.W., Greaney, K.T., Prochnow, J.E., & Arrow, A.W. (2013). Why the New Zealand national literacy strategy has failed and what can be done about it: Evidence from the progress in international reading literacy study (PIRLS) and Reading Recovery monitoring reports. *Australian Journal of Learning Disabilities, 18(2),* 139–180.

Turnbull, K., Reid, G.J., & Morton, J.B. (2013). Behavioral sleep problems and their potential impact on developing executive function in children. *Sleep, 36(7),* 1077.

Twain, M. (1897). *Following the Equator: A Journey Around the World.* Hartford, CT, The American Publishing Co. Retrieved 1 April 2016 from www.gutenberg.org/ebooks/2895

United Nations Human Rights, Office of the High Commissioner (1975). *Declaration on the Rights of Disabled Persons.* www.ohchr.org/EN/ProfessionalInterest/Pages/RightsOfDisabledPersons.aspx

Valicenti-McDermott, M., Burrows, B., Bernstein, L., Hottinger, K., Lawson, K., Seijo, R., Schechtman, M., Shulman, L., & Shinnar, S. (2014). Use of Complementary and Alternative Medicine in children with autism and other developmental disabilities: Associations with ethnicity, child comorbid symptoms, and parental stress. *Journal of Child Neurology, 29(3),* 360–367.

Vanderheiden, G.C. (2002). A journey through early augmentative communication and computer access. *Journal of Rehabilitation, Research and Development, 39(6)*, Supplement, 39-53.

Vandewater, E.A., Barr, R.F., Park, S.E., & Lee, S-J. (2010). A US study of transfer of learning from video to books in toddlers. *Journal of Children and Media, 4(4)*, 451-467.

Verdu, E.F., Armstrong, D., & Murray, J.A. (2009). Between celiac disease and irritable bowel syndrome: The "no man's land" of gluten sensitivity. *American Journal of Gastroenterology, 104(6)*, 1587-1594.

Victorian Ombudsman (2014). *Investigation into Disability Abuse Reporting.* Retrieved 21 January 2016 from www.ombudsman.vic.gov.au/Investigations/Investigation-into-disability-abuse-reporting

Virues-Ortega, J., Julio, F., & Pastor, R. (2013). The TEACCH program for children and adults with autism: A meta-analysis of intervention studies. *Clinical Psychology Review, 33(8)*, 940-953.

Vohra, S., Johnstone, B.C., Kramer, K., & Humphreys, K. (2007). Adverse events associated with pediatric spinal manipulation: A systematic review. *Pediatrics, 119(1)*, 275-283.

Vriezinga, S.L., Schweizer, J.J., Koning, F., & Mearin, L.L. (2015). Coeliac disease and gluten-related disorders in childhood. *Nature Reviews: Gastroenterology and Hepatology*, 12(9), 527-536.

Walker, N. (2012). What is Autism? In J. Bascom (Ed.), *Loud Hands: Autistic People, Speaking* (pp. 154-162). Washington, DC: The Autistic Press.

What Works Clearinghouse (2010). Løvaas model of applied behavior analysis. Retrieved 15 January 2016 from www.ies.ed.gov/ncee/wwc/reports/ece_cd/lovaas_model/index.asp

What Works Clearinghouse (2015). WWC Intervention Report: Lindamood Phoneme Sequencing (LiPS ®). Retrieved 28 August 2016 from http://ies.ed.gov/ncee/wwc/pdf/intervention_reports/wwc_lindamood_111015.pdf

Wheldall, K. & Bradd, L. (2010). Classroom seating arrangements and classroom behaviour. In K. Wheldall (Ed.) *Developments in Educational Psychology, 2nd edition* (pp. 181-195). Abingdon: Routledge.

Wickström, G. & Bendix, T. (2000). The "Hawthorne effect"—what did the original Hawthorne studies actually show? *Scandinavian Journal of Work, Environment & Health, 26(4)*, 363-367.

Weitlauf, A.S., McPheeters, M.L., Peters, B., Sathe, N., Travis, R., Aiello, R... (2014). Therapies for children with Autism Spectrum Disorder. *Behavioral Interventions Update. Comparative Effectiveness Review No. 137.* Rockville, MD: Agency for Healthcare Research and Quality.

Willcutt, E.G., Doyle, A.E., Nigg, J.T., Faraone, S.V., & Pennington, B.F. (2005). Validity of the executive function theory of attention-deficit/hyperactivity disorder: A meta-analytic review. *Biological Psychiatry, 57(11)*, 1336-1346.

White, P., Chant, D., Edwards, N., Townsend, C., & Waghorn, G. (2005). Prevalence of intellectual disability and comorbid mental illness in an Australian community sample. *Australian and New Zealand Journal of Psychiatry, 39(5)*, 395-400.

Whittingham, K., Sofronoff, K., Sheffield, J., & Sanders, M.R. (2009). Stepping Stones Triple P: An RCT of a parenting program with parents of a child diagnosed with an autism spectrum disorder. *Journal of Abnormal Child Psychology, 37(4)*, 469–480.

Wieder, S. & Greenspan, S.I. (2003). Climbing the symbolic ladder in the DIR model through floor time/interactive play. *Autism, 7(4)*, 425–435.

Williams, A.L., McLeod, S. & McCauley, R.J. (Eds) (2010). *Interventions for Speech Sound Disorders in Children*. Baltimore, MD: Paul H. Brookes Publishing Co.

Wilkes, G.A. (1985). *A Dictionary of Australian Colloquialisms, 2nd edition*. Sydney, NSW: Sydney University Press.

Wilson D.B., MacKenzie, D.L., & Mitchell, F.N. (2005). Effects of correctional boot camps on offending. *Campbell Systematic Reviews*, 6. DOI: 10.4073/csr.2005.6

Wilson, K.P. (2013). Incorporating video modeling into a school-based intervention for students with autism spectrum disorders. *Language, Speech, and Hearing Services in Schools, 44(1)*, 105–117.

Wilson, P., Rush, R., Hussey, S., Puckering, C., Sim, F., Allely, C. S., ... & Gillberg, C. (2012). How evidence-based is an 'evidence-based parenting program'? A PRISMA systematic review and meta-analysis of Triple P. *BMC Medicine, 10(1)*, 1–16.

Winner, M.G. (2000). *Inside Out: What Makes a Person with Social Cognitive Deficits Tick?* San Jose, CA: Think Social Publishing.

Winner, M.G. (2013). *Why Teach Social Thinking*? San Jose, CA: Think Social Publishing.

Winner, M.G. & Crooke, P.J. (2009). Social Thinking: A training paradigm for professionals and treatment approach for individuals with social learning/social pragmatic challenges. *Perspectives on Language Learning and Education, 16*, 62–69.

Winner, M.G. & Crooke, P. (2014). Executive functioning and social pragmatic communication skills: Exploring the threads in our social fabric. *SIG 1 Perspectives on Language Learning and Education, 21*, 42–50.

Wiseman, F.K., Alford, K.A., Tybulewicz, V.L., & Fisher, E.M. (2009). Down syndrome: Recent progress and future prospects. *Human Molecular Genetics, 18(R1)*, R75–R83.

World Health Organization (2003). *Global Strategy for Infant and Young Child Feeding*. Geneva: WHO.

World Health Organization (2012). *Health Topics: Oral Health*. Retrieved 5 February 2016 from www.who.int/mediacentre/factsheets/fs318/en/.

World Health Organization (2016). *International Classification of Diseases (ICD)*. Retrieved 8 February 2016 from www.who.int/classifications/icd/en/

Yeager, D.S. & Dweck, C.S. (2012). Mindsets that promote resilience: When students believe that personal characteristics can be developed. *Educational Psychologist, 47(4)*, 302–314.

Zimmerman, F.J., Christakis, D.A., & Meltzoff, A.N. (2007). Associations between media viewing and language development in children under age two years. *Journal of Pediatrics, 151(4)*, 364–368.

Zuberer, A., Brandeis, D., & Drechsler, R. (2015). Are treatment effects of neurofeedback training in children with ADHD related to the successful regulation of brain activity? A review on the learning of regulation of brain activity and a contribution to the discussion on specificity. *Frontiers in Human Neuroscience, 9*, 135.

Index

AAC, Augmentative and Alternative
    Communication 149-154, 159, 166-169,
    182, 185, 307
ABA; Applied Behaviour Analysis; Behaviour
    Analyst 73, 74, 75-77, 82-84, 118
Accelerating typical development; hothousing
    15, 19, 29, 299
    Baby Einstein™ 20-21, 26
    Baby Sign Language 24, 27-30, 339
    Brainy Baby® 20, 22-23, 339
    Brainy Child 20, 24, 268, 339
    HEGL/Heguru™ 24, 26-27, 331, 338
    Glenn Doman™ 25, 49, 268, 338
    Jones Geniuses Accelerated Education 21-22
    Mercury Learning Systems 20, 24, 339
    Music for Babies™ 21
    Shichida™ 24-26, 198, 268, 331, 339
    Teach Your Baby to Read 20
    The Infant Learning Company 22
    The Kiddly Company 22
    WeeHands™ 27-29, 339
Acquired brain injury (ABI) 113, 151, 154, 181
Activities of daily living (ADL) 92, 94, 271
Ad hominem 333
Alternative medicine (see Complementary
    and alternative medicine)
Amygdala 98, 107
Amyotrophic Lateral Sclerosis 279
Anecdotal evidence 2
Animal Assisted Intervention (AAI);
    Animal Assisted Therapy 71, 94-98, 338
    Companion animals 95
    Dolphin therapy 95, 97-98, 313, 314, 322, 339
    Hippotherapy (Equine assisted therapy) 74, 96, 97, 339
    Man and Beast 96
    Marine mammals 98
    Pet therapy 96
    Riding for the Disabled 95
    Service animals 95, 96
    Therapy animals 95
Anthroposophy 8, 94
    Camphill Movement 81, 94, 338
    Karl Koenig 94
    Rudolf Steiner 7, 94
    Waldorf/Rudolf Steiner 94, 247-248
Whole Language 7, 9, 76, 178, 226-228, 233, 247, 296, 339
Applied Behaviour Analysis (ABA) 27, 82-84, 118, 140
Apps 20, 48, 242, 247
Apraxia (see Childhood Apraxia of Speech; CAS)
Arrowsmith Program™ 7, 9, 178, 234-236, 237, 240, 318, 331, 339
Articulation (see Speech; Articulation)
Assessment 4, 54, 70, 112, 115-116, 140-141, 147, 151, 170, 172, 176-177, 206-207, 308, 321
    ADHD 33-38, 57
    ASD 70, 72, 74, 83, 84, 85, 91, 101, 140
    Executive control 31
    Focus 31-32, 36, 108, 200
    Audiological 170, 202, 211
    Auditory processing 216
    Down syndrome 196-197
    Dysarthria 181
    Dyslexia; reading 230-231, 249
    Dysphagia 264
    In-person assessment 172, 194
    OT 126
    Oral motor; non-speech tasks 191
    Psychological 111
    RTI 42
    Reports 14, 177
    Self-, DIY-, online- assessments; self-test 17, 53
    Sensory integration 207, 324
Asperger syndrome 59, 66-67, 280
Astrological Psychology (Psychological
    Astrology) 94, 98-99, 173, 338
    94, 98-99, 173, 338
Attention 31-32, 36-38, 129
    Executive control 31
    Focus 31-32, 36, 108, 200
    Joint 59, 88, 129, 147
Attention Deficit Hyperactivity Disorder
    (ADHD) 7, 33-57
    Practice Guidelines 38
Audiologist/Audiology 164, 171, 191, 202, 203, 206, 207, 211, 213, 303, 305, 306
Auditory Integration Treatments 71, 78, 177-178, 209-213, 296, 313, 331, 339
    ASHA Position Statement on 213
    Johansen Individualized Auditory

Stimulation 177, 211, 331, 339
Music for Babies™ 21
Samonas™ Sound Therapy 209-210, 213, 323, 331, 339
The Berard AIT Method 177, 209-210, 212, 213, 331, 339
The Listening Program® 21, 178, 209, 210, 331, 339
Therapeutic Listening™ 178, 331, 339
Tomatis® 178, 209-213, 313, 318, 331, 339
Auditory mechanism 201
Autism Speaks 65, 66, 68
Autism Spectrum Disorder (ASD) 34, 59-104, 151, 181, 205, 263, 321
Balanced literacy/Balanced instruction (see Literacy; Reading; Spelling; Handwriting; Typing)
Behaviour; conduct 105-148
   ADHD 7, 33-57
   Anxiety 79, 95, 110-116, 142, 146, 150, 151, 196, 249, 262
   Attunement 131, 135
   Behaviours of concern 218
   Cognitive-behaviour therapy (CBT) 110, 118, 142-145
   Conduct disorder 111, 136
   Corporal punishment 122-123, 131
   Crying; Controlled crying; Crying it out 105, 118, 120, 135, 172, 338
   DSM-5 33, 34, 59, 70, 111, 204, 268, 269
   Depression 79, 110-111, 114, 142, 144, 146, 262
   Externalizing disorders 109-111
   Family therapy 146, 172-173, 303
   Four P's 113-114
   Internalizing disorders 109-111
   Oppositional defiant disorder (ODD) 34, 111
   Parenting programs 131, 132-133, 136-137
   Pharmacological therapies 110
   Psychiatry 111, 112
   Psychoeducation 115, 137
   Self-efficacy 55-56, 132, 135
   Self-regulation 32, 43-44, 89, 104-108, 119-120
   Self-soothing 106, 119-121
   Smacking; slapping 82, 106, 121-123, 131, 339
   Stimming; self-stimulatory behaviours 81, 129, 298
   Temperament 109, 113
   Triple-P Positive Parenting 131-134, 338
   Tuning into Kids 135-136
Behaviour as a form of communication 130
Behavioural and emotional attunement 131, 135
Behavioural optometrist/Optometry 6, 178, 242, 331, 339
Belief 11, 14, 17, 23, 53, 56-57, 73, 132, 143, 144, 161, 166, 264, 277-278, 289, 315, 321
Best practice 11, 86, 304, 306, 321
Big Pharma 57, 166, 241
Body Work 8, 339
Boot Camp 125, 339
Brain
   Acquired brain injury (ABI) 113, 151, 154, 181
   Amygdala 98, 107
   Brain-based learning 51-52, 268, 294-295, 339
   Frontal lobes 108
   Imaging 235-236, 237, 294
   Left-brain- Right-brain- Whole-brain learning 23, 25, 27, 29-30, 51-53, 323, 339
   Limbic system 107-108
   Prefrontal region 32, 107-108
   "Re-wiring" the brain 55, 57, 237
   Scans 58, 237
   Training 9, 27, 48
   Traumatic brain injury 193
Brain Gym® (Educational Kinesiology) 9, 49-51, 318, 331, 339
Camphill 85, 94, 338
Casein 66, 263-264, 272, 281, 284-286, 313, 339
Casuistry 319-320, 321, 326, 327, 332
Case vignettes
   Abbie 114-115, 299
   Guy 2-3
   Jack 62-64, 65, 262-263, 299
   Kim 199-200, 204, 299
   Pattie 118, 299
   Robert-Louis 299, 323, 325, 330-331
   Tomás 299, 322, 324
Celebrity-Based Practice 5
Central Auditory Processing Disorder (CAPD) 199, 200, 203-217
Celebrity endorsement 7, 17, 256, 263, 278, 313
Central Executive 33
Cerebellar Developmental Delay (CDD) 17, 336
Cerebral Palsy 36, 49, 113, 126, 151, 153, 154-156, 181, 261, 271-272

Index

Chelation 66, 79, 276-280, 287, 313, 314, 323, 331, 339
   Amalgam illness 17, 288
   Mercury 277, 313
Childhood Apraxia of Speech; CAS 15, 178-179, 180-181, 187, 189, 193, 274, 315
   CASANA 189
   Elad Vashdi Apraxia VML Method 187-190, 318, 331, 339
Chiropractic 6, 8, 79, 127, 173, 198, 242, 248, 265, 313, 323, 331, 339
Circle Time 110, 137-139
Classical music
   Mozart 20, 210
   Music for Babies™ 21
   Musical training 214-215
Cleft lip and palate 17, 179, 191, 193, 261, 270
Clinical reasoning; clinical thinking 205, 319
Cluttering 194
Cochrane Collaboration; Cochrane Review 37, 38, 147, 158, 182, 212, 213, 231
Coeliac disease 263, 266, 284, 285, 286
   Gluten-sensitivity autoimmune disorder 286
Cogmed Working Memory Training 45-49, 339
Cognitive Behaviour Therapy (CBT) 110, 118, 142-145
Cognitive bias 163, 314-317
   Authority Effect 316, 324
   Backfire Effect 124, 315-316, 330
   Bandwagon Effect 4, 296, 316, 340
   Belief Bias 315
   Blind-spot Bias 314
   Confirmation Bias 3, 163, 315
   Dunning-Kruger Effect 314, 315
   Expectancy Bias 45, 288, 295
   Hawthorne Effect 295
   IKEA (not-invented-here) Effect 316, 322
   Pygmalion Effect 295
   Rosenthal Effect 295
   Self-serving Bias 315
Complementary and Alternative Medicine (CAM) 127, 248, 273
Concentration Deficit Disorder 35
Conditioning
   Classical 107, 117, 118
   Operant 44, 67, 83, 117, 118
Continuing Professional Development (CPD) 75, 191, 265, 303, 306, 316, 317, 321-322, 324-325, 328
Control group 298

Coriander (cilantro) 280
Counselling 8, 80, 94, 131, 144, 172
Cranial osteopathy 121, 127, 248, 313
Craniosacral therapy 8, 79, 121, 177, 248, 265, 339
Critical thinking 332
DSM-5 33, 34, 59, 70, 111, 204, 268, 269
Diagnosis 112, 204, 207, 320
   Diagnostic labels: Pros and cons 16
   Home diagnosis; DIY diagnosis; self-diagnosis 17, 169, 246
   No diagnosis; Diagnostic uncertainty 300-301
   Symptom cluster 15
Developmental Language Disorder; Language Disorder (DLD) 15, 166, 176-178, 199, 204, 206-207, 224, 304-305
Developmental Verbal Dyspraxia; DVD (see Childhood Apraxia of Speech; CAS)
Diet; dietary supplements; complementary medicine
   Alkaline diet 280-281, 338
   Apraxia Diet (see Speech Diet)
   Bioindividual nutrition 282, 339
   Blue-green algae; Chlorella; Green algae 257, 280, 287
   Body ecology diet 7, 281, 282, 339
   Candida diet 280-281, 282, 313, 339
   Casein free diet 66, 263, 264, 281, 339
   Chlorella 280
   Coeliac disease 263, 266, 284, 285, 286
   Coriander (cilantro) 280
   Deepak Chopra 276
   Essential fatty acids; Omega-3 fatty acids; fish oil 8, 9, 80, 173, 274, 275-276
   FODMAPs; low FODMAPS diet 263-264, 338
   GAPS nutritional protocol 7, 17, 282, 284, 287, 339
   GFCF diet 71, 263, 264, 284-286, 331, 33
   Hemsley and Hemsley 7, 256, 263, 284
   Homeopathy 6-8, 79-80, 94, 127, 173-175, 195, 198, 229, 242, 248, 258-259, 313-314, 339
   Irritable bowel syndrome (IBS) 263, 283
   Juice Plus+ 7, 339
   Kefir 281, 339
   Non-celiac gluten sensitivity 263
   Nourish Life SPEAK; SPEAK 276
   NutriiVeda 276, 340

Omega-3 fatty acids 79-80, 266, 274, 275-276
Probiotics 281, 284
Rainbow diet 287, 338
Specific carbohydrate diet (SCD) 80, 282-283, 287, 339
Speech Diet 276, 338
Spiritual Nutrition 287, 339
Succussion 174
Dietician; Dietitian 3, 173, 254, 263, 264, 266, 272, 286, 289
Nutritionist 6, 254, 256, 257, 282
Digraph 223
Disease mongering 240-241
Depression 67, 79, 110, 111, 142, 143, 144, 146, 262
Do-it-yourself Intervention (see Manualized intervention)
Doctors
   Doctorate; AuD, DPhil, EdD, PhD 4, 294
   Dr Credible 19, 29
   Dr Phil 128, 267
   Dr Poo 257
   Family Doctor 8, 116, 139
   General Practitioner (GP) 8, 116, 177, 286
   Paediatrician 79, 116, 140, 141, 172, 261, 266, 286
Dore Achievement Centres; DDAT; Dore Treatment 298, 336
Dosage 116, 325
Dysarthria 153, 155, 178, 179, 181-182, 183, 185, 195, 197
Dyslexia (see Literacy; Reading; Spelling)
Dysphagia 260-263, 264, 270, 307, 337
Dyslexia Dyspraxia Attention Treatment (DDAT); Wynford Dore 298, 336
Education; Educators (see Teaching)
Einstein, Albert 20-21
Electroencephalogram (EEG) 43-45
Eminence-based Practice 5
Epilepsy 43, 55, 80, 95, 96, 113, 116, 140, 314
Etalon 195, 331, 339
Ethics 10, 76, 164
   AAC ethics 150, 154, 157-162, 164, 169
   Animal ethics 95, 98
   Code of Ethics 4, 76, 254
   Ethical dilemmas 304-305, 308-309, 317-320, 320-333
   Ethical eating 289
   Ethical practice and responsibilities 48, 76, 84, 154, 169, 184-185, 306

Research ethics 166, 288, 298
Unethical conduct 78, 83, 98, 162, 165, 214
Every Student Succeeds Act (ESSA) 326, 327
Evidence Based Education (EBE) 11-12, 13, 225, 230, 244, 250, 252-2§53
Evidence Based Practice (EBP, E³BP) 5, 10-13, 70, 77, 97, 146, 147, 185, 329, 331-332, 258, 325-326
Executive control 31-32
Facilitated Communication (FC) 7, 71, 76, 78, 154-166, 169, 296, 313, 314, 315, 337, 339
   Amy Sequenzia 66, 67
   Andrew Solomon 69
   Ari Ne'eman 67
   "Assisted Communication" 155
   Discredited 78, 157, 161, 331
   Douglas Biklen 66, 69, 157, 159, 163
   Rapid Prompting Method (RPM) 66, 78, 150, 164, 337, 338
   Rosemary Crossley 154-156, 158
   Saved by Typing 150
   Soma® RPM 78, 337
   Supported Typing 67, 78, 150, 337, 339
   The Real Experts 65, 66
   Type to Communicate 339
Fad 1, 2, 4, 35, 69, 74, 75-77, 163, 171, 194, 197, 252, 263, 264, 336
Faith 156-157, 165-166, 241, 289, 316
Family; Family life; Parents 3, 10, 30, 68-69, 78, 93, 128-131
   Boundaries 128, 132, 135, 299, 300, 310, 317
   Far from the Tree 65, 68-69
   Pressure from family and friends 30, 296, 299-300
   Priorities 12
   Scapegoat 173
   Relationships 30, 119, 299-300
   Family Therapy 146, 172-173
Five big ideas of literacy instruction (see Literacy; Reading; Spelling; Handwriting; Typing)
Five from Five Literacy Project (see Literacy; Reading; Spelling; Handwriting; Typing)
Fluency (see Stuttering; Stammering; Cluttering)
Feuerstein Instrumental Enrichment 48, 313, 340
Functional (idiopathic) 180
Genetics 61
Global developmental delay 15
Grapheme 221, 222, 229

Index

Grandparent 3, 103, 106, 139, 197, 260, 290, 299
Greenfield, Susan 55
Growth Mind-set 55-57, 338
Guru 255, 256, 265, 266
Handwriting 249
HRH Prince Charles 7
Health and Care Professions Council (HCPC) 3, 304
Henry Spink Foundation 313-314
Holistic Medicine (see Complementary and Alternative Medicine)
Home schooling 22, 167-16
Hope 13, 48, 64, 163, 165, 288, 302, 336, 34
Homeopathy 6-8, 79-80, 94, 127, 173-175, 195, 198, 229, 242, 248, 258-259, 296, 313-314, 331, 339
Hothousing (see Accelerating typical development)
Hyperbaric oxygen chamber 79, 313, 339
ICF Framework 9
ICF-CY 74
IQ (Intelligence Quotient) 266-268, 268-270, 295
   Intellectual disability (ID) 15, 58, 61, 94, 268, 271-272
   Learning disability 15, 94, 268
   "Mental retardation" 268
Ichimankai 27
Idiopathic 113, 180
Individualized Education Plan (IEP) 90
Information literacy 310, 312, 314
Institutes for the Achievement of Human Potential 25, 49, 77
Integrative Medicine (see Complementary and Alternative Medicine)
International Communication Project (ICP) 163-164
Internet (and see Social Media; Websites) 9-10, 164, 180-181, 191, 207, 234, 258, 310-314
Intelligence Quotient (see IQ)
Interventions
   Affinity Therapy 78, 79, 338
   Arrowsmith Program™ 7, 9, 178, 234-236, 237, 240, 318, 331, 339
   Auditory Integration Treatments/Training 71, 78, 177-178, 207-214, 296, 313, 331, 339
   Autism Seminars for Families 78, 93, 338
   Baby Einstein™ 20, 21, 26
   Bioindividual Nutrition® 282, 339
   Boot Camp 125, 33
   BrainGym® 25, 49, 268
   Brainy Baby® 20, 22-23, 339
   Brain Building and Kinetic Learning 96
   CEASE Therapy 79, 339
   Camphill 81, 94, 338
   Crispiani Method 247, 339
   DIR®; DIRFloortime® 78, 84-85, 338
   EarlyBird and EarlyBird Plus programs 78, 93
   Disney Therapy 78-79, 338
   Dolphin therapy 95, 97-98, 313, 315, 322, 339
   Early Start Denver Model (ESDM) 92-93
   Facilitated Communication (FC) 7, 71, 76, 78, 154-166, 169, 296, 313, 314, 315, 337, 339
   Feuerstein Instrumental Enrichment 48, 313, 340
   Functional Communication Training 71, 78, 81, 85
   GemIIni™ 100-101, 331, 339
   Glenn Doman™ 25, 338
   Hanen Programs® 75, 78, 93, 338
   Horse Boy method (Horseboy method) 96
   Interactive Metronome® 178, 209, 239, 318, 331, 339
   Irlen® Lenses and Overlays 16, 178, 241-242, 314, 318, 339
   Kill Your Lisp 187, 190, 195, 339
   Kill Your Stutter 190, 195, 339
   Kip Online 178, 339
   Learning Experiences-An Alternative Program for Preschoolers and Parents (LEAP) 77, 78, 90-91, 338
   Løvaas Method 67, 77, 81-82, 313, 339
   Lumosity 48
   Moor House School and College 177
   Neurolinguistic Programming™ NLP™ 127, 340
   Non-speech Oral Motor Treatments; NS-OMT 9, 186, 190-191, 316, 318, 321, 323, 331, 340
   Oral Placement Therapy 190, 340
   PECS™ 71, 75, 78, 81, 85-87, 90, 150, 338
   PROMPT© 75, 186, 265, 318, 331, 338
   Positive Behaviour Support (PBS) 71, 78, 90, 93
   Psychodynamic interventions 80
   Psychological astrology 94, 98-99, 338
   Rainbow diet 287, 338
   Relationship Development Intervention® (RDI™) 75, 78, 94, 101-102, 338

Reading Recovery™ (RR) 9, 178, 232, 318, 331, 339
SCERTS® Model 91, 338
Samonas™ Sound Therapy 209-210, 323, 331, 339
Schuhfried CogniPlus and NeuroMite 47-48
Sensory Integration Therapy 76, 78, 125-12, 140, 324, 339
Shichida™ 24-27, 198, 268, 331, 339
Social Stories® 62, 78, 81, 87-88, 338
Social Thinking® 72, 78, 81, 88-90, 322, 338
Son-Rise Program® 64, 94, 102, 282, 331, 339
Speech Buddies™ 187, 192-193, 338
TEACCH® 78, 81, 91-92, 338
Talking Mats 166-167, 338
TalkTools® 74, 75, 186, 191, 625, 308-309, 318, 331, 339
Therapeutic Listening™ 178, 331, 339
Therapeutic Touch Therapy 76, 339
Tomatis® 178, 209, 212-213, 318, 331, 339
Toy Libraries 142
Traditional Chinese Medicine 8
Triple-P 131-136, 338
Tuning into Kids 131, 135, 338
Vocal Science™ 173, 339
VML Method; Verbal Motor Learning; Elad Vashdi 187-190, 318, 331, 339
WeeHands™ 27-29, 339
Journals; Journal articles 4-5, 8, 64, 75, 167, 236, 289, 292-294, 312, 326
  Jeffrey Beall 293-294, 341
  Open Access 38, 46, 107, 225, 233, 293-294, 312, 332
  Pay walled 296, 309, 311-312
  Predatory 293-294
Lactation consultant 260, 264
Language 152, 175-178, 199, 202-203
Late talkers 176
Leaky gut 285
  Opioid-Excess Theory 285, 340
Learning disability (see Specific Learning Disability; see Intellectual Disability)
Learning styles 53-54, 56, 268, 339
Left-brain, Right-brain, Left-brain-right-brain 9, 339
  Brain balancing 24, 268
  Olfactory stimulation kit 24
  Shichida™ 24-27, 198, 268, 331, 339
  Whole brain teaching 51, 52, 339

Limbic system 52, 107-108
Literacy; reading; spelling; handwriting; typing
  Alphabetic principle 221-22, 229
  Children of the Code 230-231
  "Dyslexia" 229-231
  Handwriting 249
  Instructional casualties 230, 252
  National Inquiries into Reading 70, 227, 228-229, 244, 251, 253
  Reading -Disorder -Difficulties -Disability 15, 35, 41-43, 178, 206, 230, 241, 248, 249-253
  Reading theories and methods
    Arrowsmith™; Arrowsmith Program™ 7, 9, 178, 234-236, 237, 240, 318, 331, 339
    Balanced Literacy (Balanced Instruction) 228-229, 339
    Behavioural Optometry 242, 331, 339
    Brain Gym® 9, 25, 49, 268, 318, 331, 339
    Cellfield™ 9, 178, 237-238, 318, 331, 339
    Choral Reading (Echo Reading) 251
    Dolch Words 229
    Dyslexia Diet 248
    Dyslexie font 242, 248, 339
    Fast ForWord 238-239, 331, 340
    Five big ideas of reading instruction 223-225
    Five from Five Literacy Project 225,
    Interactive Metronome® 178, 209, 239, 318, 331, 339
    Institute for Multisensory Language Education 242, 244
    Irlen® Lenses (Coloured Lenses and Overlays) 16, 178, 240-242, 313, 314, 339
    Lindamood-Bell 244-246, 250, 338
    MultiLit®; MiniLit 251-252
    Multi-Cueing (aka Searchlights) 227, 339
    Orthography 223,
    Orton Gillingham 242-244, 338
    Phonics-based instruction 222, 224-227, 250
    RIP IT UP Reading© 246, 338
    Systematic synthetic phonics 225, 228-229, 243, 252-253
    Reading Recovery™ 9, 178, 232, 318, 331, 339
    Sight Words 229
    Spalding 242

Steiner Education/Waldorf Education
247-248
Switch On Reading 9, 232, 339
Three Cueing approach (Searchlights)
227, 339
Whole Language (WL) 7, 9, 76, 178,
226-228, 233, 247, 296, 339
Made-up conditions
Amalgam Illness 17, 278-280, 288
Cerebellar Developmental Delay (CDD)
17, 336
Functional Disconnection syndrome 17, 288
Gameboy Disease 17
Gluten Allergy 263
Gut and Physiology Syndrome (GAPS) 17,
282, 284
Gut and Psychology Syndrome (GAPS) 17,
282, 284
Irritable Baby Syndrome 17
Irlen® Syndrome 17, 240-242, 288, 314
Magnetic Field Deficiency syndrome 8, 17,
76
Meares-Irlen Syndrome 241
Multiple Chemical Sensitivity 17, 288
Non-celiac gluten sensitivity 263
Nonverbal Learning Disability 17
Retained Neonatal Reflexes™ 17, 36, 288
Retained Reflex Syndrome 17, 36
Scotopic Sensitivity Syndrome (Visual
Stress) 323, 241
Sensory Integration Disorder 17, 126, 288
Wilson's Temperature syndrome 17, 288
Magic six weeks 321, 323
Magical thinking 18, 291
Majority World 305-306, 307-308
Manualized intervention 72
Mark Twain 316-317
Medications 37-38, 79, 116-117, 261
Mental illness 95, 102, 279
Miracle Mineral Solution (MMS) 79, 286, 339
Morneau Shepell 27
Motor Neurone Disease 153
Multilingualism 324
MultiLit® 251-252
Multiple Intelligences 56-57, 270, 339
Multi-cueing (aka Searchlights) 227, 339
MUSEC Briefings 86, 238, 302
Music Therapy 71, 146-147
Musical Training 214-215
OPERA Hypothesis 214

Mutual Recognition Agreement (MRA) 163,
306, 322
National Health Service (NHS) 305
Nature (journal) 4, 5, 61
Natural Medicine (see Complementary and
Alternative Medicine)
Neurodiversity 61, 62, 65, 67, 83, 103
Neurofeedback 37, 43-45, 178, 338
Neuromyths 23, 52-53
Neuropsychology 46, 48, 169, 324
Neuroscience 52, 55, 235, 237, 246, 247,
294-295, 324
NeuroTribes 62, 65, 66, 67, 103
Neurotypical (NT) 62
No Child left Behind Act (NCLB) 42, 326
Nobel Laureate 7
Non-speech Oral Motor Treatments; NS-OMT
9, 186, 190-192, 318, 321, 323-324, 331, 340
Oral Placement Therapy OPT 190, 340
TalkTools® 74, 75, 186, 191, 625, 308-309,
318, 331, 339
Nutritionist 6, 254, 256, 257, 282
Occupational Therapy (OT) 13, 67, 97
Opportunity cost 9, 47, 127, 211, 244, 297, 301,
331
Oral health 3, 265-266, 270-273, 289
Panacea 72, 104, 287-288
Parenting 1, 14, 45, 106, 117-118, 121-122,
128-131, 132-137, 148, 299-300
Peer review 4-5, 7, 246
Pencil and paper activities 48-49, 150, 249
Pharmacy/Pharmacist 3, 13, 117, 142, 174, 258,
Phone 178
Consonant 178, 182, 183, 184, 197, 214,
221, 223
Vowel 178, 182, 183, 197, 221
Phoneme 178, 221, 222, 229
Phonics-based reading instruction (see Literacy;
Reading; Spelling; Handwriting; Typing)
Placebo 6, 44-45
Placebo effect 288, 295
Sugar pill 174, 288
Polypharmacy 116-117
Practice-based research (PBR) 89
Professionals; Mainstream professionals 1, 3-5,
9, 74
Professional Associations and Societies (see also
Client advocacy)
American Library Association 310
American Psychiatric Association 33, 58, 111, 204, 268

American Psychological Association 67, 146
American Physical Therapy Association 188
Association of Health Care Journalists 9
Australian Music Therapy Association 146
Australian Psychological Society 146, 304
British Chiropractic Association 8
British Dietetics Association 254
British Psychological Society 146
Chinese International Speech-Language and Hearing Association 308
Dietitians Association of Australia 254
Guild of Health Writers 9
International Association of Animal-Human Interactions Organizations 95
Pharmaceutical Society of Australia 258
Society for Children as Money-spinners 19, 30
Professional Associations (MRA signatories) 3-5, 75, 322, 328-329, 332
   ASHA 75, 77, 88, 98, 162, 163, 180, 188-190, 213, 305-306, 322, 328, 332
   IASLT 75, 163, 305-306, 322, 328
   NZSTA 75, 163, 305-306, 322, 328
   RCSLT 75, 163, 180, 304, 305-306, 322, 325-326, 328
   SAC-OAC 75, 163, 305-306, 322, 328
   SPA 5, 75, 150, 162, 163, 189, 305-306, 322, 328
Prognosis 176, 323
Progressive neurological disorders 261
Pseudoscience ix, 1, 2, 8, 16-18, 29, 52, 54, 74, 75-77, 89, 94-104, 165-166, 173-175, 177-178, 187-193, 194-195, 197-198, 248, 257, 258-259, 273-288, 291-292, 313-314, 329, 331, 336
"Pseudoscience alert" 97, 100, 257, 282, 283
Psychologist/Psychology 2, 3, 6, 9, 10, 13, 17, 39, 48, 56, 57, 68, 69, 71,73, 75, 76, 78, 81, 83, 84, 86, 88, 90, 101, 110-112, 115, 117, 124, 131, 132, 140, 158, 172, 177, 178, 203, 204, 206, 207, 228, 230, 241, 264, 267, 269, 270, 284, 288, 295, 301, 303, 315, 324.
Psychological Astrology 98-99, 173
Rare diseases, conditions and disorders 16
   National Organization for Rare Disorders (NORD) 16
Reading (see Literacy; Reading; Spelling; Handwriting; Typing)
Rebounder; rebounding 276, 281
Red flag(s) 112, 115, 140, 211, 233, 236, 237, 287

Research; Scientific research 5-6
   Juried literature 4, 101, 235, 265, 311
   Literacy 233, 309, 310, 324
   Literature 4-5, 76, 133, 296-297, 329
   Method; Methodology 5-6, 167, 267, 298
   Peer review 4-5, 7, 246
   Pre-registration of research/clinical trials 133
Response to Intervention; Three-tiered RTI approach 41-43
Restorative conferencing 137-139
Schuhfried Education 47-48
Screen-time 54-55
Searchlights (aka Multi-cueing) 227, 339
Second opinion 231
Self-stimulatory behaviours (stimming; stim) 81, 129, 298
Sensory Integration Therapy (SIT) 76, 78, 125-127, 140, 324, 339
   Sensory Integration Disorder 17, 126, 288
   Weighted vests 9, 126, 339
Severe communication impairment 115-117, 149, 154, 156, 160-161, 163, 165, 168
Sex; Sexuality 68, 109,
Sexual abuse/assault/harassment 40, 117, 122, 146, 160-162, 165
Short tongue (see Tongue-tie; Ankyloglossia)
Side-effects 38, 110, 124, 144
Significant other 3, 169
Skepticism (Scepticism); Skeptics 97, 255, 292 301-302
   Ben Goldacre 257
   Carl Sagan ix
   Dead Cat Hettie 257
   Edzard Ernst ix, 8, 121, 273
   Foxx and Mulick 69, 75-76, 93
   James Randi 8
   Neurobollocks 295
   Rogue's Gallery of harms 10
   Simon Chapman 174
   Simon Singh 8
Sleep 41, 55, 79, 118-121, 172, 259, 270, 285
Sluggish Cognitive Tempo 35
Smacking/slapping – see Behaviour
Social Media 3, 7, 17, 25, 27, 55, 98-99, 149, 165, 286, 295-296, 302, 311, 312, 315, 328
   Facebook 265, 295-297, 322, 337
   Twitter 296, 312, 336
      @catnutritionist 257
      @PamelaSnow2 15

@SimonChapman6 174
@Speech_Woman 15
@TxChoices 15, 336
Social Stories® 62, 78, 81, 87-88, 338
Solution-Focused Brief Therapy (SFBT) 145
Special Education; Special Educators 11, 50, 69, 71, 73, 75-76, 147, 157, 166, 177, 191, 238, 251, 298, 302, 331
Specific Learning Disability 7, 126, 230, 336
Speech; Articulation 169, 178, 179, 181, 182, 183, 185, 186, 193, 307
Speech Language Pathologist/Speech Language Therapist 3, 7. 9. 10, 14, 54, 69-77, 81, 86, 88, 90,91, 98, 112, 140, 149, 151, 153, 154, 159, 161, 164, 169, 171, 172, 176, 177, 180-182, 184-199, 202, 203, 206, 216, 221, 228, 213, 240, 244, 246, 252, 260, 261, 264, 265, 289, 301, 303-309, 311, 312, 315, 317-324, 327-330, 332
Stimming 81, 129, 298
Succussion 174
Swallowing 116, 171, 175, 197, 259-261, 277, 304, 306, 307
Stuttering; Stammering 2, 171, 179, 190, 193-195, 307
   Anna Deeter: Etalon 195, 331, 339
   Kill Your Stutter; Kill That Stutter 190, 195, 339
   McGuire Program 7, 195, 331, 339
   McGuire Speech Helper Software 195
Super food 16, 287
Supported typing (see AAC; Facilitated communication)
Symptom cluster 15
Syndrome 15-16, 179, 300
   Angelman syndrome 61, 307
   Asperger/Asperger's syndrome 58
   Down syndrome 15, 17, 61, 68, 98, 113, 115, 261, 181, 191,193, 195-198
   Foetal Alcohol Spectrum Disorder (FASD) 181, 261, 307
   Food Protein-Induced Enterocolitis syndrome (FPIES) 261, 266
   Fragile X syndrome 15, 61, 181, 307
   Irritable bowel syndrome (IBS) 263, 283
   Klinefelter syndrome 15, 61
   Landau-Kleffner syndrome 61
   Locked-in syndrome 153
   Made-up syndromes 17, 76, 240-241, 282-283, 288
   Prader-Willi syndrome 15, 61, 261, 266, 307
   Rett syndrome 15, 61
   Velo-cardio-facial syndrome 307
   Williams syndrome 15, 61, 307
   Zellweger syndrome 240
Teachers
   Camphill 94
   English teacher 20, 172, 178, 304-305
   Preschool teachers 37, 90-91, 177
   Professional development (PD) 52, 54, 56, 57
   RTI 42
   Reading 217-253
   School teachers 3, 4, 9, 11, 12, 23, 31-32, 40, 114-115, 118, 177, 199-207
   Teacher pre-service education 40, 52, 54, 108
   Teacher-report 37
Teams 141, 300
   Inter-disciplinary team 59, 74, 84, 112, 113, 230, 303
   Multidisciplinary team 74, 91, 92, 139, 140, 189, 26, 303
   Team dynamics 321
   Team morale 310
   Transdisciplinary team 70, 73, 74, 84, 91, 140, 303, 321
   Treatment team 93
Testimonials 5, 17, 19, 21, 48, 50, 51, 56, 90, 102, 127, 140, 186, 189, 193, 200, 212, 236, 297, 332, 338
Toddlers-in-Mortarboards 19, 30
Tongue-tie; Ankyloglossia 17, 179, 264-265
Toy library 142
Traumatic brain injury (TBI) 193
Type to Communicate (see AAC; Facilitated Communication)
Underlying representation 178, 221
Vaccination 2-3, 166, 277, 316
   Anti-vaccination; anti-vax; anti-vaxxer 3, 66, 79, 94, 278, 280, 284, 296, 337
   Andrew Wakefield 66, 68, 277, 337
   Donald Trump 278
   Homeopathic "vaccination" 79, 175, 296, 331, 339
   MMR 2-3, 277, 316
   Sherri Tenpenny 278
Voice disorders; vocal load; vocal nodules; voice therapy 172-174
Volunteers 264, 307, 308-309, 328

Websites
    Association of Healthcare Journalists 9
    Autism Speaks 65
    Bad Science 257
    Croakey Blog 8
    Guild of Health Writers 9
    Google; Google™ 9, 155, 206, 280, 293-294, 296, 302, 312
    Google Scholar™ 36, 236, 296-297, 312
    Huffington Post: Healthy Living 9
    NHS News Pages 9
    LinkedIn™ 27
    National Autism Center 70
    ResearchGate 297
    Sci-Hub 312
    Science Daily 9
    Smart Talkers 99
    Speech-Language-Therapy dot com 234
    The Conversation 9
    The Snow Report 234
    Thinking Person's Guide to Autism 65
    W3C® 311
    Wikipedia® 25, 48, 104, 312
    YouTube™ 9
Weaning; Baby-led; Spoon feeding 260
Weighted vests 9, 16, 126, 339
White paper 70, 240, 292
Working Memory 32-33, 45, 48, 152, 200, 202, 216, 249
World Health Organization 74, 260, 270
Xlens 178, 340
Yeast 79, 80, 279, 280, 281, 340
Z-vibe 191
Zellweger syndrome 240
Zinc 174, 272